The Challenge of Pain

The Challenge of Pain

Ronald Melzack
and Patrick D. Wall

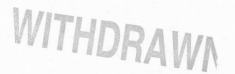

Basic Books, Inc., Publishers   New York

To the memory of our parents

Contents

Preface

Pain is one of the most challenging problems in medicine and biology. It is a challenge to the sufferer who must often learn to live with pain for which no therapy has been found. It is a challenge to the physician or other health professional who seeks every possible means to help the suffering patient. It is a challenge to the scientist who tries to understand the biological mechanisms that can cause such terrible suffering. It is also a challenge to society which must find the medical, scientific and financial resources to relieve or prevent pain and suffering as much as possible.

Pain is such a common experience that we rarely pause to define it in ordinary conversation. Yet no one who has worked on the problem of pain has ever been able to give it a definition which is satisfactory to all of his colleagues. Pain has obvious sensory qualities, but it also has emotional and motivational elements. It is usually caused by intense, noxious stimulation, yet it sometimes occurs spontaneously without apparent cause. It normally signals physical injury, but it sometimes fails to occur even when extensive areas of the body have been seriously injured; at other times it persists after all the injured tissues have healed and becomes a crippling problem that may require urgent, radical treatment.

We consider ourselves extremely privileged to have taken part in a genuine scientific revolution in the past two decades. Until the middle of this century, pain was considered primarily to be a symptom of disease or injury. We now know that chronic, severe pain is a problem in its own right that is often more debilitating and intolerable than the disease process which initiated it. The problem of pain was therefore transformed from a mere symptom to be dealt with by the various medical specialities to a speciality in its own right which is now one of the most exciting, rapidly advancing fields of science and medicine.

When we proposed the gate-control theory in 1965, we hardly dreamed of the explosion in research studies and new therapeutic approaches that followed. It was our unexpected good fortune that the theory came at a time when the field was ripe for change. A small number of original thinkers fought hard to replace the old concept of a specific pain pathway by a more dynamic conception in which pain is determined by many factors in addition to injury – by personality, culture, and other activities in the nervous system at the time of injury. This small band of courageous men hammered away at the established, traditional theory. Goldscheider, Head, Leriche, Livingston, and Noordenbos all proposed exciting new ideas. But despite occasional lip-service to their ingenuity, the field continued unchanged, holding tenaciously onto Descartes' idea, proposed in 1664, that pain is like a bell-ringing alarm system whose sole purpose is to signal injury of the body.

In the 1960s, a wave of new facts and ideas (that had evolved gradually) was beginning to crest, and the gate-control theory rode in on the wave of the times. No one was more astounded at its success than we were. Naturally, acceptance was not immediate or total, but in spite of continuing controversy about details, the *concept* that injury signals can be radically modified and even blocked at the earliest stages of transmission in the nervous system is virtually universally accepted. Happily, the main beneficiary has been the suffering person. The new concept provided the foundation and framework for a host of novel, exciting approaches to the treatment of pain.

This book contains four major sections. The first section describes the psychological and clinical aspects of pain and outlines the scope of the challenges of pain. The second section presents the physiological evidence regarding pain, which continues to grow at a breathtaking pace. The third section examines the major theories of pain in terms of their ability to explain pain phenomena and their implications for the control of pain. The final, fourth section describes the exciting new approaches to pain control and the rapidly evolving conception that the terrible suffering of patients with chronic pain, such as those due to cancer or nerve injuries, need an entirely new approach characterized by the pain clinic and the hospice.

We are grateful to many colleagues and friends who have worked with us and helped us in our attempts to understand pain. Their names appear in the pages of this book and in the bibliography. We are also grateful to Carol Stokes-Rogolino and Julia O'Connor who provided outstanding secretarial assistance in preparing this book.

Part One
The Puzzle of Pain

'... physicians too readily claim that *pain is a reaction of defence, a fortunate warning, which puts us on our guard against the risks of disease* ... Reaction of defence? Against whom? Against what? Against the cancer which not infrequently gives little trouble until quite late? Against heart afflictions, which always develop quietly? ... One must reject, then, this false conception of beneficient pain.'

René Leriche, 1939

1
Pain and Injury: the Variable Link

The link between pain and injury seems so obvious that it is widely believed that pain is always the result of physical damage and that the intensity of pain we feel is proportional to the severity of the injury. In general, this relationship between injury and pain holds true: a pinch of a finger usually produces mild pain while a door slammed on it is excruciating; a small cut hurts a little, while a laceration can be agonizing. However, there are many instances in which the relationship fails to hold up. For example, about 65% of soldiers who are severely wounded in battle and 20% of civilians who undergo major surgery report feeling little or no pain for hours or days after the injury or incision (Beecher, 1959). In contrast, no apparent injury can be detected in about 70% of people who suffer from chronic low back pain (Loeser, 1980). Clearly, the link between injury and pain is highly variable: injury may occur without pain, and pain without injury.

This is the essence of the puzzle of pain. Why are pain and injury not always related? What activities of the nervous system intervene between injury and pain perception that make the relationship so variable? We shall begin to answer these questions by describing some extreme examples of the variability of the link between injury and pain. These examples challenge our intuitive feelings about pain and reveal the subtlety of the mechanisms which we will need to explain. Each example also contains clues for the control of pain.

Injury without pain

People who are born without the ability to feel pain provide convincing testimony on the value of pain (Sternbach, 1968).

Many of these people sustain extensive burns, bruises and lacerations during childhood, frequently bite deep into the tongue while chewing food, and learn only with difficulty to avoid inflicting severe wounds on themselves. The failure to feel pain after a ruptured appendix, which is normally accompanied by severe abdominal pain, led to near death in one such man. Another man walked on a leg with a cracked bone until it broke completely.

The best documented of all cases of congenital insensitivity to pain is Miss C., a young Canadian girl who was a student at McGill University in Montreal. Her father, a physician in western Canada, was fully aware of her problem and alerted his colleagues in Montreal to examine her. The young lady was highly intelligent and seemed normal in every way except that she had never felt pain. As a child, she had bitten off the tip of her tongue while chewing food, and had suffered third-degree burns after kneeling on a hot radiator to look out of the window. When examined by a psychologist (McMurray, 1950) in the laboratory, she reported that she did not feel pain when noxious stimuli were presented. She felt no pain when parts of her body were subjected to strong electric shock, to hot water at temperatures that usually produce reports of burning pain, or to a prolonged ice-bath. Equally astonishing was the fact that she showed no changes in blood pressure, heart rate, or respiration when these stimuli were presented. Furthermore, she could not remember ever sneezing or coughing, the gag reflex could be elicited only with great difficulty, and corneal reflexes (to protect the eyes) were absent. A variety of other stimuli, such as inserting a stick up through the nostrils, pinching tendons, or injections of histamine under the skin – which are normally considered as forms of torture – also failed to produce pain.

Miss C. had severe medical problems. She exhibited pathological changes in her knees, hip and spine, and underwent several orthopaedic operations. Her surgeon attributed these changes to the lack of protection to joints usually given by pain sensation. She apparently failed to shift her weight when standing, to turn over in her sleep, or to avoid certain postures, which normally prevent inflammation of joints.

The condition of the joints that Miss C. suffered from, because of her failure to feel pain, is called the 'Charcot joint'. It has long been known that if the nerves which normally innervate a joint are missing or defective, a condition develops in which the joint surface is damaged and the ligaments and other tissues are stretched. This happens particularly to those joints which are frequently subject to minor injuries in everyday life – ankles, knees, wrists and elbows. All of us quite frequently stumble, fall or wrench a muscle during ordinary activity. After these trivial injuries, we limp a little or we protect the joint so that it remains unstressed during the recovery process. This resting of the damaged part is an essential part of its recovery. But those who feel no pain go on using the joint, adding insult to injury. Apparently this is eventually sufficient to produce the Charcot joint with its severely eroded tissues. Dead or dying tissue is the perfect culture medium for bacteria and is the most likely place for infection to develop. Because blood flow is impaired by the injuries, the tissue is isolated from the body's own defence mechanisms. The infection is then free to extend into nearby bone and eventually into marrow, producing osteomyelitis where even the most powerful antibiotics cannot penetrate from the bloodstream. These are the conditions that led to Miss C.'s death.

Miss C. died at the age of twenty-nine of massive infections that could not be brought under control. During her last month, she complained of discomfort, tenderness and pain in the left hip. The pain was relieved by analgesic tablets. There is little doubt that her inability to feel pain until the final month of her life led to the 'extensive skin and bone trauma that contributed in a direct fashion to her death' (Baxter and Olszewski, 1960, p.381).

Astonishingly, careful examination of Miss C.'s nervous system by several experts failed to reveal any abnormality. The nerve endings and specialized receptors in her skin and joints appeared completely normal, as did her nerves, spinal cord, and brain. Clearly, however, her nervous system was abnormal in some unknown way. Somewhere, the injury signals that normally ascend to the brain through the spinal cord were blocked at one or more of the many junctions (synapses) through which they pass. We will examine the possibilities in later chapters.

While Miss C.'s case is the most thoroughly documented one, there are reports of several families with the same problem. In fact, there is strong evidence that some forms of this condition are inherited. However, it is now clear that congenital insensitivity to pain may be due to many causes (Comings and Amromin, 1974). In some cases, as in Miss C.'s, the cause remains a mystery; but in other cases there is evidence of neurological damage. Even this is puzzling, though. In one form of insensitivity, examination of small pieces of excised nerve (nerve 'biopsies') showed that the large fibres in nerves are highly abnormal. In other cases, the small fibres in nerves are damaged or missing. This form occurs almost solely in Jewish families and is known as dysautonomia (or the Riley-Day syndrome). It is a tragic disease because all physical development is abnormal and these people rarely live to adulthood. One form of pain insensitivity is accompanied by the inability to sweat. In still another form, the nerve roots that fan out from a peripheral nerve and enter the spinal cord are damaged (sensory radicular neuropathy). Other kinds of insensitivity to pain are associated with severe mental retardation.

The importance of pain for survival becomes clear when we consider what happens to people who are insensitive to pain (Comings and Amromin, 1974). One woman, for example, reported only a 'tight feeling' during an appendicitis attack and was saved when her family doctor, who knew of her condition, suspected the worst and admitted her to hospital. After the operation, she had no pain but reported 'a pulling sensation' in the region of the fresh scar. Throughout her life, this woman had sustained numerous cuts and burns without feeling pain. Her mouth was scarred from blisters as a result of drinking beverages that were too hot, and her hands were calloused from frequent burns. During two pregnancies, she reported 'a funny, feathery feeling' rather than pain.

Her seven-year-old daughter had the same condition. At the age of three she broke her arm and at five she broke her nose, and felt no pain at any time. At seven, after taking a bath, 'she leaned over and her buttocks pressed up against a grated bathroom heater; she was branded with five large crosshatches over the buttocks but felt no pain'. Interestingly, during a careful neurological examination, it was found that the girl felt no pain when pinpricked on all parts of her body except a small circular area over the lower (lumbar) spine. Yet all the tests indicated no other neurological abnormality in any of the areas insensitive to pain. This girl had one brother who had a mild form of insensitivity and two sisters who perceived pain normally.

Consider another family, some of whose members were normal in every respect except that they felt no pain. The mother was once near death from eclampsia during pregnancy – an extremely dangerous condition of unknown origin – because she did not have a severe headache, which is an early warning signal followed by other symptoms including convulsions. She was saved from death by sheer luck and a fast-thinking doctor who immediately recognized the symptoms despite the absence of the headache. Because of her condition, the woman was especially alert to signs of disease in her children. Indeed, one child developed appendicitis and peritonitis without any pain, and was saved by his mother's prompt reaction to his casual remark about a 'stiff stomach' (Sternbach, 1968).

These drastic consequences are relatively rare. Most people who are insensitive to pain learn, with difficulty, to avoid damaging themselves severely. However, they survive because they have language to communicate a problem. The report to a doctor of unusual symptoms by the pregnant woman with eclampsia, or the remark by her son of a 'stiff stomach' saved their lives. Animals, who have no such verbal communication, would have died. It is amply clear, then, that pain plays an important role in survival.

But there is still a puzzle. Even in normal people, injuries sometimes occur without pain. A recent study (Melzack, Wall and Ty, 1982) found that thirty-seven per cent of the people who arrived at the emergency clinic of a large urban hospital with a variety of injuries, including amputated fingers, major lacerations of the skin and fractured bones, reported that they did not feel any pain until many minutes – even hours – after the injury. Why? How is it that a finger can be chopped off in an accident and no pain be felt? What happens to the nerve signals from the hand to the brain that makes them fail to evoke pain? There is no certain answer. But it is now known that there are biological mechanisms that set a limit on pain.

Pain without injury

Lesch-Niehan disease is a rare congenital disorder which seems to be the opposite of congenital insensitivity to pain. The children appear normal at birth but they fail to thrive, both mentally and physically. They begin to exhibit self-mutilation, which is the major characteristic of the disease. With cries and appearances of great anguish, the child suddenly and viciously attacks some part of himself, acting as though it was the source of intolerable pain. It is necessary to restrain these children for their own protection. They do not attack others. Postmortem examination of their brains shows no anatomical abnormalities. The disease is tentatively explained as due to a failure to develop one of the essential enzymes which regulate metabolism (enzymeopathy). These children are particularly affected by a class of chemicals – the xanthines – which includes caffeine. In experiments designed to test the chronic effects of extremely large doses of caffeine in rats, it was found that the animals would start to bite viciously at their feet and limbs as though they felt that they were injured.

Pain disproportionate to severity of injury

Those who have experienced the passing of a kidney stone describe it as painful beyond any expectation that pain can reach such an intensity. The kidney may, under certain conditions, concentrate some components in the urine so that these compounds precipitate out and form small kidney stones (renal calculi). Small pieces of these stones break off and pass into the ureter that leads from the kidney to the bladder. In size, they are often not more than twice the size of the normal diameter of the ureter. Pressure of urine builds up behind the plug formed by the stone, tending to drive it into the ureter. As a result, the muscle in the ureter wall goes into localized strong contraction. This band of contraction moves down the ureter to produce peristaltic waves to drive the stone down. During this process, agonizing spasms of pain sweep over the patient so that the toughest and most stoical of characters usually collapses. The patient is pale, with a racing pulse, knees drawn up with a rigid abdominal wall and motionless. Even crying out is restrained because all movement exaggerates the pain. As the stone passes into the bladder, there is immediate and complete relief, leaving a dazed and exhausted patient. The reason for describing this condition here is that in mechanical terms it is a rather trivial event. Furthermore it occurs in a structure which is poorly innervated when compared to any equal volume of skin. In spite of the minor nature of the actual event and the relatively small number of nerve impulses which are sent to the spinal cord, the effect in terms of pain is gigantic.

Pain after healing of an injury

Nerve injury of the shoulder is becoming increasingly common because motorcycles are widely accessible and all too often their power is far greater than the skill of their riders. On hitting an obstruction, the rider is catapulted forwards and hits the road at about the speed the bike was travelling. The wearing of crash helmets has effectively decreased head injuries; but the next vulnerable point to hit the road is often the shoulder, which is violently wrenched down and back. The arm is supplied by a network of nerves – the brachial plexus – which leaves the spinal cord at the level of the lower neck and upper chest, and funnels into the arms.

In the most severe of these injuries, the spinal roots are avulsed – that is, ripped out of the spinal cord – and no repair is possible. In 1979, well over a hundred brachial plexus avulsions occurred in England alone. C.A., aged twenty-five, an air-force pilot, suffered such an accident. After eight months he had completely recovered from the cuts, bruises and fractures of his accident. There had been no head injury and he was alert, intelligent and busy as a student shaping a new career for himself. His right arm was completely paralysed from the shoulder down and the muscles of the arm were thin. In addition, the limp arm was totally anaesthetic, so that he had no sensation of any stimuli applied to it. On being questioned, he stated that he could sense very clearly an entire arm, but it had no relationship to his real arm. This 'phantom' arm seemed to him to be placed across his chest while the real paralysèd arm hung at his side. The phantom never moved and the fingers were tightly clenched in a cramped fist with the nails digging into the palm. The entire arm felt 'as though it was on fire'. Nothing has helped his condition and he finds that he can control the pain only by absorbing himself in his work.

On first hearing such a story, anyone might reasonably conclude that the man is not sane. In fact, such patients often decide not to mention their condition except to very special friends, possibly to some medical staff. Wynn Parry (1980) studied a hundred consecutive cases of this type of brachial plexus avulsion and found ninety-five to be in severe pain with very similar descriptions of their phantoms and their pain. We shall return to this subject later to consider the causes of the pain. It is introduced here to show that pain may persist long after all possible healing has occurred. Even the most damaging stimulation of the arm is incapable of producing pain, yet pain is constantly felt even though no injury is occurring.

Damage of peripheral nerves in the arms or legs, by gunshot wounds or other injuries, is also sometimes accompanied by excruciating pains that persist long after the tissues have healed. These pains may occur spontaneously for no apparent reason. They have many qualities, and may be described as burning, cramping or shooting. Sometimes they are triggered by innocuous stimuli such as gentle touches or even a puff of air. Spontaneous attacks of pain may take minutes or hours to subside, but may occur repeatedly each day for years after the injury. The frequency and intensity of the spontaneous pain-attacks may increase over the years, and the pain may even spread to distant areas of the body. The initial cause of these pains is sometimes far more subtle than peripheral nerve damage. Minor injuries may give rise to astonishingly severe pain. In these cases, Livingston (1943, p.110) notes:

The onset of symptoms may follow the most commonplace of injuries. A bruise, a superficial cut, the prick of a thorn or a broken chicken-bone, a sprain or even a post-operative scar may act as the causative lesion. The event which precipitates the syndrome may appear both to the patient and the physician as of minor consequence, and both have every reason to anticipate the same prompt recovery that follows similar injuries. This anticipation is not realized and the symptoms tend to become progressively worse.

One of these cases was described by Livingston (1943, p.109):

Mrs G. E. A., aged fifty-eight, was referred for treatment of periodic pain in her right foot . . . Three years previously she fell and injured this foot. The outer side of the foot at the base of the toes turned 'black and blue', but X-ray plates did not reveal any fractures. As the ecchymosis (discoloration) cleared she noted that the outer three toes 'felt dead'. Later she began to have periodic pains 'like a toothache' in these toes and during such attacks all three would be extremely sensitive to touch. The attacks continued with increasing frequency and severity, sometimes occurring several times a day, and occasionally skipping a day or two, but never longer . . . The subjective feeling of 'deadness' seemed to increase just before an attack began – next she experienced a sensation of swelling in the toes beginning at their bases on the plantar (sole) surface and spreading to involve all three toes to their junction with the foot. At its height she said the toes felt 'as if bursting and on fire'. During the attack she was unable to tolerate the lightest touch to the toes.

Nothing of significance was found in physical examination. She received ten injections of a 2 per cent novocaine solution into the (bottom) of the foot at the base of the toes. Each injection was followed by a period of complete relief from attacks, and these intervals of freedom became increasingly long as the treatment progressed. (After the) last injection . . . there has been no recurrence of pain.

Not all cases end as happily as this one. Sometimes the pain persists and becomes so unbearable that the patient may undergo successive surgical operations.

Pain: good and evil

These prolonged, agonizing pains inevitably force us to examine the purpose and value of pain. From the cases described so far, it is evident that pain can serve three purposes. First, the pain that occurs *before* serious injury, such as when we step on (or pick up) hot, sharp, or otherwise potentially damaging objects, has real survival value. It produces immediate withdrawal or some other action that prevents further injury. Second, the pains that prevent further injury serve as the basis for learning to avoid injurious objects or situations which may occur at a later time. The larger the animal's brain, the more easily such learning occurs, and it generalizes to other situations. In man, the learning involves language and the use of other symbols, so that even people who are insensitive to pain can limit the extent of damage so that survival is possible. Third, pains due to damaged joints, abdominal infections, diseases, or serious injuries set limits on activity and enforce inactivity and rest, which are often essential for the body's natural recuperative and disease-fighting mechanisms to ensure recovery and survival.

However, there are pains, such as those after brachial plexus avulsion or amputation of a limb that serve no useful purpose. A person who has a leg removed because of a circulatory problem may suffer excruciating phantom limb pain for years, perhaps the remainder of his life, but gains nothing from the pain. Pain such as this now becomes a problem in its own right. It is no longer the symptom of a disease but becomes a serious medical syndrome that requires attention for its own sake. Chronic pain can even be detrimental to survival in man. The pain can be so terrible, so feared, that people would sooner die than continue living with it. Suicide among patients who suffer prolonged, unremitting pain is not uncommon. In cases such as these, the pain serves no biologically useful purpose. It is as though some normally adaptive mechanism has run amok and, like the dangerous criminal whose mind may be brilliant but warped, needs to be isolated, contained and treated. Leriche (1939, p.23), a brilliant surgeon who spent much of his life attempting to relieve suffering, contemplated this aspect of pain:

Defence reaction? Fortunate warning? But as a matter of fact, the majority of diseases, even the most serious, attack us without warning. When pain develops . . . it is too late . . . The pain has only made more distressing and more sad a situation already long lost . . . In fact, pain is always a baleful gift, which reduces the subject of it, and makes him more ill than he would be without it.

The puzzle

The kinds of cases we have examined so far – ranging from the inability to feel pain in spite of injury to spontaneous pain in the absence of injurious stimulation – represent the extremes of the full spectrum of pain phenomena. They demonstrate that the link between pain and injury is often highly variable and unpredictable. We do not yet have a satisfactory explanation for either type of case. Instead we must resort to speculation and theory: the best possible guess on the basis of the available evidence.

It was once thought that the mechanisms that subserve pain would be entirely revealed if we applied noxious stimuli to the skin and then mapped the pathways taken by nerve impulses through the spinal cord and brain. Unfortunately, pain mechanisms are not as simple as this. When the skin is pinched or crushed, for example, it is true that receptors with very high thresholds are stimulated, but so are receptors with much lower thresholds which are ordinarily activated by gentle touch or vibration. The same is true for extreme heat, or cold, or any other noxious stimulus. Painful stimuli, in other words, are usually extremes of other natural stimuli, and they tend to activate receptors that may also be involved in eliciting other sensations such as tickle, touch, warmth or cold. A noxious stimulus, moreover, brings about a variety of other changes, such as increased sweating and blood flow at the skin, and these too would contribute to the afferent (sensory) information going to the brain. How, then, is the neurophysiologist to know which portion of the afferent pattern is related to pain? Or is it all related to pain? The critical question is this: does the brain examine just a specific message ascending along specific fibres, or does it monitor *all* the input and make a decision in terms of the sheer number of nerve impulses in all active fibres?

The answer to this question represents the key to the puzzle of pain. It therefore has profound implications for its treatment. It was long hoped that we need only find the pathways in the nervous system that send pain messages from the body to the brain, and pain could be eliminated simply by cutting the pathways. There are many forms of pain, however, that defy this simple solution. Attempts to stop spontaneous pains by cutting pathways in the spinal cord or the brain produce as many failures as successes (Sunderland, 1978). Other kinds of pain are more amenable to surgical treatment. Pain produced by cancer in the lower part of the body is totally relieved by spinal cord surgery in about fifty per cent of patients, and is partially relieved in another twenty-five per cent. But the remainder – about one out of four – continue to suffer (Nathan, 1963). Even those who are helped sometimes report that they now have intense 'girdle pains' at the level of the operation – pains which they did not have before (Noordenbos, 1959). In a few cases, the pain after surgery may be worse than the pain for which the patients were treated (Drake and McKenzie, 1953).

An important aim of pain research is the successful treatment of pathological pain. The clinical syndromes which result from peripheral nerve injury bewilder the scientist who tries to understand them. Still worse, the failure to solve the problems they present means prolonged suffering and tragedy to many patients. People who face death due to a malignant disease such as cancer also face the prospect of extreme pain. Those who sustain brain damage as a result of a stroke may suffer severe pain (often called 'central pain') for the rest of their lives. The pain may continue unabated until the end. Pain, then, is more than an intriguing puzzle. It is a terrible problem that faces all humanity and urgently demands a solution.

The field of pain research and theory has developed rapidly in recent years. These developments have come from many disciplines, including psychology, physiology and clinical medicine. As a result of this progress, exciting new techniques have been proposed for the treatment of pain. The purpose of this book is to describe the research and the theories, as well as the pursuit of new directions aimed at the control of pain.

2
The Psychology of Pain

It is evident, from the cases we have examined so far, that pain can occur without injury and injury without pain. It may be argued that these are extreme examples based on people who have pathological conditions of the nervous system. However, the absence of a fixed, predictable relationship between pain and injury is also frequently evident in day-to-day events. Psychological and anthropological studies have shown that, in higher species at least, pain is not simply a function of the amount of bodily damage alone. Rather, the amount and quality of pain we feel are also determined by our previous experiences and how well we remember them, by our ability to understand the cause of the pain and to grasp its consequences. Even the culture in which we have been brought up plays an essential role in how we feel and respond to pain.

When compared with vision or hearing, the perception of pain seems simple, urgent and primitive. We expect the nerve signals evoked by injury to 'get through', unless we are unconscious or anaesthetized. But experiments and clinical observations show that pain is not always perceived after injury even when we are fully conscious and alert. Thus a knowledge of pain perception goes beyond the problem of injury and the sensory signals of pain. The study of pain perception can help us to understand the enormous plasticity of the nervous system and the individual differences that make each of us respond to the world in a unique fashion (Melzack, 1961).

A vast amount of study has been devoted to the perception of pain, especially in the last decade, and from it is emerging a concept of pain that is quite different from the older views on the subject. The evidence shows that pain is much more variable and modifiable than many people have believed in the past. Pain differs from person to person, culture to culture. Stimuli that produce intolerable pain in one person may be tolerated without a whimper by another. In some cultures, moreover, initiation rites and other rituals involve procedures that we associate with pain, yet observers report that these people appear to feel little or no pain. Pain perception, then, cannot be defined simply in terms of particular kinds of stimuli. Rather, it is a highly personal experience, depending on cultural learning, the meaning of the situation, and other factors that are unique to each individual.

Cultural determinants

Cultural values are known to play an important role in the way a person perceives and responds to pain. One of the most striking examples of the impact of cultural values on pain is the hook-hanging ritual still in practice in parts of India (Kosambi, 1967). The ceremony derives from an ancient practice in which a member of a social group is chosen to represent the power of the gods. The role of the chosen man (or 'celebrant') is to bless the children and crops in a series of neighbouring villages during a particular period of the year. What is remarkable about the ritual is that steel hooks, which are attached by strong ropes to the top of a special cart, are shoved under his skin and muscles on both sides of the back (Figure 1). The cart is then moved from village to village. Usually the man hangs on to the ropes as the cart is moved about. But at the climax of the ceremony in each village, he swings free, hanging only from the hooks embedded in his back, to bless the children and crops. Astonishingly, there is no evidence that the man is in pain during the ritual; rather, he appears to be in a 'state of exaltation'.

There are many examples of comparable procedures in other cultures. In East Africa, men and women undergo an operation – entirely without anaesthetics or pain-relieving drugs – called 'trepanation', in which the scalp and underlying muscles are cut in order to expose a large area of the skull. The skull is then scraped by the doktari as the man or woman sits calmly, without flinching or grimacing, holding a pan under the chin to catch the dripping blood. Films of this procedure are extraordinary to watch because of the discomfort they induce in the observers which is in striking contrast to the apparent lack of discomfort in the people under-

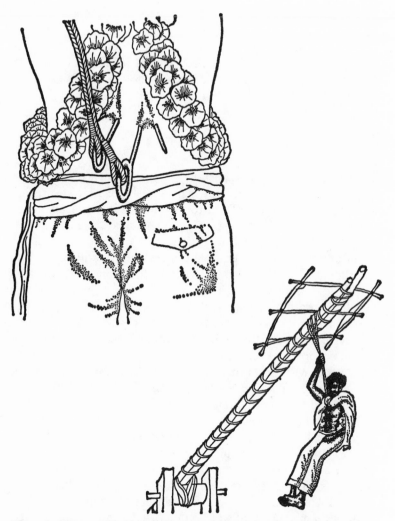

Figure 1. The annual hook-swinging ceremony practised in remote Indian villages. *Top* shows two steel hooks thrust into the small of the back of the 'celebrant', who is decked with garlands. The celebrant is later taken to a special cart which has upright timbers and a cross-beam. *Bottom* shows the celebrant hanging on to the ropes as the cart is moved to each village. After he blesses each child and farm field in a village, he swings free, suspended only by the hooks. The crowds cheer at each swing. The celebrant, during the ceremony, is in a state of exaltation and shows no sign of pain.
(from Kosambi, 1967, p. 105)

going the operation. There is no reason to believe that these people are physiologically different in any way. Rather, the operation is accepted by their culture as a procedure that brings relief of chronic pain. The expectation of relief, the trust in the skill of the doktari as well as other psychological factors appear to alter the experience of pain.

Pain thresholds

It is often asserted that variations in pain experience from person to person are due to different 'pain thresholds'. However, there are several thresholds related to pain and it is important to distinguish among them. Typically, thresholds are measured by applying a stimulus such as electric shock or radiant heat to a small area of skin and gradually increasing the intensity. Four thresholds can be measured by this technique: (a) sensation threshold (or lower threshold) – the lowest stimulus value at which a sensation such as tingling or warmth is first reported; (b) pain perception threshold – the lowest stimulus value at which the person reports that the stimulation feels painful; (c) pain tolerance (or upper threshold) – the lowest stimulus level at which the subject withdraws or asks to have the stimulation stopped; (d) encouraged pain tolerance – the same as (c) but the person is encouraged to tolerate higher levels of stimulation.

There is now evidence that all people, regardless of cultural background, have a uniform *sensation threshold.* Sternbach and Tursky (1965) made careful measurements of sensation threshold, using electric shock as the stimulus, in American-born women belonging to four different ethnic groups: Italian, Jewish, Irish, and Old American. They found no differences among the groups in the level of shock that was first reported as producing a detectable sensation. The sensory conducting apparatus, in other words, appears to be essentially similar in all people so that a given critical level of input always elicits a sensation.

Cultural background, however, has a powerful effect on the *pain perception threshold.* For example, levels of radiant heat that are reported as painful by people of Mediterranean origin (such as Italians and Jews) are described merely as warmth by Northern

Europeans (Hardy, Wolff and Goodell, 1952). Similarly, Nepalese porters on a climbing expedition are much more stoical than the occidental visitors for whom they work: even though both groups are equally sensitive to changes in electric shock, the Nepalese porters require much higher intensities before they call them painful (Clark and Clark, 1980).

The most striking effect of cultural background, however, is on *pain tolerance levels*. Sternbach and Tursky (1965) report that the levels at which subjects refuse to tolerate electric shock, even when they are encouraged by the experimenters, depend, in part at least, on their ethnic origin. Women of Italian descent tolerate less shock than women of Old American or Jewish origin. In a similar experiment (Lambert, Libman and Poser, 1960), in which Jewish and Protestant women served as subjects, the Jewish, but not the Protestant, women increased their tolerance levels after they were told that their religious group tolerated pain more poorly than others.

These differences in pain tolerance reflect different ethnic attitudes towards pain. Zborowski (1952) found that Old Americans have an accepting, matter-of-fact attitude towards pain and pain expression. They tend to withdraw when the pain is intense, and cry out or moan only when they are alone. Jews and Italians, on the other hand, tend to be vociferous in their complaints and openly seek support and sympathy. The underlying attitudes of the two groups, however, appear to be different. Jews tend to be concerned about the meaning and implications of the pain, while Italians usually express a desire for immediate pain relief.

Just how far people can push themselves to tolerate pain is indicated by the Sun Dance 'self-torture' ceremonies of the North American Plains Indians. Each young man who participated in the ceremonies around the sacred Sun Dance pole first had two incisions made with a sharp knife on each side of his chest. Skewers were then inserted through one of the incisions, pushed under the skin and out of the other incision. Wissler (1921, p.264), who observed the ceremony, describes the subsequent events:

This being done to each breast, with a single skewer for each, strong enough to tear away the flesh, and long enough to hold the lariats fastened to the top of the sacred pole, a double incision was made on the back of the left shoulder, to the skewer of which was fastened an Indian drum. The work being pronounced good by the persons engaged in the operation, the young man arose, and one of the operators fastened the lariats (to the skewers) giving them two or three jerks to bring them into position.

The young man went up to the sacred pole, and while his countenance was exceedingly pale, and his frame trembling with emotion, threw his arms around it, and prayed earnestly for strength to pass successfully through the trying ordeal. His prayer ended, he moved backward until the flesh was fully extended, and placing a small bone whistle in his mouth, he blew continuously upon it a series of short sharp sounds, while he threw himself backward, and danced until the flesh gave way and he fell. Previous to his tearing himself free from the lariats, he seized the drum with both hands and with a sudden pull tore the flesh on his back, dashing the drum to the ground amid the applause of the people. As he lay on the ground, the operators examined his wounds, cut off the flesh that was hanging loosely, and the ceremony was at an end. In former years the head of a buffalo was fastened by a rope on the back of the person undergoing the feat of self-immolation, but now a drum is used for that purpose.

From two to five persons undergo this torture every Sun Dance. Its object is military and religious. It admits the young man into the noble band of warriors whereby he gains the esteem of his fellows, and opens up the path to fortune and fame.

In contrast to these studies, which demonstrate *variability* in pain tolerance, other psychophysical experiments are aimed at revealing a mathematically precise relationship between the measured stimulus input and the intensity of sensation reported by the subject. Stevens, Carton and Shickman (1958) asked subjects to estimate the magnitudes of a series of electric shocks of varying intensity by assigning a number to each that expressed the subjective intensity of the shock. They found that the stimulus–sensation relationship is best described as a mathematical power function, a fact which has been confirmed by several other investigators. The actual value of the exponent, however, varies from study to study (Sternbach and Tursky, 1964). A similar orderly, predictable relationship between the intensity of electric shocks and the perceived intensity of the sensory and 'unpleasantness' components of pain has also recently been found using verbal descriptors and hand-grip force to express the perceived intensities (Gracely, 1979).

Psychophysical studies that find a mathematical relationship between stimulus intensity and pain intensity are often cited (Beecher, 1959; Mountcastle, 1980) as supporting evidence for the assumption that pain is a primary sensation subserved by a direct communication system from skin receptors to pain centre. A simple psychophysical function, however, does not necessarily reflect equally simple neural mechanisms. Activities in the central nervous system, such as memories of earlier cultural experience, may intervene between stimulus and sensation and invalidate any simple psychophysical 'law'. The use of laboratory conditions that minimize such activities or prevent them from ever coming into play reduces the functions of the nervous system to those of a fixed-gain transmission line. It is under these conditions that psychophysical functions prevail.

Past experience

The evidence that pain is influenced by cultural factors leads naturally to an examination of the role of early experience in adult behaviour related to pain. It is commonly accepted that children are deeply influenced by the attitudes of their parents towards pain. Some families make a great fuss about ordinary cuts and bruises, while others tend to show little sympathy towards even fairly serious injuries. There is reason to believe, on the basis of everyday observations, that attitudes towards pain acquired early in life are carried on into adulthood.

The influence of early experience on the perception of pain has also been demonstrated experimentally. Melzack and Scott (1957) raised Scottish terriers in isolation cages from infancy to maturity so that they were deprived of normal environmental stimuli, including the bodily knocks and scrapes that young animals get in the course of growing up. They were surprised to find that these dogs, at maturity, failed to respond normally to a variety of noxious stimuli. Many of them poked their noses repeatedly into a flaming match, and endured pinpricks with little evidence of pain. They invariably withdrew reflexively from the flame or pinprick and oriented to the stimuli, but few of them showed strong emotional arousal or behavioural withdrawal. In contrast, the litter-mates of these dogs that had been reared in a normal environment recognized potential harm so quickly that the experimenters were usually unable to touch them with the flame or pin more than once.

This astonishing behaviour of dogs reared in isolation cannot be attributed to an inability to feel pain. Intense electric shock elicited strong emotional excitement and the dogs made obvious attempts to escape from it. But the low levels of observable emotional disturbance evoked by fire or pinprick suggests that their perception of pain was highly abnormal.

This abnormal behaviour may be due, in part at least, to a failure to attend selectively to noxious stimuli when they are presented in an unfamiliar environment in which all stimuli are equally attention-demanding. It is apparent (Melzack, 1965, 1969) that young animals partly learn which environmental stimuli are important and which are not. The results suggest, therefore, that the significance – or meaning – of environmental stimuli acquired during early experience plays an important role in pain perception. It is important to note that heredity may determine the extent to which early experience influences later behaviour. Beagles raised in isolation cages are not as severely disturbed as Scotties or mongrels and are capable of behaving more normally towards flaming matches and pinpricks (Melzack, 1965).

The importance of early experience in determining pain perceptiion and response is especially evident in studies of monkeys raised in isolation. In several experiments, infant monkeys were raised in individual cages that kept them isolated from the normal experience of encounters with damaging objects, or elders who slap or bite in the attempt to teach the youngsters how to live in a normal social environment. The resulting behaviour was disastrous. These monkeys, when released into a normal environment, often engaged in suicidal attacks against older and stronger monkeys. They also viciously bit their own limbs. These acts of self-destruction by the monkeys 'have on occasion resulted in broken bones and torn skin and blood vessels. After being repaired, many of these animals fail to profit from their experiences, continuing to bite themselves and to attack larger animals who inflict new wounds . . .' (Lichstein and Sackett, 1971, p.340).

Meaning of the situation

There is considerable evidence to show that people also attach variable meaning to pain-producing situations and that the meaning greatly influences the degree and quality of pain they feel. During the Second World War, Beecher (1959) observed the behaviour of soldiers severley wounded in battle. He was astonished to find that when the wounded men were carried into combat hospitals, only one out of three complained of enough pain to require morphine. Most of the soldiers either denied having pain from their extensive wounds or had so little that they did not want any medication to relieve it. These men, Beecher points out, were not in a state of shock, nor were they totally unable to feel pain, for they complained as vigorously as normal men at an inept vein puncture. When Beecher returned to clinical practice after the war, he asked a group of civilians who had surgical wounds similar to those received by the soldiers whether they wanted morphine to alleviate their pain. In contrast with the wounded soldiers, four out of five claimed they were in severe pain and asked for a morphine injection.

Beecher (1959, p.165) concluded from his study that:

The common belief that wounds are inevitably associated with pain, and that the more extensive the wound the worse the pain, was not supported by observations made as carefully as possible in the combat zone ... The data state in numerical terms what is known to all thoughtful clinical observers: there is no simple direct relationship between the wound *per se* and the pain experienced. The pain is in very large part determined by other factors, and of great importance here is the significance of the wound ... In the wounded soldier (the response to injury) was relief, thankfulness at his escape alive from the battlefield, even euphoria; to the civilian, his major surgery was a depressing, calamitous event.

A similar study (Carlen, Wall, Nadvorna and Steinbach, 1978) of Israeli soldiers with traumatic amputations after the Yom Kippur War provided comparable observations. Most of the wounded men spoke of their initial injury as painless and used neutral terms such as 'bang', 'thump' or 'blow' to describe their first sensation. They often volunteered their surprise that the injury did not hurt. These men were fully aware of the sad consequences of losing a limb, and some spoke of feeling guilt at letting down their comrades, annoyance at allowing the injury to occur, and misery about the future. Although these soldiers were depressed rather than euphoric, the meaning of the situation was clear: the battle was over for them, they escaped alive, and they were going to hospitals far from the battlefront.

The importance of the meaning associated with a pain-producing situation is made particularly clear in conditioning experiments carried out by Pavlov (1927, 1928). Dogs normally react violently when they are given strong electric shocks to one of the paws. Pavlov found, however, that if he consistently presented food to a dog after each shock, the dog developed an entirely new response. Immediately after a shock the dog would salivate, wag its tail and turn eagerly towards the food dish. The electric shock now failed to evoke any responses indicative of pain and became instead a signal meaning that food was on the way. This type of conditioned behaviour was observed as long as the same paw was shocked. If the shocks were applied to another paw, the dogs reacted violently. Pavlov reports that similar results were obtained in other experiments in which intense pressure or heat were used as the conditioned stimuli. This study shows convincingly that stimulation of the skin is localized, identified and evaluated *before* it produces perceptual experience and overt behaviour. The meaning of the stimulus acquired during earlier conditioning modulates the sensory input before it activates brain processes that underlie perception and response.

There are more familiar examples of the role played by personal evaluation of the situation. Abdominal sensations that are assumed to be gas cramps and are usually ignored may be felt as severe pain after learning that a friend or relative has stomach cancer. The pain may persist and get worse until a doctor assures the person that nothing is wrong. It may then vanish suddenly. Still another example is the frequent observation by dentists that patients who arrive early in the morning, complaining of a terrible toothache that kept them awake all night, sometimes report that the pain disappeared when they entered the dentist's office. They may even have difficulty remembering which tooth had hurt. The presence or absence of pain in these patients is clearly a function of the meaning of the situation: the pain was unbearable when help was unavailable, and diminished or vanished when relief was at hand.

Attention, anxiety and distraction

If a person's attention is focused on a potentially painful experience, he will tend to perceive pain more intensely than he would normally. Hall and Stride (1954) found that the simple appearance of the word 'pain' in a set of instructions made anxious subjects report as painful a level of electric shock they did not regard as painful when the word was absent from the instructions. Thus the mere anticipation of pain is sufficient to raise the level of anxiety and thereby the intensity of perceived pain. Similarly, Hill, Kornetsky, Flanary and Wikler (1952a and b) have shown that if anxiety is dispelled (by reassuring a subject that he has control over the pain-producing stimulus), a given level of electric shock or burning heat is perceived as significantly less painful than the same stimulus under conditions of high anxiety.

In contrast to the effects of attention on pain, it is well known that distraction of attention away from pain can diminish or abolish it. Distraction of attention may partly explain why boxers, football players and other athletes sometimes sustain severe injuries during the excitement of the sport without being aware that they have been hurt.

The common observation that pain is diminished when attention is wilfully directed toward other events, such as exciting games, books or films has provided a simple 'home-made' remedy for pain. Every sufferer of chronic pain has learned to force himself to concentrate on activities that become so absorbing that pain is not felt or is greatly diminished. A well-known actress, for example, reports that her intense arthritic pain vanishes the moment her part begins on stage and returns as soon as it is over (Glyn, 1971). People who suffer severe pain after brachial plexus lesions (see Chapter 1) report that the most effective way to reduce their pain is to absorb themselves in their work (Wynn Parry, 1980).

A study of the effects of music and 'white noise' (a wide range of sound frequencies) on pain shows that people learn quickly to use the auditory inputs to decrease their pain. In this experiment (Melzack, Weisz and Sprague, 1963), the subjects had a hand immersed in ice-water, which produces a deep, aching, severe pain that few people can tolerate for more than a few minutes. However, when the subjects were given an opportunity to listen to music and white noise, they did not just passively sit back and listen to them. Instead, they tapped their feet, sang out loud, and continually turned the volume control buttons on the audio-apparatus in the attempt to distract their attention away from the pain.

Distraction of attention, however, is effective only if the pain is steady or rises slowly in intensity (Melzack, Weisz and Sprague, 1963). If radiant heat is focused on the skin, for example, the pain may rise so suddenly and sharply that subjects are unable to control it by distraction. But when the pain rises slowly, people may use auditory stimulation to distract their attention from it. They often find that the pain actually levels off or decreases *before* it reaches the anticipated intolerable level (Figure 2). Distraction stratagems employing music and noise are used effectively by some people to control pain produced by dental drilling and extraction (Gardner and Licklider, 1959).

Feelings of control over pain

In the course of growing up, we learn early in life that pain has a unique aspect to it: after an injury, such as a burned finger or a cut knee, the pain persists without possibility of escape. A severely burned patient can only scream out or weep as layers of dead skin are carefully removed (debridement) – an agonizing process. The procedure is repeated frequently and the patient dreads these horrible experiences. Yet there is no escape for the patient. It is possible to walk away from unpleasant sights, sounds or smells, but once the body is injured, there is no escape.

It is, of course, possible to avoid some kinds of pain. Touching a hot stove or stepping on a sharp stone often produces a sudden movement that may limit or prevent injury. It is also possible to change the level of pain by giving people the *feeling* that they have control over it even though, in fact, they do not. When burn

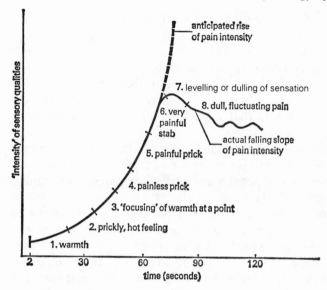

Figure 2. Idealized curve of sensory qualities produced by radiant heat, based on reports of subjective sensation. The subject anticipates a continuing rise in pain intensity which, instead, begins to fall after reaching a peak. Distraction stratagems enable people to tolerate the pain through level 6 on the curve, thereby prolonging their pain tolerance.
(from Melzack, Weisz and Sprague, 1963, p.239)

patients are allowed to participate in the debridement of their burned tissues, they claim that the process is more bearable. Several studies have established the effects and conditions that play a role in the sense of control over pain.

Rats, like people, are more disturbed by pain they cannot control. In one study, two groups of rats were shocked while they were eating. One group could 'control' (or terminate) the shock by jumping up, while the animals in the other group received the shock regardless of what they did. Although both groups received the same amount of shock during each testing session, the rats that had 'control' of the shock were less disturbed and ate more (Mowrer and Viek, 1948). A similar study showed that rats which had no control over the electric shocks had consistently greater rises in blood pressure than rats which *were* given 'control'. The input – the actual amount and intensity of shock – was the same for both groups, but the disruptive effects were significantly different (Hokanson *et al.*, 1971). In a comparable experiment, human subjects who were given a 'sense of control' over electric shocks, by being told how to respond to them, rated the shocks as much less painful than a group of people who received the shocks and were told that there was nothing they could do to avoid them (Bowers, 1968).

These laboratory studies have important implications for pain in real-life situations. It is now apparent that the severity of post-surgical pain is significantly reduced when patients are taught how to cope with their pain. Patients who were scheduled to undergo major surgery to remove the gall bladder, uterus or portions of the digestive tract were given detailed information about the pain they would feel after the operation and how they could best cope with it. They were told where they would feel pain, how severe it could be, how long it could last, and that such pain is normal after an operation. They were also shown how to relax by using breathing and relaxation stratagems. Finally, they were told that total relaxation is difficult to achieve and that they should request medication if they were uncomfortable. The results showed that patients who received these instructions reported significantly less pain and asked for many fewer medications during recovery than a comparable group of patients who received no instructions (Egbert *et al.*, 1964).

It was originally thought that the information alone is sufficient psychological preparation to reduce the uncertainty and anxiety associated with major surgery. However, it is evident that knowledge, in this case, may only increase the anxiety because of the certain expectation of pain and various discomforts. The essential ingredient is providing the patient with skills to cope with the pain and anxiety – at the very least, to provide the patient with a sense of control. Recent studies have shown that simply giving patients information about their pain tends to make them focus on the discomforting aspects of the experience, and their pain is magnified rather than reduced. However, when the patients are taught skills to cope with their pain, such as relaxation or distraction strategies, the pain is less severe (Langer *et al.*, 1975). Other studies have shown that the amount of post-surgical pain is directly proportional to the amount of anxiety perceived by the patient (Martinez-Urrutia, 1975). Achieving a sense of control, then, appears to diminish both anxiety and pain. This simple psychological fact has important implications: not only are post-surgical pain levels reported to be significantly less severe, but the amount of medication is reduced by half and the amount of time spent in the hospital is reduced by two to three days (Egbert *et al.*, 1964).

Suggestion and placebos

The influence of suggestion on the intensity of perceived pain is clearly demonstrated by studies of the effectiveness of placebos. Clinical investigators (Beecher, 1959) have found that severe pain, such as post-surgical pain, can be relieved in some patients by giving them a placebo (usually some non-analgesic substance such as a sugar or salt solution) in place of morphine or other analgesic drugs. About thirty-five per cent of the patients report marked relief of pain after being given a placebo. This is a strikingly high proportion because morphine, even in large doses, relieves severe pain in only about seventy-five per cent of patients.

Because suggestion, even in the subtlest form, may have a powerful effect on pain experience, the use of the 'double-blind' technique is essential in the evaluation of drugs. When this technique is used, both the experimental drug and the placebo are labelled in such a way that neither the patient nor the physician knows which one has been administered. Only then can the effect of the drug be evaluated in comparison with a physiologically neutral control chemical agent. The remarkably powerful effect of a placebo in no way implies that people who are helped by a placebo do not have real pain; no one will deny the reality of post-surgical pain. Rather, it illustrates the powerful contribution of suggestion to the perception of pain.

It is generally assumed that the suggestion itself is sufficient to produce the entire placebo effect. However, the placebo may also decrease anxiety because it makes the patient believe that something is being done to relieve the pain. Both effects probably always occur together. Whatever the explanation, it is clear that the physician may often relieve pain significantly by prescribing placebos to influence cognitive processes as well as by treating the injured areas of the body (Benson and Epstein, 1975).

A surprising recent discovery about placebos is that their effectiveness is always about fifty per cent of that of the drug with which it is being compared, even in double-blind experiments (Evans, 1974). That is, if the drug is a mild analgesic such as aspirin, then the pain relief produced by the placebo is half that of the aspirin. If it is a powerful drug such as morphine, the placebo has greater pain-relieving properties, again about fifty per cent of that of morphine. How is this possible? Anyone who has conducted a double-blind experiment quickly learns the answer. The experimenter has expectations of the power of the drug being tested and his enthusiasm is conveyed, implicitly or explicitly, to the subject. If the drug is new and especially effective, then certain patients are helped considerably at the beginning of the study, and the experimenter (or research assistant) is inevitably excited. Then, even though the 'double-blind' is maintained, the excitement is conveyed to the patient. The magnitude of the placebo effect, therefore, is about half the *assumed* strength of the analgesic drug being administered under double-blind conditions. This shows clearly that the psychological context – particularly the physician's and the patient's expectations of pain relief – contains powerful therapeutic value in its own right in addition to the effects of the drug itself (Evans, 1974).

There are large individual differences in susceptibility to placebos, and studies have been carried out to determine some of the factors that are involved (Evans, 1974). These studies have revealed that placebos are more effective for severe pain than for mild pain, and are more effective when the patients are under great stress and anxiety than when they are not. Is it possible, then, that the placebo effect can simply be attributed to a reduction in anxiety? Experiments show that the reduction of anxiety may account for some – but not all – of the placebo effects (McGlashan *et al.*, 1969). Placebo-induced analgesia is not significantly related to suggestibility, hypnotic susceptibility, or anxiety induced specifically by pain or the therapeutic situation (which is known as 'state-anxiety'). However, placebo effects occur more powerfully in people who have chronic generalized anxiety (personality 'trait-anxiety'). Nevertheless, even in people with high trait-anxiety, placebos are effective when pain levels are high rather than low. Apart from trait-anxiety levels, no consistent differences have been found to distinguish between placebo reactors and non-reactors.

Several studies also show that placebo effects and medication effects interact and may be addictive. One study (Lasagna *et al.*, 1954) demonstrated that a standard dose of morphine was only 54% effective in placebo non-reactors but was 95% effective in placebo reactors. Clearly, then, drug effects are dramatically enhanced in those people who are fortunate enough to be placebo reactors. The *kind* of pain is also an important factor. Most kinds of pain are relieved in 35% of patients. However, 52% of people suffering headaches are helped by placebos; it is possible that this may be due to a particularly strong role of anxiety in such sufferers.

There are other fascinating factors in the placebo response. Two placebo capsules, for example, are more effective than one capsule, and large capsules are better than small ones. A placebo is more effective when injected than when given by mouth, and is more potent when it is accompanied by strong suggestion that a powerful analgesic has been given. In short, the greater the implicit and explicit suggestion that pain will be relieved, the greater the relief obtained by the patient. Unfortunately, however, patients tend to get less and less relief from repeated administration of placebos.

It is clear, then, that placebo effects provide a remarkably powerful form of therapy for many medical problems. They are effective not only for pain but also for anxiety and depression as well as a variety of medical complaints in which psychological factors play a role. It is important to maximize these effects so that they contribute as much as possible to the relief of pain and suffering.

Hypnosis

The manipulation of attention together with strong suggestion are both part of the phenomenon of hypnosis. The hypnotic state eludes precise definition. But, loosely speaking, hypnosis is a trance state in which the subject's attention is focused intensely on the hypnotist while attention to other stimuli is markedly diminished. After people are hypnotized they can, with appropriate suggestion, be cut or burned yet report that they did not feel pain (Hilgard and Hilgard, 1975). They may say that they felt a sharp tactile sensation or strong heat, but they maintain that the sensations never welled up into pain. Evidently a small percentage of people can be hypnotized deeply enough to undergo major surgery entirely without anaesthesia. For a larger number of people hypnosis reduces the amount of pain-killing drug required to produce successful analgesia.

Self-hypnosis or auto-suggestion may be related to the state of meditation observed in mystics or other profoundly religious people. Deep meditation, or prolonged, intense focusing of attention on inner feelings, thoughts or images, may produce a state similar to hypnotic analgesia. Indian fakirs have frequently been observed to walk across beds of hot coals, or lie on a bed of nails or cactus thorns without evidence of pain. It is possible that the fakirs develop highly calloused skin. But this cannot be the whole explanation. It is more likely that they enter a trance-like state as a result of deep meditation. (In other cultures, the same effect may be achieved by a prolonged period of singing, drumming and dancing.) The human ability to voluntarily direct attention towards inner feelings, thoughts or images, and to block out all extraneous environmental inputs may also explain the observations (Huxley, 1952) that men and women who were burned at the stake for their religious beliefs were sometimes observed to experience what can only be described as ecstasy (although others were certainly in agony). It is possible, of course, that the meaning of the situation also played an important role in the behaviour of these people. The prospect of certain salvation of the soul or an imminent meeting with their Maker may have contributed to the transformation of the somatic input evoked by the flames so that it evoked ecstasy rather than agony.

Despite the long history of hypnotism, which goes back hundreds of years under different names such as animal magnetism and mesmerism, very little is known about its mechanisms. Still worse, most of its major features are highly controversial. For example, there is a vigorous (sometimes vicious) debate on the nature of hypnosis: is it a special state of consciousness known as a 'trance state' or is it merely a trait of responsiveness to strong suggestion? There is no resolution yet to this question (Sheehan and Perry, 1976).

Nevertheless, anyone who has observed the behaviour of people who have been hypnotized realize that this is an especially interesting phenomenon. Under hypnosis, people sustain pain, during demonstrations or experiments, at levels at which they would normally cry out and withdraw. Major surgery on every part of the body has been carried out on hypnotized patients. There are countless articles describing these procedures as well as reports that hypnosis is effective in relieving severe clinical pains, such as phantom limb pain. Although excellent studies of hypnotic analgesia have been carried out with experimentally induced pains (Hilgard and Hilgard, 1975), there are as yet no convincing studies, using the necessary control groups, of clinical pain. The evidence so far is observational or 'anecdotal'.

Even though the precise nature of hypnosis remains a mystery, there are several features of it that are important in understanding the psychological contributions to pain. It is known, for example, that not all people can be hypnotized. About 30% of people can reach a state of deep hypnosis, 30% reach a moderate state, and another 30% achieve a drowsy-light state. About 10% of people are not susceptible at all. These figures are interesting because, broadly, they resemble the proportions of placebo reactors and non-reactors. However, there is strong evidence that the lack of responsiveness to pain in hypnotized subjects is more than a placebo effect. An elegantly designed experiment (McGlashan *et al.*, 1969) has shown that pain perception and pain tolerance levels are strikingly increased during hypnosis, but only the pain perception threshold is raised after administration of a placebo. In fact, this study demonstrated that the hypnotic procedure itself has a placebo effect, but also has an additional effect that raises pain threshold and tolerance still further.

The most exciting discovery about hypnotic analgesia in recent years is the phenomenon of the 'hidden observer'. Many highly hypnotizable people are able to respond to commands under hypnosis by 'automatic writing', in which one of the hands writes answers to specific questions but the person is not aware of it. In experiments on hypnotic analgesia, in which pain is produced by immersion of an arm and hand in ice-water, the subjects are told that there is a part of the mind of which they are unaware – metaphorically called the 'hidden observer' – which can communicate with the hypnotist by automatic writing by the other hand. Hilgard (1973, p.398) describes the sequence of events:

We initially tried this procedure with a young woman highly experienced in hypnosis. In the normal non-hypnotic state, she found the experience of the circulating ice-water very painful and distressing. In the hypnotic analgesic state, she reported that she felt no pain and was totally unaware of her hand and arm in the ice-water; she was calm throughout. All the while that she was insisting verbally that she felt no pain in hypnotic analgesia, the dissociated part of herself was reporting through automatic writing that *she felt the pain just as in the normal non-hypnotic state.* Subsequent experiments with her and with additional subjects have similarly reported no conscious pain but some pain reported in automatic writing, at a level usually below that of the full pain in the normal non-hypnotic condition.

The results suggest that the intense cold evokes activity simultaneously in at least two areas of the brain. Hypnosis appears to be able to 'dissociate' one from the other, which implies that hypnotic suggestion given by the hypnotist is able to modify or suppress signals in one area but not in the other. These experiments reflect the complexity of pain mechanisms and lead us away from the concept that pain is subserved by a direct pathway that transmits 'pain impulses' faithfully from the skin to a pain centre in the brain.

While hypnosis is a fascinating research technique, it is important to recognize its limitations as a clinical therapy. Like the placebo, repeated hypnosis by a professional may become less and less effective, and exert its effects for shorter durations. Furthermore, only a relatively small percentage of people can be deeply hypnotized (Perry, 1980). However, people who tend to resist the traditional hypnotic instructions in which the hypnotist plays a dominating (sometimes overpowering) role are less resistant when they are taught to hypnotize themselves ('self-hypnosis') so that they always feel fully in control of the situation. With self-hypnosis instructions (Hilgard and Hilgard, 1975) or gentle guidance from the hypnotist (Barber, 1979), people feel less vulnerable and are more open to suggestion. Whether these procedures achieve a 'trance state' is open to debate. But they do achieve a relaxed, comfortable state. The decreased tension and anxiety, together with the suggestion and distraction, are all conducive to psychological control over pain.

Psychogenic pain

Because psychological factors play such a powerful role in pain, several clinical pain syndromes have been labelled as 'psychogenic', with the implication that the primary cause of the pain is psychological. That is, the person is presumed to be in pain because he needs or wants it. A typical case has been reported by Freeman and Watts (1950, pp.354 –5):

A woman of hysterical temperament began at the age of sixteen to complain of abdominal pain so persistently that she accumulated a series of twelve to eighteen abdominal operations, with what might be termed progressive evisceration. Following a trivial head injury, she complained so bitterly of pain in the head that a subtemporal decompression was performed. From 1934 to 1936 she was confined to bed because of agonizing pain in the back and limbs. Examination showed swollen knuckles, tender knee joints with contracture, and roentgenograms of the spine revealed lipping of the vertebrae. When we saw her for the first time, she appeared uneasy, would not give her history and began wincing and overbreathing before the bed covers were turned down. She lay constantly on her left side and cried out if any attempt was made to turn her on her back. She defended herself with her right hand from any examination of her back, and when the right hand was restrained and the region of the sacrum was gently stroked, she screamed and trembled violently. On account of exaggeration of the complaints with very little anatomic substrate, a diagnosis of conversion hysteria with polysurgical addiction was made.

The concluding sentence of this case history suggests that the patient suffered pain primarily because of psychological needs, and that she became addicted to multiple surgical operations as a way of satisfying her needs. This woman, Freeman and Watts (1950) report, then underwent a frontal lobotomy (to cut the neural connections between the frontal cortex and thalamus). The operation did not entirely relieve her pain, but she was not bothered by it as much and was able to live a useful life.

A sympathetic analysis of this kind of patient is presented by Sternbach (1970, p.182):

Such patients may acquire thick hospital charts over the years, as they have one operation after another and make the rounds from doctor to doctor. It is tempting to label them 'hysterics' or 'crocks', but such labels do not help them nor add to our understanding. Naming, as we know, is not explaining. Now it turns out that psychiatric studies of such patients have found them to be depressed. The depression may result from loss, as in inadequate grief reactions, or it may result from intropunitive reactions, as happens when anger is not appropriately directed outwardly. In chronic conditions such patients become 'pain-prone'. You must understand that these people are not faking or malingering; they have real pain by any measure we can devise, and their suffering is manifest. But neurological models do not adequately describe them, at least not yet as well as psychiatric ones do. The tactics of treating such patients are those that will relieve depression. This may consist of psychotherapy, which encourages a complete response of mourning or which enables the patient to learn that it is safe and appropriate to express anger directly. Or, if the patient is manipulating or controlling his family with his symptom, family therapy may be necessary to change the system. Or, if therapy is not appropriate for the particular patient, then antidepressant medications, or mood elevators, can be very successful. In fact, for these people with persistent or recurrent pain with no apparent organic basis, analgesics may only worsen their symptoms, whereas antidepressants do much to alleviate them.

It is clear that we must recognize the psychological contribution to pain, but we must maintain a balanced view of it. Psychological factors contribute to pain, and pain may be helped by using psychological approaches. But there are, as we shall see, other contributions. This does not deny the existence of patients who need their pain, and whose lives derive meaning from it. Such patients complain of terrible pain yet discontinue certain types of therapies because of minor unpleasantness, such as an injection or the taste of a particular drug. However, even when psychological factors appear to play a major role, there is often tissue pathology which can also be treated. In such cases, the physical as well as the psychological symptoms require treatment.

Perhaps the most convincing evidence that chronic pain is usually the cause rather than the result of neurotic symptoms derives from studies of patients who are eventually relieved of their pain. Typically, these patients, while they are suffering chronic pain, show evidence of psychological disturbance on the Minnesota Multiphasic Personality Inventory (MMPI). In particular, they have elevated scores on the scales for hysteria, depression and hypochondriasis. Some investigators have argued that these personality characteristics lead to pain or to susceptibility to chronic pain after minor injuries that would have little effect on people who do not have these characteristics. A chronic emotional problem is assumed to become manifest as chronic pain. However, the evidence points in the other direction: that pain produces the elevations in these emotional characteristics. In one study, it was found that patients who had pain of more than six months' duration – due to spinal injuries, post-herpetic neuralgia and other problems – showed significant decreases in several indices of psychological disturbance when their pain was abolished by successful surgery. The results, the authors conclude, 'support the hypothesis that the neuroticism associated with chronic pain is the result of it, and may be reversible when the pain is reduced or abolished' (Sternbach and Timmermans, 1975, p.177). Comparable decreases in several key MMPI scales (hysteria, depression, hypochondriasis and anxiety) occur after successful treatment with a variety of therapies (Sternbach, 1974).

Similarly, patients suffering several forms of chronic pain – including headache, colitis and abdominal pain – were found to have lower self-esteem than pain-free control groups. However, after these patients underwent several therapeutic procedures that significantly reduced their pain, they showed a striking improvement in their self-esteem ratings (Elton *et al.*, 1978). It is evident from studies such as these that it is unreasonable to ascribe chronic pain to neurotic symptoms. The patients with the thick charts are all too often prey to the physician's innuendoes that they are neurotic and that their neuroses are the cause of the pain. While psychological processes contribute to pain, they are only part of the activity in a complex nervous system. All too often, the diagnosis of neurosis as the cause of pain hides our profound ignorance of many aspects of pain mechanisms.

Implications of the psychological evidence

Taken together, the psychological data refute the concept that the intensity of noxious stimulation and the intensity of perceived pain have a one-to-one relationship. A stimulus may be painful in one situation and not in another. The same injury can have different effects on different people or even on the same person at different times. The data indicate that psychological variables may intervene between stimulus and perception and produce a high degree of variability between the two. In most instances, to be sure, a simple relationship holds: the harder the slam of a hammer on the thumb, the greater the pain is likely to be. The exceptions, however, illuminate the nature of the underlying mechanisms. The apparent simplicity of a psychophysical relationship does not mean that the underlying physiological mechanisms are equally simple. Their complexity is indicated by the role of early experience, meaning, and culture on pain perception. These data represent pieces of the puzzle which must play a key role in the development of any satisfactory theory of pain.

Pain, we now believe, refers to a category of complex experiences, not to a single sensation produced by a specific stimulus. We are beginning to recognize the many different qualities of sensory and affective experience that we simply categorize under the broad heading of 'pain'. We are more and more aware of the plasticity and modifiability of events occurring in the central nervous system. Livingston (1943, 1953) long ago argued against the classical conception that the intensity of pain sensation is always proportional to the stimulus. He proposed instead that pain, like all perceptions, is 'subjective, individual and modified by degrees of attention, emotional states and the conditioning influence of past experience'. Since that time we have moved still further away from the classical assumption that noxious stimulation invariably produces pain, that the pain has only one specific quality, and that it varies only in intensity.

The psychological evidence strongly supports the view of pain as a perceptual experience whose quality and intensity are influenced by the unique past history of the individual, by the meaning he gives to the pain-producing situation and by his 'state of mind' at the moment. We believe that all these factors play a role in determining the actual patterns of nerve impulses that ascend from the body to the brain and travel within the brain itself. In this way pain becomes a function of the whole individual, including his present thoughts and fears as well as his hopes for the future.

The recognition, in recent years, that psychological processes play a major role in pain has led to the development of a wide variety of psychological techniques to fight pain. These include relaxation therapy, biofeedback, and exciting new approaches to the use of hypnosis. These methods will be described and evaluated in Chapter 15. Not only does each of these procedures produce some degree of pain relief in some people, but the use of several techniques in combination has led to increasing success in the battle against some of the most vicious, intractable forms of chronic pain.

3
The Varieties of Pain

The French novelist, Marcel Proust, noted that 'Illness is the doctor to whom we pay most heed: to kindness, to knowledge we make promises only: pain we obey.' Pain is by far the most common reason for a patient to seek help from a physician. When he first feels the pain, he may restrict his activity, waiting for it to pass. If the pain persists, he may try such common remedies as rubbing the painful area, applying heat or ice, or simply resting. These universal first-aid procedures should not be dismissed as purely symbolic or magical remedies because otherwise they would not be practised universally. Any satisfactory explanation of pain must include an understanding of these remedies and we shall return to them.

If the pain rises to an intolerable level, or if it persists unabated, or keeps recurring, the sufferer goes to a physician. The doctor first listens to the patient, to the history of the development of his pain, and to the words he uses to describe and locate his pain. From his experience and training the doctor has by now classified the pain; he then goes into action to locate and define the nature and the extent of damaged tissue which he thinks is the cause of the pain.

In this simple, common consultation it is evident that there have been three quite separate processes. First, the patient has his reasons for seeking help. Second, the words he uses are aimed at convincing the doctor that he has pain and needs help. The pain may be particularly difficult to describe because the patient's ordinary language is rarely adequate to describe unusual sensations. Third, the doctor has an educated bias about how he expects his findings to match the patient's words. It can readily be seen that each of these three processes contains a multiplicity of possible variables so that the path from complaint to diagnosis and to treatment is always tortuous and needs to be followed with care and patience.

The time-course of pain

Transient pain. Pains of brief duration are usually recognized as having little consequence and rarely produce more than fleeting attention. A mild burn, a stubbed toe, the prick of a hypodermic, or a bang on the shin may produce pain for several seconds or minutes and then vanish. Little or no damage has been done and there is rarely any accompanying anxiety. The person may curse out loud, rub the area, and continue with whatever task occupied him before the injury or near-injury occurred. These momentary, transient pains are often felt as two pains. Anyone who has dropped a heavy book on his foot or accidentally put a hand on a hot stove usually feels a 'first' pain, which is relatively mild and well localized. From experience, however, we know that a 'second' pain will arrive shortly – and when it does, it wells up in our consciousness and obliterates all thought. It may rapidly decrease in intensity, or perhaps throb or feel like a series of shooting stabs for several minutes until it gradually fades away. All of these pains are characteristic of minor injuries.

When pain persists, however, we know that the injury was probably severe. The hot stove may actually have damaged the skin so that a blister will form. The book dropped on a toe may have broken it. The persistent abdominal pain may portend an inflamed appendix, an ulcer, or some other damage that we usually expect to remain, in varying degrees, until healing begins. These pains are generally known as *acute pains* – they are intense and usually diminish and disappear when healing is well under way. Sometimes, however, the pain persists even after healing is apparently complete. This may occur after injuries as innocuous as stabbing the finger on a rosebush-thorn or long after an operation which has proceeded without incident and all tissues appear to have healed normally. These persistent pains – *chronic pains* – often have tragic consequences.

Acute pain. The characteristics of acute pain are the combination of tissue damage, pain and anxiety. It is a transitional period between coping with the cause of the injury and preparing for recovery. The transitional nature of acute pain is shown by the direction of the anxiety in man after injury. Anxiety occurs in a spectrum from specific to free floating. The specific anxieties are aimed in three directions: to the past, the present and the future. The past and completed act which caused the injury may be highly defined but the reaction is prolonged and diffuse. For the wounded soldier, the man who fired the shot is the specific object of fear and threat but the victim is alerted to a more general awareness of the threatening nature of the world.

Present anxieties relate to treatment in progress. Here in particular there is a balance between private suffering and public display, which is subject to personality and social factors. The citizen of Oslo and of Naples has learned each in his different way about socially accepted and expected behaviour and about the acceptable quality of medical care. The patient calls for help with words and actions in his personal and national language.

Mixed in with anxiety about the past and present, there is the obvious fear of future consequences. Death or prolonged suffering are possibilities. The assessment of this threat and therefore the degree of anxiety will depend on personality, experience, knowledge, religion and trust. While the backward directed anxiety represents a diversion from the injury, the present and future directed anxieties concentrate on the damage. Acute pain and acute anxiety of the latter types are completely coupled. The treatment of one is the treatment of the other. There is no justification for considering the two states as independent variables. They appear as two aspects of the same phenomenon. Both were triggered by damage to tissue but are more related to treatment and recovery processes than to the injury itself. The acute state of injury in animals shows some of the same aspects as those seen in man. Arousal, agitation and aggressiveness suggest an irrational continuation of the actual fight-flight period and a diffusing of assessment of threat. The helping hand is bitten and the familiar home becomes a threatening prison from which escape is mandatory.

Acute pain, then, encompasses the unpleasantness of past injury and the hope of future recovery. Once relative safety from the source of injury has been achieved, a new form of behaviour begins which is related to promoting recovery. The need for the initiation of this behaviour is signalled by pain. In the transitional stage from injury to the beginning of recovery, anxiety is a cardinal feature. The anxiety is directed at assuring safety from the original damage, at assuring the best conditions for the initiation of treatment and recovery, and at the possible future consequences of the damage.

Chronic pain. One of the major advances in the field of pain in recent years has been the recognition that chronic, persistent pain is a distinct medical entity different from acute pain in many respects. Chronic pain, which persists after all possible healing has occurred or, at least, long after pain can serve any useful function, is no longer simply a symptom of injury or disease. It becomes a pain *syndrome* – a medical problem in its own right which requires urgent attention. Chronic pain becomes debilitating and often produces severe depression. Most important for diagnosis, treatment and prognosis is the recognition that treatments which are normally effective for most kinds of acute pain are not necessarily effective for chronic pain. Pain, which is normally associated with the search for treatment and optimal conditions for recovery, now becomes intractable. Patients are beset with a sense of helplessness, hopelessness and meaninglessness. The pain becomes evil – it is intolerable and serves no useful function. We are especially indebted to Bonica (1953, 1974) for the recognition of chronic pain as a distinct medical entity that requires special investigation and treatment; chronic, intractable pain presents a special challenge to the physician or health professional.

In chronic pain, the patient's behaviour changes during the months after the onset of his pain in the acute stage. Pain and complaint are unremitting and often a more and more elaborate search for treatment becomes a major activity. In other respects, the patient shows all aspects of a deepening depression. Movement is restricted, thought is slow and attention to the outside world is limited. There is loss of appetite, constipation, loss of libido, change of sleep pattern and disturbance of family and social relations. As this pattern of sick behaviour predominates, the original signs of injury may disappear or resolve to some minimal scar. Here we have a mismatch between the amount of pain and the amount of injury. Needless to say, relatives and doctors begin to express their frustration at being unable to help, by suspecting that 'there is nothing wrong'. This is an expression of the dualistic thinking of our society: a pain is a mental process associated with a body process – damaged tissue. If pain seems disproportionate to the apparent damage, the external observer becomes suspicious. 'Nothing wrong' in the obviously suffering person implies that nothing is wrong with the body and therefore the disease is of the mind. The patient is then examined to determine if there is some psychological cause for his sick behaviour. Has he been rewarded for his sick behaviour? Is he gaining some secondary benefit by getting more love and attention than previously, by avoiding the tensions of ordinary life, by getting a pension or an insurance settlement? These thoughts may begin to dominate people's thinking about the patient and may soon lead to abandoning the patient. These patients, in their search for treatment, frequently take high doses of several drugs and sometimes become narcotic addicts. Especially in rich societies, they seek and get multiple surgical operations, often repeats of previously unsuccessful surgery. Recently we have learned to recognize that chronic pain rarely has not a single cause but is instead the result of multiple, interacting causes. A variety of subtle physical and psychological factors all interact and contribute to chronic pain.

An understanding of chronic pain and new methods to relieve it are two of the salient challenges which provide the focus for most of this book.

The language of pain

Anyone who has suffered severe pain and tried to describe the experience to a friend or to the doctor often finds himself at a loss for words. Virginia Woolf, in her essay 'On Being Ill' touches on precisely this point: 'English,' she writes, 'which can express the thoughts of Hamlet and the tragedy of Lear, has no words for the shiver and the headache ... The merest schoolgirl, when she falls in love, has Shakespeare and Keats to speak for her; but let a sufferer try to describe a pain in his head to a doctor and language at once runs dry.'

The reason for this difficulty in expressing pain experience, actually, is not because the words do not exist. As we shall soon see, there is an abundance of appropriate words. Rather, the main reason is that, fortunately, they are not words which we have occasion to use often. There is another reason: the words may seem absurd. We may use descriptors such as splitting, shooting, gnawing, wrenching or stinging, but there are no 'outside', objective references for these words. If we talk about a blue pen or a yellow pencil we can point to an object and say 'that is what I mean by yellow' or 'the colour of the pen is blue'. But what can we point to to tell another person precisely what we mean by smarting, tingling, or rasping? A person who suffers terrible pain may say that the pain is burning and add, with embarrassment (and tears) that 'it feels as if someone is shoving a red-hot poker through my toes and slowly twisting it around.' These 'as if' statements are often essential to convey the qualities of the experience.

If the study of pain in people is to have a scientific foundation, it is essential to measure it. If we want to know how effective a new drug is, we need numbers to say that the pain decreased by some amount. Yet, while this is important to know, we also want to know whether the drug specifically decreased the burning quality of the pain, or if the especially miserable, tight, cramping feeling is gone. There is now a way to get this kind of information.

Until recently, the methods that were used for pain measurement treated pain as though it were a single, unique quality that varies only in intensity. The most common of these methods is the use of words such as 'mild', 'moderate', and 'severe', and subjects (or patients) are asked to choose the word that best describes the intensity of their pain. Another method consists of a five-point scale which ranges from 1 = mild pain to 5 = unbearable pain, and subjects are asked to choose the most appropriate number. In this way, some quantitative measure of pain is obtained. Still another method is the use of fractions, so that subjects who have received injections of analgesic drugs such as morphine are asked whether their pain is $\frac{1}{3}$, $\frac{1}{2}$, or $\frac{2}{3}$ of what it was before the injection. Yet another method is the 'visual analogue scale'. The patient or subject is presented with a line which is 10 centimetres long and has the numbers 0 and 10 at

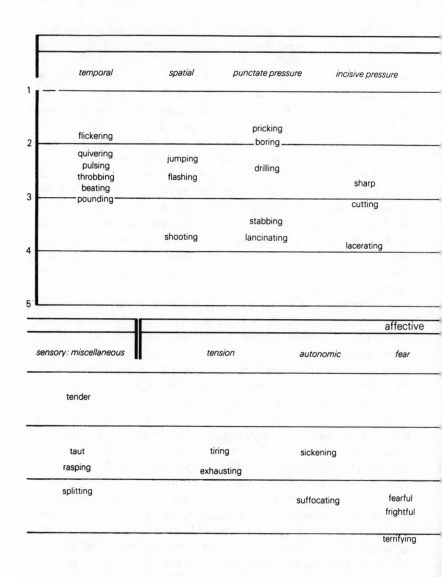

Figure 3. Spatial display of pain descriptors based on intensity ratings by patients.
The intensity scale values range from 1 (mild) to 5 (excruciating)
(from Melzack and Torgerson, 1971, p.50)

sensory				
constrictive pressure	traction pressure	thermal	brightness	dullness
			tingling itchy	dull
pinching			smarting	sore
pressing gnawing	tugging pulling	hot	stinging	hurting aching
cramping				
		burning		heavy
	wrenching	scalding		
crushing		searing		

punishment	affective-evaluative-sensory: miscellaneous	anchor words	evaluative	
		mild		1
		discomforting	annoying	2
			troublesome	
		distressing	miserable	3
	wretched			
punishing gruelling	blinding		intense	
cruel		horrible		4
vicious killing			unbearable	
		excruciating		5

either end. He is told that one end represents no pain and the other represents the worst pain imaginable, and is then asked to make a mark on the line which represents the intensity of his pain. A ruler is then used to get a numerical measure of pain intensity, such as 7cm, or units of pain intensity. These simple methods have all been used effectively in hospital clinics, and have provided valuable information about the relative effectiveness of different drugs.

All of these methods specify only intensity. It is clear, however, that to describe pain solely in terms of intensity is like specifying the visual world only in terms of light flux without regard to pattern, colour, texture, and the many other dimensions of visual experience.

Clinical investigators have long recognized the varieties of pain experience. Descriptions of the burning qualities of pain after peripheral nerve injury, or the stabbing, cramping qualities of visceral pains frequently provide the key to diagnosis and may even suggest the course of therapy. The layman is equally aware of the many qualities and dimensions of pain. An evening of radio, television or newspaper commercials makes us aware of the splitting, pounding qualities of headaches, the gnawing, nagging pain of rheumatism and arthritis, the cramping, heavy qualities of menstrual pain, and the smarting, itching qualities apparently well known to sufferers of haemorrhoids. Despite the frequency of such descriptions, and the seemingly high agreement that such adjectives are valid descriptive words, there are few studies of their use and meaning.

Melzack and Torgerson (1971) have made a start towards the specification of the qualities of pain. In the first part of their study, subjects were asked to classify 102 words, obtained from patients and from articles on pain, into smaller groups that describe different aspects of the experience of pain. On the basis of the data, the words were categorized into three major classes and sixteen subclasses. The distribution of a portion of the words is shown in Figure 3. The classes are:

1 Words that describe the *sensory qualities* of the experience in terms of temporal, spatial, pressure, thermal, and other properties.

2 Words that describe *affective qualities*, in terms of tension, fear, and autonomic properties that are part of the pain experience.
3 *Evaluative* words that describe the subjective overall intensity of the total pain experience.

Each subclass, which was given a descriptive label, consists of a group of words that were considered by most subjects to be qualitatively similar. Some of these words are undoubtedly synonyms, others seem to be synonymous but vary in intensity, while many provide subtle differences or nuances (despite their similarities) that may be of importance to a patient who is trying desperately to communicate to a physician.

The second part of the study was an attempt to determine the pain intensities implied by the words within each subclass. Groups of doctors, patients, and students were asked to assign an intensity value to each word, using a numerical scale ranging from least (or mild) pain to worst (or excruciating) pain. When this was done, it was apparent that several words within each subclass had the same relative intensity relationships in all three sets. For example, in the spatial subclass, 'shooting' was found to represent more pain than 'flashing', which in turn implied more pain than 'jumping'. Although the precise intensity values differed for the three groups, all three agreed on the positions of the words relative to each other. The scale values of the words assigned by patients are shown in Figure 3.

The measurement of pain

Because of the high degree of agreement on the intensity relationships among pain descriptors by subjects who have different cultural, socio-economic, and educational backgrounds, it has been possible to develop a questionnaire (Figure 4) to determine the properties of different pain syndromes (Melzack, 1975a). In addition to the three major classes of pain descriptors, the questionnaire includes a fourth class of miscellaneous words arranged in four subclasses. It also contains the overall Present Pain Intensity (PPI). The PPI is recorded as a number from 0 to 5, in which each number is associated with the following words: 0, no

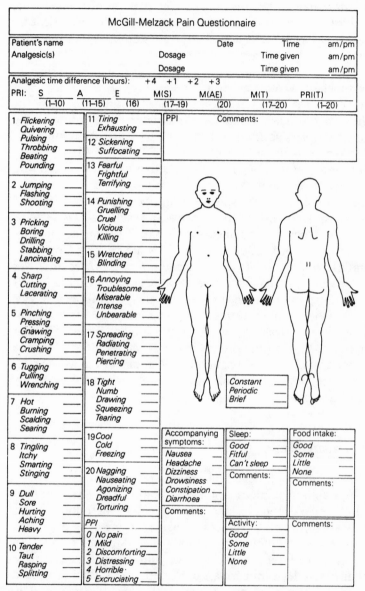

McGill-Melzack Pain Questionnaire

Patient's name				Date		Time	am/pm
Analgesic(s)			Dosage			Time given	am/pm
			Dosage			Time given	am/pm

Analgesic time difference (hours): +4 +1 +2 +3

PRI: S ___ A ___ E ___ M(S) ___ M(AE) ___ M(T) ___ PRI(T) ___
      (1–10) (11–15) (16) (17–19) (20) (17–20) (1–20)

1 Flickering ___
  Quivering ___
  Pulsing ___
  Throbbing ___
  Beating ___
  Pounding ___

2 Jumping ___
  Flashing ___
  Shooting ___

3 Pricking ___
  Boring ___
  Drilling ___
  Stabbing ___
  Lancinating ___

4 Sharp ___
  Cutting ___
  Lacerating ___

5 Pinching ___
  Pressing ___
  Gnawing ___
  Cramping ___
  Crushing ___

6 Tugging ___
  Pulling ___
  Wrenching ___

7 Hot ___
  Burning ___
  Scalding ___
  Searing ___

8 Tingling ___
  Itchy ___
  Smarting ___
  Stinging ___

9 Dull ___
  Sore ___
  Hurting ___
  Aching ___
  Heavy ___

10 Tender ___
   Taut ___
   Rasping ___
   Splitting ___

11 Tiring ___
   Exhausting ___

12 Sickening ___
   Suffocating ___

13 Fearful ___
   Frightful ___
   Terrifying ___

14 Punishing ___
   Gruelling ___
   Cruel ___
   Vicious ___
   Killing ___

15 Wretched ___
   Blinding ___

16 Annoying ___
   Troublesome ___
   Miserable ___
   Intense ___
   Unbearable ___

17 Spreading ___
   Radiating ___
   Penetrating ___
   Piercing ___

18 Tight ___
   Numb ___
   Drawing ___
   Squeezing ___
   Tearing ___

19 Cool ___
   Cold ___
   Freezing ___

20 Nagging ___
   Nauseating ___
   Agonizing ___
   Dreadful ___
   Torturing ___

PPI
0 No pain ___
1 Mild ___
2 Discomforting ___
3 Distressing ___
4 Horrible ___
5 Excruciating ___

PPI Comments:

Constant ___
Periodic ___
Brief ___

Accompanying symptoms:
Nausea ___
Headache ___
Dizziness ___
Drowsiness ___
Constipation ___
Diarrhoea ___
Comments:

Sleep:
Good ___
Fitful ___
Can't sleep ___
Comments:

Food intake:
Good ___
Some ___
Little ___
None ___
Comments:

Activity:
Good ___
Some ___
Little ___
None ___

Comments:

Figure 4. McGill Pain Questionnaire, adapted for a study of narcotic drugs. Descriptors fall into four major groups: sensory, 1 to 10; affective, 11 to 15; evaluative, 16; and miscellaneous, 17 to 20. The rank value for each descriptor is based on its position in the word set. The sum of the rank values is the 'pain rating index' (PRI). The 'present pain intensity' (PPI) is based on a scale of 0 to 5.

pain; 1, mild; 2, discomforting; 3, distressing; 4, horrible; 5, excruciating. The average scale values of these words, which were chosen from the evaluative category, are approximately equally far apart, so that they represent equal scale intervals and thereby provide 'anchors' for the specification of overall pain intensity (Melzack and Torgerson, 1971).

The descriptor-lists of the McGill Pain Questionnaire are read to a patient with the explicit instruction that he choose *only* those words which describe his feelings and sensations at that moment. Two major indices are obtained. The first is the Pain Rating Index (PRI), which is the sum of the rank values of the words chosen, based on the positions of the words in each category or 'subclass' in Figure 4. The PRI score can be computed separately for the sensory (subclasses 1–10), affective (subclasses 11–15), evaluative (subclass 16), and miscellaneous (subclasses 17–20) words, in addition to providing a total score (subclasses 1–20). The second is the Present Pain Intensity (PPI) which measures overall pain intensity on a scale of 0 to 5.

The McGill Pain Questionnaire is still an experimental tool and will undoubtedly be revised and refined as it continues to be used. There has been some controversy, for example, regarding the evaluative category – whether it is distinctly different from the affective category. Some studies (Van Buren and Kleinknecht, 1979) suggest that it is not, but a recent well-designed experiment (Prieto *et al.*, 1980) indicates that it is. There are also discussions on the exact composition of the word lists. Some portion of the words may eventually have to be arranged in different combinations. However, there is unanimous agreement that most of the words that comprise the language of pain fall into at least two distinct categories – sensory and affective. Universal agreement on a finer-grained analysis requires additional research. For the time being, the McGill Pain Questionnaire in its present form is a useful measuring tool.

The varieties of pain experience

Because pain is a private, personal experience, it is impossible for us to know precisely what someone else's pain feels like. No man

Table 1. Descriptions characteristic of clinical pain syndromes.

Menstrual pain (N = 25)	Arthritic pain (N = 16)	Labour pain (N = 11)	Disc disease pain (N = 10)	Toothache (N = 10)	Cancer pain (N = 8)	Phantom limb pain (N = 8)	Post-herpetic pain (N = 6)
Sensory							
Cramping (44%)	Gnawing (38%)	Pounding (37%)	Throbbing (40%)	Throbbing (50%)	Shooting (50%)	Throbbing (38%)	Sharp (84%)
Aching (44%)	Aching (50%)	Shooting (46%)	Shooting (50%)	Boring (40%)	Sharp (50%)	Stabbing (50%)	Pulling (67%)
		Stabbing (37%)	Stabbing (40%)	Sharp (50%)	Gnawing (50%)	Sharp (38%)	Aching (50%)
		Sharp (64%)	Sharp (60%)		Burning (50%)	Cramping (50%)	Tender (83%)
		Cramping (82%)	Cramping (40%)		Heavy (50%)	Burning (50%)	
		Aching (46%)	Aching (40%)			Aching (38%)	
			Heavy (40%)				
			Tender (50%)				

Affective

Tiring (44%) Sickening (56%)	Exhausting (50%)	Tiring (37%) Exhausting (46%) Fearful (36%)	Tiring (46%) Exhausting (40%)	Sickening (40%)	Exhausting (50%)	Tiring (50%) Exhausting (38%) Cruel (38%)	Exhausting (50%)

Evaluative

	Annoying (38%)	Intense (46%)	Unbearable (40%)	Annoying (50%)	Unbearable (50%)		

Temporal

Constant (56%)	Constant (44%) Rhythmic (56%)	Rhythmic (91%)	Constant (80%) Rhythmic (70%)	Constant (60%) Rhythmic (40%)	Constant (100%) Rhythmic (88%)	Constant (88%) Rhythmic (63%)	Constant (50%) Rhythmic (50%)

Note that only those words chosen by more than one third of the patients are listed, and the percentages of patients who chose each word are shown below the word. The word 'rhythmic' is one of three words 'rhythmic/periodic/intermittent' used in different versions of the McGill Pain Questionnaire (Melzack, 1975).

can possibly know what it is like to have menstrual cramps or labour pain. Nor can a psychologically healthy person know what a psychotic patient is feeling when he says he has excruciating pain. But the McGill Pain Questionnaire provides us with an insight into the qualities that are experienced.

One of the most exciting discoveries made with the McGill Pain Questionnaire is that each kind of pain is characterized by a distinctive constellation of words (Dubuisson and Melzack, 1976). The questionnaire was administered to patients suffering from one of eight pain syndromes: post-herpetic neuralgia, phantom-limb pain, metastatic carcinoma, toothache, degenerative disc disease, rheumatoid or osteoarthritis, labour pain, and menstrual pain. A statistical analysis of the data showed that each type of pain has unique qualities which are described by a distinctive set of words. Table 1 presents the words that characterize the eight syndromes – that is, words that were chosen by more than 33 per cent of the patients in each group. Later studies of pain due to tooth extraction (Van Buren and Kleinknecht, 1979), cancer (Graham *et al.*, 1980) and labour (Melzack *et al.*, 1981) have noted the remarkable consistency in the choice of words by patients suffering the same or similar pain syndromes. The words chosen by patients in these studies are strikingly similar to the lists of words in Table 1.

The McGill Pain Questionnaire provides information about the intensity of pain as well as the qualities of the pain. Since the PRI total score provides an index of overall pain intensity, it is possible to compare the relative intensity (or severity) of pains on the basis of this measure. For example, Figure 5 shows the average pain intensity reported by women during labour with their first baby (primiparas) and those in labour for a second, third or later child (multiparas). The graph shows clearly that the intensity scores are higher for primiparas (Melzack *et al.*, 1981). Figure 5 also shows the mean PRI scores obtained in an earlier study of several pain syndromes observed at an out-patient Pain Clinic in a general hospital. It is evident that the average PRI scores for labour pain are higher than the range of the average scores recorded for the other forms of pain. While the data do not warrant strong statements that one pain is worse than another, it can nevertheless be concluded that labour is, at least, among the

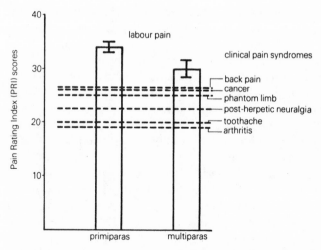

Figure 5. Average total Pain Rating Index (PRI) scores obtained from primiparous and multiparous women during labour. The average total PRI scores for several pain syndromes observed in an out-patient pain clinic are shown for comparison.
(from Melzack, Taenzer, Feldman and Kinch, 1981)

most severe pains that have been recorded with the McGill Pain Questionnaire.

While labour pain is extremely high on the average, there is a wide range in the levels of pain experienced by different women. Among primiparas, 23% report pain scores in the top third of the range of PRI scores, while only 11% of multiparas report pain at this high level. These data are consistent with the number of women who describe their pain as 'horrible' or 'excruciating' on the Present Pain Intensity (PPI) index: 25% of primiparas and 9% of multiparas report pain at 'horrible-excruciating' levels. In contrast, 24% of multiparas report pain scores in the lower third of the range while only 9% of primiparas report scores at these low levels.

Language and diagnosis

We have already noted that major kinds of pain are characterized by distinct constellations of words. Sometimes a few words can be the basis of diagnosis by a physician. An eye specialist who is told by a patient on the telephone that the pain in his eye is a 'dull ache' may diagnose a serious condition which can produce blindness, and the ophthalmologist may ask the patient to see him immediately. A severe 'burning' pain in the chest may be the clue for a possible heart attack. A persistent 'gnawing' in the fingers may mean arthritis. It is not surprising, then, that the descriptors chosen by patients can be used for diagnosis. This kind of research has already begun, with the help of computers, and is extremely promising.

In a recent study, the descriptors chosen by patients with one of eight different pain syndromes – those in Table 1 – were fed into a computer which had to make a diagnosis on the basis of the words alone (Dubuisson and Melzack, 1976). The computer made a correct classification in seventy-seven per cent of the cases. When the sex of the patient and the location of the pain were also included, the classification was correct in one hundred per cent of the cases. It is evident, then, that there are appreciable and quantifiable differences in the way various types of pain are described, and that patients with the same disease or pain syndrome tend to use remarkably similar words to communicate what they feel.

Descriptor patterns can also provide the basis for discriminating between two major types of low back pain. Some patients have clear physical causes such as degenerative disc disease, while others suffer low back pain even though no physical causes can be found. Leavitt and Garron (1980) have used a modified form of the McGill Pain Questionnaire in which the pain descriptors are presented in random order and patients can check off any words without the constraint of the intensity order in which they usually appear. They found that patients with physical – 'organic' – causes use distinctly different patterns of words from patients whose pain has no detectable cause and is labelled as 'functional'. On the basis of their research, they found that a particular group of descriptors – squeezing, nagging, exhausting, dull, sickening, troublesome, throbbing, tender, intermittent, numb, shooting, punishing, tiring – were especially important in distinguishing between the two groups. They then compared the diagnosis – 'organic' versus 'functional' – made on the basis of the word patterns alone, with the diagnosis made by surgeons on the basis of elaborate clinical and laboratory findings. Their results showed that the pain descriptors correctly identified 220 out of 253 cases. This represents an accuracy rate of 87 per cent which, astonishingly, is higher than the success rates attained with the complex, highly respected Minnesota Multiphasic Personality Inventory (MMPI).

These results, taken together, point to the value of verbal descriptors in the measurement and diagnosis of different pain syndromes. The field is new and is developing rapidly, and although the 'ultimate' pain questionnaire has not yet been developed, new research will lead to increasingly accurate tools with greater predictive powers.

Towards a definition of pain

Despite the importance of pain in medicine and biology, it is astonishing to discover that the word 'pain' has never been defined satisfactorily. Consider three recent attempts at a definition. The first (Mountcastle, 1980, p.391) states unequivocally that 'pain is that sensory experience evoked by stimuli that injure or threaten to destroy tissue, defined introspectively by every man as that which hurts'. This definition is unsatisfactory and misleading. No one can deny a link between pain and real or threatened tissue damage, but the link is so variable (as we have already seen) that pain cannot be defined exclusively in terms of tissue damage. Pain may occur in the absence of injury or long after an injury has healed. In several pain syndromes (which we will describe in the next chapter), severe pain is evoked by gentle stimulation of normal skin. The converse – the occurrence of injury without concomitant pain – is so common that it makes nonsense of definitions that rigidly link injury and pain. The definition also states that pain, introspectively, is 'that which hurts'. But this too makes no sense. If pain is a hurt, then how does one define a hurt? Presumably as a pain. The definition is circular and does not advance our knowledge of pain mechanisms. By designating tissue damage as the exclusive cause of pain, the definition ignores most of the clinical and psychological evidence on pain, and fails to incorporate the affective, motivational, and cognitive dimensions of pain as an integral part of the experience.

The second definition (Sternbach, 1968, p.12) defines pain as an abstract concept that refers to '(1) a personal, private sensation of hurt; (2) a harmful stimulus which signals current or impending tissue damage; (3) a pattern of responses which operate to protect the organism from harm'. This definition is wrong on all three counts. To define pain as a 'sensation of hurt' is, as we have just seen, a circular argument that fails to advance our understanding. To define pain as 'a harmful stimulus' is equally wrong. It confuses the cause with the experience, the physical event with the complex psychological process. Finally, protective responses may occur without pain and pain may be experienced without protective responses. Multiple complex neural factors intervene between experience and response, and one cannot be defined in terms of the other.

The third definition is much better, but still falls short of being acceptable. Merskey *et al.* (1979) define pain as 'an unpleasant sensory and emotional experience associated with actual or potential tissue damage, or described in terms of such damage'. The great merits of this definition are its explicit recognition of the loose association between injury and pain, and its inclusion of the emotional dimension of pain experience in addition to its sensory dimension. The problem it encounters lies in the word 'unpleasant'. Pain, to be sure, is unpleasant; but it is much more. The unpleasant – or 'negative-affective' – dimension of pain is really comprised of multiple dimensions. It is the kind of 'unpleasantness' that makes people scream, fight, undergo crippling, disfiguring operations, or commit suicide. What is missing in the word 'unpleasant' is the misery, anguish, desperation and urgency that are part of some pain experiences. The qualities of 'unpleasantness' are complex and comprise multiple dimensions that have yet to be determined.

Pain research, it appears, has not yet advanced to the stage at which an accurate definition of pain can be formulated. However, the continuing debate on a definition of pain is a sign of the vigour, excitement and rapid development of the field. Even in the physical sciences, the basic concepts of 'matter' and 'energy' are still being continually re-defined, yet no one can deny the incredible advances of modern-day physics and chemistry.

The diversity of pain experiences explains why it has been impossible, so far, to achieve a satisfactory definition of pain. The word 'pain' represents a *category* of experiences, signifying a multitude of different, unique experiences having different causes, and characterized by different qualities varying along a number of sensory and affective dimensions.

The analysis of the language of pain in the preceding sections points the way towards a definition of pain. It suggests that pain may be defined in terms of a multidimensional space comprising several sensory and affective dimensions. The space comprises those subjective experiences which have both somatosensory and negative-affective components and that elicit behaviour aimed at stopping the conditions that produce them. If injury or any other noxious input fails to evoke negative affect and aversive drive (as in the cases described earlier of the soldier at the battlefront or Pavlov's dogs) the experience cannot be called pain. Conversely, anxiety or anguish without concomitant activity in the somatic afferent system is not pain. The 'pain' of bereavement or the 'heartache' of the scorned lover do not legitimately fall within this definition, although both psychological states may *contribute* to pain by modulating the afferent input.

The evaluative words in Figure 3 reflect the capacity of the brain to evaluate the importance or urgency of the overall situation. These words represent judgements based not only on sensory and affective qualities, but also on previous experiences, capacity to judge outcome, and the meaning of the situation. Thus, by reflecting the total circumstances at a given time, they serve to locate the position of the pain experience within the multidimensional space for the particular individual.

At present, we must be content with guidelines *toward* a definition rather than a definition itself. We must recognize that the value of any contemporary definition is heuristic – to reflect past advances and to point the direction for new attacks on the puzzle of pain. Too much remains to be learned about pain mechanisms before we can define pain with precision. In particular, not until we understand the perplexing phenomena of clinical pain syndromes can we hope to achieve a satisfactory definition.

4
Clinical Aspects of Pain

Valuable clues about the nature of pain have derived from the study of complex pain syndromes. In particular, three syndromes, *phantom limb pain*, *causalgia*, and the *neuralgias*, have been studied in detail and present unusual features that are difficult to explain. These types of pain, which begin as signals of serious bodily damage, may persist, spread, and increase in intensity, so that they become maladies in their own right. In each case, the pain may become far worse than that associated with the original injury. In this chapter we will examine the major features of these syndromes and their implications for understanding pain.

Phantom limb pain

Phantom limb pain is one of the most terrible and fascinating of all clinical pain syndromes. Its description by Ambroise Paré in 1552 captures the sense of awe and mystery it evokes in people who hear about it for the first time:

Verily it is a thing wonderous strange and prodigious, which will scarce be credited, unless by such as have seen with their eyes, and heard with their ears, the patients who have many months after the cutting away of the leg, greviously complained that they yet felt exceeding great pain of that leg so cut off.

When Admiral Lord Horatio Nelson lost an arm in battle, he wrote to a friend that he could still sense his missing arm and that he took this as evidence for the existence of his eternal soul. Whatever one may think of this conclusion, one wishes that all patients were as fortunate in experiencing a phantom limb without additional complications. Unfortunately, the lives of many amputees become dominated by some sensory aspect of their missing limb.

There is a natural tendency for physicians to subdivide amputees into two groups: those with and those without chronic complaints. However, the relative proportion of amputees in each group inevitably varies among studies depending on the definition of the words 'chronic' and 'complaint'. Feinstein, Luce and Langton (1954) state that thirty-five per cent of amputees suffer at some time from pain in their phantoms. Carlen *et al.* (1978) examined 73 Israeli soldiers 1–6 months after traumatic amputations in the Yom Kippur War, and made every effort not to select a particular group with or without complaint. All of the amputees experienced phantom limb sensations and sixty-seven per cent had felt phantom limb pain, which was usually transient. The massive survey of American patients reported by Sherman *et al.* (1980) included 29,000 amputees, of whom about 2,000 experienced phantom limb pain. The reports in the survey came from a variety of departments (46% from physical medicine, 15% from orthopaedic surgery, 22% from surgery, 14% from anaesthesiology, and 3% from psychiatry), and the patients were treated with 43 different types of therapy. This widespread scatter of departments and therapies shows clearly that there is a general failure to understand the disorder.

Carlen *et al.* (1978) suggest that it would be unwise or premature, in seeking the origin of pain after amputation, to divide the patients into two rigid groups: those with or without pain complaints. There is also a dangerous tendency to subdivide patients according to a presumed origin of the pain, such as stump versus phantom or psychiatric versus organic. While these may be felt necessary for practical clinical situations, it would be foolhardy to accept these categories as implying a proven set of independent origins of the pain. The possibility remains that the patients lie along a continuous spectrum in which all share all of the phenomena in varying degrees. The most sensible approach for the scientist in this situation is to stand back without joining a particular diagnostic or therapeutic school, and to describe the phenomena as seen in man and animals.

The painless phantom
Most amputees report feeling a phantom limb almost immediately after amputation of an arm or leg (Simmel, 1956). The

phantom limb is usually described as having a tingling feeling and a definite shape that resembles the real limb before amputation. It is reported to move through space in much the same way as the normal limb would move when the person walks, sits down, or stretches out on a bed. At first, the phantom limb feels perfectly normal in size and shape – so much so that the amputee may reach out for objects with the phantom hand, or try to get out of bed by stepping on to the floor with the phantom leg. As time passes, however, the phantom limb begins to change shape. The arm or leg becomes less distinct and may fade away altogether, so that the phantom hand or foot seems to be hanging in mid-air. Sometimes, the limb is slowly 'telescoped' into the stump until only the hand or foot remain at the stump tip.

Amputation of a limb, however, is not essential for the occurrence of a phantom. We have already seen (p.21) that people report a phantom arm after an avulsion of the brachial plexus. Furthermore, a painless phantom is often reported by subjects or patients who have a local anaesthetic block of a sufficiently large part of the body. This has been described in detail by Simmel (1962) for patients who received a block of the lower spinal cord and by Melzack and Bromage (1973) for patients who received a block of the brachial plexus. We have all experienced a version of this in dental anaesthesia when we notice that the anaesthetic lip is apparently swollen and attracts our attention so that we may touch the lip repeatedly and inspect it in the mirror. One of us experienced a phantom arm after a block of the brachial plexus (Melzack and Bromage, 1973), and the other experienced a phantom hand when his radial, ulnar and median nerves were blocked at the wrist (Wall, Nathan and Noordenbos, 1973). In both cases, the hand felt clearly enlarged as though it were a boxing glove and the feeling was so striking that it held the centre of attention until the anaesthetic wore off. This emphasizes the second meaning of the word 'phantom', which the Oxford English Dictionary describes as 'a haunting thought or an illusion which repeatedly recurs in the mind'. It is wrong to imagine that the patient's initial phantom is a vague sensation; it appears as a startling reality.

This phantom must be produced by a lack of nerve impulses

from the limb or hand since local anaesthetics (such as lidocaine) do not generate nerve impulses. It is true that when a nerve is cut through in the absence of a local anaesthetic there is a violent injury discharge in all types of fibres (Wall, Waxman and Basbaum, 1974). But this excitation decreases rapidly and the cut nerve becomes silent until new nerve endings begin to sprout. This implies that the central nervous system must sense the lack of normal input. Furthermore, the 'normal' phantom can be generated within seconds after completion of the block of nerves. We know of no mechanism that can so quickly transport the anaesthetic agent from the area of injection to the central nervous system. We must therefore assume that the mechanism results from a loss of nerve impulses.

However, it is now apparent that the input does not need to be totally blocked for a phantom to appear; rather it has to be reduced below some critical level. In studies of phantom limbs after anaesthetic block of the brachial plexus, strikingly vivid phantom arms were felt even when the block was incomplete (Melzack and Bromage, 1973). In one subject, partial voluntary movement and sensation remained in the fingers after the block, yet the arm and hand were felt clearly to be stationed palm downwards and floating twelve inches above the hip – when in fact it had been moved by the experimenter (while the subject's eyes were closed) to a position above and behind the head (Bromage and Melzack, 1974). Phantom limb phenomena even occur when the nerves of the arm are blocked by applying a blood-pressure cuff to the upper arm and inflating it above arterial pressure. When the block is maintained for forty minutes, with the real hand hidden from vision, the phantom hand moves gradually toward the body so that it lies six inches or so away from the real hand (Gross and Melzack, 1978).

After a brachial plexus block, the phantom arm is felt as having a strong tingling or pins-and-needles feeling, in which the hand and fingers are felt especially vividly, and as occupying a definite position in space. Yet when the subject looks at the real arm, which may be distant from the perceived phantom arm, the phantom instantly 'fuses' with the real anaesthetized arm. When the eyes are then closed, the phantom usually assumes its previous position (Melzack and Bromage, 1973; Bromage and Melzack,

1974). These phenomena suggest that the phantom limb is produced by brain activities which normally underlie the body image – the neural substrate of our perception of the position of the body during movement or rest (Head, 1920). Normally, the body image is guided by sensory inputs from skin, muscles and joints. But when these inputs are reduced below a critical level, the body image becomes spontaneously active so that the limbs are felt in positions that are totally unrelated (in the absence of visual cues) to the position of the real limbs.

This suggestion that the phantom is generated by a loss of input does not mean that positive sensory signals are irrelevant. It is remarkable that, as early as 1905, Souques-Poisot observed that electrical stimulation of an amputation stump can exaggerate the phantom. Carlen *et al.* (1978) confirmed this observation, and noted that, after electrical stimulation, some patients report a striking and unpleasant exaggeration of their phantom. Our interpretation of this is that the electrical stimulation may actually inhibit the activity of spinal cord cells, so that the activity of cells which are deprived of input by the amputation is decreased still further, thereby enhancing the conditions necessary for the experience of the phantom.

The painful phantom

The distinction between a painless and a painful phantom is not a rigid one. Some amputees have so little pain or feel it so infrequently that they deny having a painful phantom. Others suffer pains periodically, ranging from several bouts a day to one each week or two. Still others have continuous pains which vary in quality and intensity. In about five to ten per cent of amputees the pain is severe and may become worse over the years. It may be occasional or continuous, and is described as cramping, shooting, burning or crushing. It may start immediately after amputation, but sometimes appears weeks, months, even years later. The pain is felt in definite parts of the phantom limb (Livingston, 1943). A common complaint, for example, is that the phantom hand is clenched, fingers bent over the thumb and digging into the palm, so that the whole hand is tired and painful.

If the pain persists for long periods of time, other regions of the body may become sensitized so that merely touching these

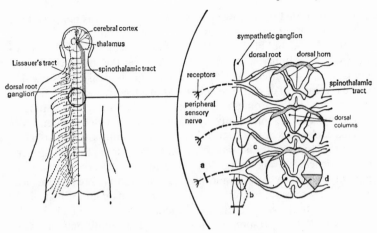

Figure 6. Traditional concept of pain and several conventional surgical procedures. *Left* is Larsell's (1951) diagram of the pain pathway: pain fibres from each dermatome enter the spinal cord, ascend a few segments (in Lissauer's tract), and connect with fibres that cross the cord and form the spinothalamic tract to the thalamus. Fibres from the thalamus project to the cortex. *Right* is a diagram of spinal cord cross sections and adjacent sympathetic ganglia, showing several neurosurgical procedures to relieve pain. a: neurectomy; b: sympathectomy; c: rhizotomy; and d: cordotomy.

new 'trigger zones' will evoke spasms of severe pain in the phantom limb (Cronholm, 1951). Pain, moreover, is often triggered by visceral inputs produced by urination and defecation (Henderson and Smyth, 1948). Even emotional upsets such as an argument with a friend may sharply increase the pain. Still worse, the conventional surgical procedures (Figure 6) often fail to bring permanent relief, so that these patients may undergo a series of such operations without any decrease in the severity of the pain.

Before we analyse the major properties of phantom limb pain we shall first examine a case history reported by W. K. Livingston (1943, pp.1–4) an outstanding surgeon and clinical observer who made important contributions to our understanding of pain:

In 1926, a physician, who had long been a close friend of mine, lost his left arm as a result of gas bacillus infection. (He had sustained a puncture wound of his left hand when a glass syringe containing the bacillus broke as he was injecting it into a guinea pig. Virulent and rapidly spreading gas gangrene made its appearance during the night and his arm was amputated the following morning.) The arm was removed by a guillotine type of amputation close to the shoulder and for some three weeks the wound bubbled gas. It was slow in healing and the stump remained cold, clammy, and sensitive ... At times the stump would jerk uncontrollably or, after a period of quiet, flip suddenly outward. He suffered a great deal of pain and submitted to a reconstruction operation and the removal of neuromas (small nodules of regenerated nerve tissue), without any relief. In spite of my close acquaintance with this man, I was not given a clearcut impression of his sufferings until a few years after the amputation, because he was reluctant to confide to anyone the sensory experiences he was undergoing. He had the impression, that is so commonly shared by layman and physician alike, that because the arm was gone, any sensations ascribed to it must be imaginary. Most of his complaints were ascribed to his absent hand. It seemed to be in a tight posture with the fingers pressed closely over the thumb and the wrist sharply flexed. By no effort of will could he move any part of the hand ... The sense of tenseness in the hand was unbearable at times, especially when the stump was exposed to cold or had been bumped. Not infrequently he had a sensation as if a sharp scalpel was being driven repeatedly, deep into ... the site of his original puncture wound. Sometimes he had a boring sensation in the bones of the index finger. This sensation seemed to start at the tip of the finger and ascend to the extremity of the shoulder, at which time the stump would begin a sudden series of clonic contractions. He was frequently nauseated when the pain was at its height. As the pain gradually faded, the sense of tenseness in the hand eased somewhat, but never in a sufficient degree to permit it to be moved. In the intervals between the sharper attacks of pain, he experienced a persistent burning in the hand. This sensation was not unbearable and at times he could be diverted so as to forget it for short intervals. When it became annoying, a hot towel thrown over his shoulder or a drink of whisky gave him partial relief.

I once asked him why the sense of tenseness in the hand was so frequently emphasized among his complaints. He asked me to clench my fingers over my thumb, flex my wrist, and raise the arm into a hammerlock position and hold it there. He kept me in this position as long as I could stand it. At the end of five minutes I was perspiring freely, my hand and arm felt unbearably cramped, and I quit. But you can take your hand down, he said.

He was prepared to submit to a posterior rhizotomy (see Figure 6), but asked my opinion as to whether or not the simpler operation of sympathectomy (Figure 6) might afford some relief. I was unable to predict the effect of a sympathectomy, and suggested that some time when his pain was particularly severe, a novocaine infiltration of the appropriate sympathetic ganglia might provide, by its temporary effect, some index of the value of sympathectomy in his particular case. The opportunity to try this did not occur until early in 1932. On that occasion I was visiting at his home when a particularly bad attack of pain came on. We went at once to the hospital and carried out a novocaine injection of the upper thoracic sympathetic ganglia of both sides. Following the injection the stump was found to be warm and dry, and the pain in the phantom limb gone. To our mutual surprise, he felt that he could voluntarily move each of his phantom fingers. This freedom of movement and complete relief of pain persisted the following day, and when I finished my visit we agreed that the test seemed to indicate that a surgical sympathectomy should be worth doing. It was arranged that he should come to my home city in the next few weeks for this operation.

He did not come, nor did I hear from him for three months. I found then that he had remained entirely free from pain and discomfort in the phantom extremity . . . He stated that this was the first time he had been free from pain in the phantom hand since the day of amputation. Though he was delighted with the result, he interpreted it as proof of the purely psychic origin of his pains and as confirmation of his fear that he was suffering from a psychoneurosis. He could not see why an injection with novocaine, the effect of which should wear off in a few hours, could possibly confer relief from pain of months' duration. I did not know 'why' it could, but previous experiences with similar injections for other pain syndromes had taught me that it sometimes does confer lasting relief.

The relief from pain persisted for many months but gradually he became aware again of an increasing tension in the phantom hand and an intolerable sensation of constriction in the shoulder, as if 'a wire tourniquet' were being constantly tightened, shutting off the circulation. He had been on a hunting trip in Canada about a month before I saw him in October 1934. The weather had been chilly and, although he wore a woollen sock over the stump, it had become very cold. He believed that the exposure had aggravated his distress. At this time the stump was extremely cold and wet, measuring 10°–12°C. colder than the same level of the opposite arm. On 12 October 1934, five ml of 2-per-cent solution of novocaine were injected near each of the upper four sympathetic ganglia of the left side. During the placing of the needles, as the second needle was inserted below the neck of the second rib, he complained of a sudden, sharp, stabbing pain in the base of his thumb. The needle was readjusted but the pain persisted. An hour after the injection, all of the digits except the thumb felt warm and relaxed. The thumb seemed to remain pressed into the palm and was the seat of a burning pain. During the night the pain spread up the arm and he slept little in spite of heavy sedation. The following day the burning sensation gradually disappeared. The hand remained warm and the digits were freely movable. For more than seven years the pains did not return. The stump remained warm and insensitive, and there were no attacks of clonic jerking. Sweating remained normal on the affected side. There were intervals in which he seemed to completely forget the phantom arm and at times he could not even voluntarily recall its image. Within recent months, however, there have been signs that trouble might be brewing again. He has had none of his former complaints but occasionally he gets a sharp and arresting twinge of pain in the stump itself.

Properties of phantom limb pain

Phantom limb pain is characterized by four major properties:

1 The pain may endure long after the healing of the injured tissues. While the pain is transient in many patients, it may persist for years or decades in others (Sunderland, 1978) so that there are still amputees from World War II who continue to struggle with their pain. In some patients the pain is clearly related to faulty regrowth of nerves in their stump, but in many the original area of damage seems completely healed. Sometimes, the pain may resemble, in both quality and location, the pain that was present before amputation (Bailey and Moersch, 1941; White and Sweet, 1969). Thus, a patient who was suffering from a wood sliver jammed under a finger nail, and at that time lost his hand in an accident, subsequently reported a painful sliver under the finger nail of his phantom hand. Similarly, lower limb amputees may report pain in particular toes or parts of the phantom foot that were ulcerated or diseased prior to amputation.

2 Trigger zones may spread to healthy areas on the same or opposite side of the body (Cronholm, 1951). Gentle pressure or pinprick on another limb or on the head (Figure 7) may trigger terrible pain in the phantom limb. There is also evidence that pain at a site distant from the stump may evoke pain in the phantom limb. Thus, amputees who develop anginal pain as long as twenty-five years after amputation may suffer severe pain in the phantom limb during each bout of anginal pain, although phantom limb pain may never before have been experienced (Cohen, 1944).

3 Prolonged relief of pain may occur after temporary *decreases*

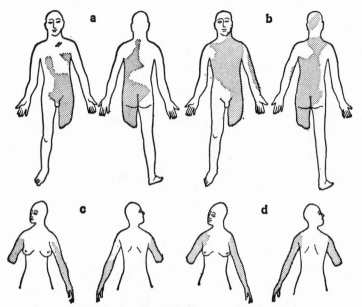

Figure 7. Cronholm's (1951) observations on stimulation sites which evoke pain sensation in the phantom limb. *Top* shows a 59-year-old man who received compound fractures of the lower left leg at the age of twenty-one: amputation was four months later. Pressure (A) or pinpricks (B) were applied to the skin. Stimulation of effective sites (crosshatched areas) produced severe shooting pains and other sensations in the phantom limb. *Bottom* shows a 34-year-old woman: amputation was at the age of fourteen. Pressure (C) or pinpricks (D) were applied to the skin. Stimulation of effective sites (crosshatched areas) produced sensations of a diffuse, unpleasant 'irritation' in the phantom hand.

of somatic input. The most obvious therapy for phantom limb pain is to decrease the input by injecting a local anaesthetic at sensitive spots or nerves in the stump. Astonishingly, these blocks may stop the pain for days, weeks, sometimes permanently, even though the anaesthesia wears off within hours (Livingston, 1943). Successive blocks may produce increasingly longer periods of relief. Similarly, an anaesthetic injected into the lower-back interspinous tissue in leg amputees produces a progressive numbness of parts of the phantom limb and prolonged, sometimes permanent, relief of pain in all or part of it (Feinstein, Luce and Langton, 1954).

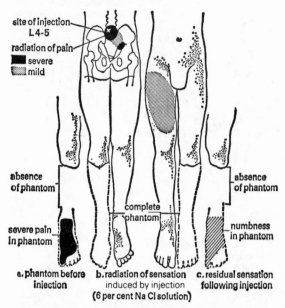

Figure 8. Observations by Feinstein, Luce and Langton (1954) on the effect of hypertonic saline injection into lumbar (L4–L5) interspinous tissues on phantom limb pain. The saline injection, in this case, produced a radiation of pain to the right hip and thigh, and sudden detailed awareness of the complete phantom limb. After injection, numbness was felt in the previously painful area. Pain relief, after this procedure, may last for days, weeks, sometimes permanently.

4 Prolonged relief of pain may occur after *increases* of the sensory input. Injection of small amounts of hypertonic saline into the interspinous tissue of amputees (Figure 8) produces a sharp, localized pain that radiates into the phantom limb, lasts only about ten minutes, yet may produce dramatic partial or total relief of pain for hours, weeks, sometimes indefinitely (Feinstein, Luce and Langton, 1954). Vigorous vibration of the stump may also produce relief of phantom limb pain (Russell and Spalding, 1950). The most recent of these techniques (Wall and Sweet, 1967) applies electrical stimulation to the stump and has become an established method for the control of pain in the phantom limb and stump (Krainick *et al.*, 1980). In a related technique, the

electrodes may be placed surgically on to the dorsal columns of the spinal cord (Figure 6). This procedure has become the most successful of the surgical therapies for phantom limb pain (Sherman *et al.*, 1980; Krainick *et al.*, 1980).

The search for causal mechanisms
The mechanisms underlying phantom limb pain have been the basis of bitter controversy. The crux of the problem has been the attempt to discover a single factor as the whole explanation. Historically, the search for *the* causal mechanism has progressed from the periphery to the central nervous system, each site on the way leading to a proposed mechanism and a particular therapy to relieve pain (Figure 6, p.77). The earliest treatment was to surgically remove the neuromas (small nodules of tangled, re-generated nerve fibres) which form after a major nerve is cut and prevented from regenerating normally. However, this procedure generally fails to relieve phantom limb pain. The next treatment was to cut the sensory roots that lead from the nerves of the stump to the spinal cord (operation C in Figure 6); yet this surgery usually fails, often replacing the original pain with worse suffering (Sunderland, 1978). Similarly, attempts to cut ascending tracts in the spinal cord which are presumed to carry the pain-evoking signals (operation D in Figure 6) fail to produce pro-longed relief and may ultimately increase pain and discomfort. Adding to the mystery of the origin of the pain, it has been found that the sympathetic nervous system plays a crucial role in some cases, by means of mechanisms which have only recently become understandable and which we will explain later (Chapter 8).

Because of the frequent failure of traditional surgical therapy, it has been suggested that the patients are in pain because of psychopathological personal needs (Kolb, 1954). It is true that patients suffering phantom limb pain often have emotional dis-turbances such as anxiety about social adjustment. Indeed the intense, unrelenting pain may itself produce marked withdrawal, paranoia, and other personality changes (Livingston, 1943). However, the hypothesis that phantom limb pain always has a psychiatric basis is untenable. It cannot explain the sudden relief produced by nerve blocks. It would be wrong to assume that the injections have only psychotherapeutic (or placebo) value, because injection of an inappropriate nerve fails to relieve pain, even though injection of the appropriate nerve in the same patient is effective (Livingston, 1943). Moreover, statistical analysis of the data presented by Ewalt, Randall and Morris (1947) indicates that patients with phantom limb pain do not have a greater incidence of neuroses than those without pain in the phantom limb. Emotional factors undoubtedly contribute to the pain but are not the major cause.

In summary, these data, taken together, indicate that phantom limb pain cannot be satisfactorily explained by any single mechanism such as peripheral nerve irritation, abnormal sympathetic activity, or psychopathology. All contribute to the pain in some way. The question is: how? The most satisfactory answer so far is that traumatic or otherwise abnormal inputs may produce a change in activity in the central nervous system itself, so that abnormal patterns of nerve impulses are triggered by cutaneous inputs and sympathetic outputs, and are modulated by brain activities.

Phantom body pain in paraplegics

Phantom body pain in paraplegic patients is the most mysterious of all pain phenomena. Paraplegia refers to the total loss of sensation and motor activity that occurs after severe damage of the spinal cord. Immediately after a serious automobile or shooting accident, a person may report that he or she has no sensation below a certain level of the body – the level of the spinal damage. Sometimes the legs feel as though they are up in the air with the toes over the head even though they are stretched out straight on the bed.

Three kinds of pain are reported by paraplegic patients: (1) *root pain* (or 'girdle pain') localized at or near the level of the cord lesion; (2) *visceral pain* which usually accompanies a distended bladder or bowel; and (3) *phantom body pain* which is felt in the areas of complete sensory loss. Because many earlier studies fail to distinguish among the three kinds of pain, the frequency of occurrence of each is difficult to determine. On the basis of the available data, however, it is estimated that five to ten per cent of paraplegic patients suffer severe phantom body pains. The patients complain of burning, tingling pains in segments of the body below the level of the lesion in which there is a complete loss of sensation to sensory stimuli. These pains are sometimes replaced by 'severe, crushing pressure, by vice-like pinching sensations, by streams of fire running down the legs into the feet and out the toes, or by a pain produced by the pressure of a knife being buried in the tissue, twisted around rapidly and finally withdrawn all at the same time' (Davis and Martin, 1947, p.486). The onset of pain may be immediate, but may also occur months or years after injury. In the most severe cases, the pain may persist for years without abating (Botterell *et al.*, 1954). The severity of pain in these patients has often led to multiple operations: rhizotomies, cordotomies and sympathectomies (Figure 6). Although claims of success have been made for one or another procedure, most operations fail to provide lasting relief.

The most striking feature of phantom body pain in paraplegics is its presence even when the spinal cord is known to be totally transected. Melzack and Loeser (1978) have recently reviewed these cases, of which the following is typical:

D.G. sustained a fracture of the upper spine in an automobile accident and was subsequently paraplegic. Although he had some muscle spasms during the first few weeks, he did not complain of significant pain. When he was seen one year later, he complained of muscle spasms in his legs, knife-like pains in the chest, burning pain in his hips and cramping pains in his abdomen. He had no sensation or voluntary motor activity below the mid-chest level. Anaesthetic blocks at the level of the spinal lesion eliminated the muscle spasms but did not change his pain. The following year, the patient was seen again and complained of three types of pain: crushing, knife-like pain in the chest; cramping pain in the abdomen; and burning pain in the hips and legs. A neurosurgical operation was then carried out to cut the pathways (cordotomy, Figure 6) that are traditionally held to carry pain signals. The cordotomies were performed on both sides above the level of spinal lesion, but the pains were unchanged. Several drugs were tried but they failed to relieve the pain. Four months later, anaesthetic blocks of the sympathetic system were performed on both sides but instead of helping, they increased the abdominal cramping and burning hip pain. New analgesic drugs were tried but they had no effect. Finally, the decision was made to remove an entire segment of spinal cord – an operation known as a cordectomy which is rarely carried out. After complete removal of about an inch of spinal cord above the level of the lesion, the patient reported that the operation relieved his back pain and some of his chest pain but did not alter his cramping abdominal pain, the burning pain in his hip or the tingling and burning pain in his legs. Eight months after the operation, the patient reported that most of his chest pain had returned, and his abdominal and leg pains were not altered. When last seen he persistently complained of cramping pain in the lower abdomen and burning, tingling pain in the hips and legs.

Patients such as this tragic man present a remarkable puzzle: they feel pain in specific areas of the trunk or the limbs below the level of a known spinal transection. The removal of a segment of spinal cord precludes any possibility of transmission from peripheral receptors to the brain through spinal cord pathways. Furthermore, activity of the sympathetic nervous system often produces sharp increases in pain (Melzack and Loeser, 1978), but sympathetic blocks or sympathectomy usually fail to relieve the pain. Finally, although these patients are often depressed, there is no evidence that the pain is produced by psychological factors.

It is clear that the pains in these unfortunate patients resemble phantom limb pain, and the neural mechanisms may also be similar. In paraplegics, even more than in amputees, there is an enormous loss of sensory input to spinal cord cells above the level of the lesion. This loss of input, there is reason to believe (Melzack and Loeser, 1978), produces highly abnormal activity in the remaining spinal cells. As we will see in later chapters, this abnormal activity is influenced by sensory inputs, autonomic outputs, and brain activities. While phantom limb pain can now be helped in a significant proportion of amputees by modulating these influences, the pains suffered by paraplegics are, sadly, less easily relieved.

Causalgia

Causalgia is a severe, burning pain that is characteristically associated with rapid, violent deformation of nerves by high-velocity missiles such as bullets (Sunderland, 1978). It is estimated to occur in 2–5% of cases of peripheral nerve injury, and is typically seen in young men who have been wounded in military combat. Causalgia persists more than six months after injury in 85% of cases, and then begins to disappear spontaneously. Nevertheless, a year after injury, about 25% still complain of pain (Echlin, Owens and Wells, 1949).

Causalgia (which means 'burning pain') exhibits many of the features of phantom limb pain as well as other unusual characteristics. Its dominant feature is the unrelenting intensity of the pain which evokes images of Dante's *Inferno*. It has been described by patients as being 'like a blaze of fire', 'like someone was pouring boiling water on the top of my foot and holding a cigarette lighter under my big toe', 'like my hand was pressed against a hot stove' (Echlin, Owens and Wells, 1949). Mitchell (1872), who coined the terms 'causalgia' and 'phantom limb pain', believed causalgia to be 'the most terrible of all tortures which a nerve wound may inflict'.

The classic description of causalgia was recorded by Mitchell (1872, pp.292–6) at the time of the American Civil War. He describes the case of Joseph Corliss, who was shot in the left arm by a bullet that entered just above the elbow, penetrated without touching the artery, and emerged through the belly of the biceps:

On the second day the pain began. It was burning and darting. He states that at this time sensation was lost or lessened in the limb, and that paralysis of motion came on in the hand and forearm. The pain was so severe that a touch anywhere, or shaking the bed, or a heavy step, caused it to increase.

The pain persisted despite healing of the wound, so that two years after the injury:

He keeps his hand wrapped in a rag, wetted with cold water, and covered with oiled silk, and even tucks the rag carefully under the flexed finger tips. Moisture is more essential than cold. Friction outside of the clothes, at any point of the entire surface, 'shoots' into the hand, increasing the burning (pain) . . . Deep pressure on the muscles has a like effect, and he will allow no one to touch his skin, save with a wetted hand, and even then is careful to exact careful manipulation. He keeps a bottle of water about him, and carries a sponge in the right hand. This hand he wets before he handles anything; used dry, it hurts the other limb. At one time, when the suffering was severe, he poured water into his boots, he says, to lessen the pain which dry touch of friction causes in the injured hand . . . He thus describes the pain at its height: 'It is as if a rough bar of iron were thrust to and fro through the knuckles, a red-hot iron placed at the junction of the palm and (thumb), with a heavy weight on it, and the skin was being rasped off my finger ends.'

The debilitating effects of such prolonged pain have been described by Mitchell (pp.196-7):

Perhaps few persons who are not physicians can realize the influence which long-continued and unendurable pain may have upon both body and mind. The older books are full of cases in which, after lancet wounds, the most terrible pain and local spasms resulted. When these had lasted for days or weeks, the whole surface became hyperaesthetic, and the senses grew to be only avenues for fresh and increasing tortures, until every vibration, every change of light, and even ... the effort to read brought on new agony. Under such torments the temper changes, the most amiable grow irritable, the soldier becomes a coward, and the strongest man is scarcely less nervous than the most hysterical girl.

Role of input from the limb

An abnormal sensory input from the areas innervated by the injured nerve is clearly implicated in causalgia (Livingston, 1943). The fact that even the gentlest touch may provoke pain makes these people withdraw from all tactile stimuli. They tend to protect the limb by placing wet clothes around it, and keep it almost immobile since any movement is usually accompanied by pain. The pain, then, limits movement, which in turn decreases the usual, patterned cutaneous and proprioceptive input from the limb. The input, therefore, is doubly abnormal as a result of the lesion of the nerve and the excessive protection of the limb.

Once the causalgic state is full-blown, the original injury is no longer the major cause of pain. The frequent failure of peripheral nerve surgery to abolish pain indicates that more is involved than simply an irritating peripheral lesion. Section of the peripheral nerve at successively higher levels, amputation of the limb, and cutting the dorsal sensory roots which enter the spinal cord, have all produced as many failures as successes. Indeed, operations have been performed for causalgic pain at nearly every site in the sensory pathway from peripheral receptors to somatosensory cortex, and at every level the story is the same: some initial encouraging results, but a disheartening tendency for the pain to return (Sunderland, 1978).

Modulation of the sensory input, however, may bring about

dramatic relief of pain. Injection of local anaesthetics into the nerves or tissues associated with the lesion may abolish pain for hours or days, and on rare occasions it never returns. Livingston (1948) reports, moreover, that the pain can be abolished if the patient is trained to tolerate sensory stimulation of the affected limb and is urged to use it normally. He encouraged his patients to place the affected arm in warm water baths, in which the water currents flowing over the limb were made increasingly vigorous over a period of weeks. Once the patient allowed the therapist's hand to touch the limb under water, he was urged to permit the therapist to massage the arm, at first gently, then more vigorously. As the pain diminished, the patient tended to use the arm, which in turn produced a more normal proprioceptive input. In this way, the causalgic pain diminished in intensity over a period of weeks.

Non-specific triggering stimuli

One of the most remarkable features of causalgic pain is the degree to which it is triggered or enhanced by a variety of non-noxious stimuli. Pain is produced by the gentlest somatic stimulation, and even by non-somatic stimuli. Sudden noises, rapidly changing visual stimuli, emotional disturbances, almost any stimulus which elicits a startle response, are all capable of making the pain worse (Livingston, 1943). When Livingston was Commander of the Peripheral Nerve Injury Ward in a United States Naval Hospital, he had to request a special order from Washington to prevent airplanes from flying in the vicinity of the hospital since the vibration and noise produced screams of agony in his causalgic patients.

Sympathetic nervous system mechanisms

The sympathetic nervous system appears to play a particularly important role in causalgia. The affected limb usually shows a variety of symptoms indicative of abnormal sympathetic activity. The hand is cold, often drips sweat, is discoloured (presumably due to vascular changes) and even the fingernails become brittle and shiny. Injection of a local anaesthetic into the sympathetic ganglia may dramatically abolish the pain as well as the abnormal sympathetic symptoms for long periods of time, sometimes permanently (Livingston, 1943). Sympathectomy, moreover, usually produces permanent relief of causalgia (Sunderland, 1978; White and Sweet, 1969).

In summary, the data show that causalgia, like phantom limb pain, is determined by several contributions: by sensory inputs from the somatic as well as the auditory and visual systems, by activity in the sympathetic nervous system, and by cognitive activities such as emotional disturbance. No one of these contributions can be considered as the sole cause. Rather, the data suggest that causalgia is brought about by changes in activity in the central nervous system, so that all avenues of input are now capable of triggering nerve impulse patterns that produce pain. Abnormal sympathetic manifestations are clearly a major source of somatic input, and appear to have a more potent role in causalgia than in phantom limb pain. Nevertheless, they represent only one source of sensory input. Cutaneous and proprioceptive inputs also evoke pain, and they too can be modulated to bring about temporary or permanent relief of pain.

The neuralgias

There are several pain syndromes associated with peripheral nerve damage that are generally categorized as neuralgic pain. Their properties are essentially similar to those of phantom limb pain and causalgia, and are characterized by severe, unremitting pain which is difficult to treat by surgical or other traditional methods. The causes of neuralgic pain include viral infections of nerves, nerve degeneration associated with diabetes, poor circulation in the limbs, vitamin deficiencies, and ingestion of poisonous substances such as arsenic. In brief, almost any infection or disease that produces damage to peripheral nerves, particularly the large myelinated nerve fibres, may be the cause of pain that is labelled as neuralgic.

Post-herpetic neuralgia
Infection by the virus *herpes zoster* (which is related to the virus that causes chicken pox) produces inflammation of one or more sensory nerves. The inflammation, which is painful, is associated with eruptions (or 'shingles') at the skin at the termination of the

nerve. The herpetic attack is itself painful, but the pain usually subsides. In a small number of people, however, the post-herpetic pain persists and may become worse. Noordenbos (1959) notes that neuralgic skin areas are not only the site of spontaneous pain (in the absence of stimulation), but are extremely hyper-aesthetic, so that the pain is aggravated by any cutaneous stimuli applied to them. Even the friction of clothes is highly un-pleasant and contact is avoided as much as possible. The pain may also be intensified by noise in the immediate vicinity or by emotional stress. This condition may last for many months or even years, and is extremely resistant to most forms of therapy including surgical treatment.

Noordenbos (1959) describes two major characteristics of post-herpetic pain. The first is the remarkable summation of stimula-tion. One of the stimuli Noordenbos used was a test-tube con-taining hot water. When the hot tube was applied to normal skin, the patient reported that it felt hot but tolerated it without dis-comfort for long periods of time. When it was then placed on the neuralgic skin area, an entirely different sequence of events occurred. There was no sensation of temperature for the first few seconds. The tube was then gradually felt as warm or tingling, slowly becoming hotter. If stimulation was continued, the patient stated that it began to burn and finally he cried out with pain and pushed the examiner's hand away. This whole sequence took from twenty seconds to as long as a full minute or longer. Noordenbos notes that if a larger surface of the hot tube was applied to the skin the entire sequence was accelerated, starting as indifferent and rapidly going through all the intermediate sen-sations to end in unbearable pain. Thus the speed of summation of input was dependent on the size of the area that was stimulated.

The second characteristic is a marked delay in the onset of pain after stimulation. This was apparent in the sequence of events Noordenbos observed after application of the hot test-tube. It was especially clear when he applied multiple gentle pin-pricks to the affected skin areas. After a distinct delay following onset of the pinpricks, the patients reported feeling intense pain that spread over large areas and then wore off slowly. The onset of pain was 'very sudden, almost explosive in character, and had an extremely unpleasant quality that differed markedly from the pain evoked in normal skin with the same stimulus' (Noordenbos, 1959, p.8).

This disease has a combination of pathologies. A substantial number of nerve fibres are destroyed and the fibre loss presumably produces a state of raised excitability in neurons in the spinal cord. The activity of these cells is assumed to produce a deep ongoing pain which is influenced by peripheral manipulation. This combination of peripheral and central pathology produces a mixture of raised thresholds, abnormal unpleasant evoked sensations, and ongoing pain.

Trigeminal neuralgia

Several neuralgic states are associated with the nerves of the head and face, and are classified on the basis of the particular nerve which is affected (White and Sweet, 1969). Trigeminal neuralgia – which is also known as 'tic douloureux' – is particularly vicious. It is characterized by paroxysmal attacks of pain that may be triggered by eating or talking, or may even occur spontaneously. The pain is extremely severe, so that these people often refuse to eat or talk, and become physically weak and depressed. These properties are described in a case history reported by Livingston (1943, pp.147–8):

Mr J.M., aged sixty-four, suffered from attacks of trigeminal neuralgia in 1932. In 1933 a competent neurosurgeon partially divided the trigeminal nerve . . . He was completely relieved of pain for three years. Then, in spite of the fact that there was numbness . . . the attacks, exactly similar in type, recurred. A second operation was carried out to divide the [nerve] more completely. Again he had a period of three years of complete relief. In 1939 the pain attacks again began, in all respects similar to his previous trouble. He was advised to submit to a third operation . . . He refused the third operation. At the time of my first examination in May 1940, he said that his pain was beyond description, in spite of large doses of hypnotics and opiates. Eating, smoking, talking, shaving, or brushing his teeth brought on the painful paroxysms. He had lost forty pounds in weight . . . Attacks could be set off by contact near the . . . nostril, near the outer margin of the lip, near the . . . eye, and at two areas in the gum on each side of his two remaining incisor teeth in the right upper jaw. Each of these sensitive points was injected several times in the course of a three weeks' treatment. Whenever he had a twinge of pain, the site from which the pain seemed to originate was infiltrated with novocaine. The attacks rapidly diminished in frequency and severity. There was a temporary exacerbation when the two incisor teeth were removed. He remained entirely free from pain from June until December. Then he had a mild recurrence requiring five injections to control. In March 1942, sharp paroxysms began again. They were relieved within two weeks by a few injections and the fitting of an upper plate.

One of the remarkable features of tic douloureux is that the paroxysmal attacks are triggered by gentle stimulation but not by intense stimuli (Kugelberg and Lindblom, 1959; White and Sweet, 1969). Severe pinches, pin jabs, or intense pressure, heat or cold applied to the trigger zones usually fail to evoke pain. When weak stimuli are used, however, paroxysms are evoked after a long summation time. Successive gentle touches for fifteen to thirty seconds may be required to fire an attack. The pain may then last for one to three minutes. These observations, together with the fact that there is a refractory period of several minutes after an attack before a new one can be evoked, led Kugelberg and Lindblom (1959) to conclude that tic douloureux is the result of abnormal central neural processes. Fortunately, tic douloureux is one of the few pain states which can often be treated simply and effectively. Tegretol (carbamazepine), a drug which is used to treat epilepsy, also relieves tic douloureux in the majority of patients (White and Sweet, 1969). Unfortunately, it appears not to be effective in the treatment of other neuralgic pain states.

We know almost nothing of the cause of this disease which occurs more commonly in older people, in cold countries, and on the right side of the face (63 per cent of 6,719 cases; White and Sweet, 1969). This condition, which is limited to the face, is not associated with a raised threshold for triggering sensation and is therefore unlike the other neuropathies. Calvin, Loeser and Howe (1977) propose that slight damage to nerve fibres may result in an unusual reverberation of nerve impulses in and out of the trigeminal nucleus in the medulla and in the damaged nerve.

In summary, the neuralgias exhibit many of the properties characteristic of phantom limb pain and causalgia. The remarkable summation of cutaneous stimulation of hyperaesthetic skin areas, the increases in pain produced by sudden auditory stimulation or by emotional disturbance, and the long delays in perception all point to abnormal activity in the central nervous system in addition to any peripheral pathology. Changes in peripheral nerves certainly exist in these syndromes. However, these changes cannot be the whole story: surgical section of the appropriate nerves right up to the point of entry into the spinal cord or brain frequently fails to relieve the pain. Rather, the data suggest that changes in central nervous system activity, perhaps initiated by peripheral factors, may underlie the summation, delays, persistence and spread of pain.

Implications of the clinical evidence

The implications of the pathological pain syndromes described above are the following:

1 *Summation.* Gentle touch, warmth, and other non-noxious somatic stimuli can trigger excruciating pain. The fact that repetitive or prolonged stimulation is usually necessary to elicit pain, together with the fact that referred pain can often be triggered by mild stimulation of normal skin, makes it unlikely that the pain can be explained by postulating hypersensitive 'pain receptors'. A more reasonable explanation is that abnormal information processing in the central nervous system allows these remarkable summation phenomena to occur.

2 *Multiple contributions.* The pain, in these syndromes, cannot be attributed to any single cause. There are, instead, multiple contributions. The cutaneous input from the affected part of the body obviously plays an important role. However, inputs that result from sympathetic activity are also important. So too are inputs from the auditory and visual systems. All of these inputs appear to act on structures in the central nervous system that summate the total activity to produce nerve impulse patterns that ultimately give rise to pain. Anxiety, emotional disturbance, anticipation and other cognitive activities of the brain also contribute to the neural processes underlying these pains. They may facilitate or inhibit the afferent input and thereby modulate the quality and severity of perceived pain.

3 *Delays.* Pain from hyperalgesic skin areas often occurs after long

delays and continues long after removal of the stimulus. Gentle rubbing, repeated pinpricks, or the application of a warm test-tube may produce sudden, severe pain after delays as long as forty-five seconds. Such delays cannot be attributed simply to conduction in slowly conducting fibres; rather, they imply a remarkable temporal and spatial summation of inputs in the production of these pain states.

4 *Persistence.* The durations of these pain states often exceed the time taken for tissues to heal or for injured nerve fibres to regenerate. Causalgia tends to disappear as regeneration occurs, but sometimes it persists for years, as does neuralgic or phantom limb pain. Furthermore, in all of these syndromes pain may occur spontaneously for long periods without any apparent stimulus. These considerations – together with the observation that pain in the phantom limb frequently occurs at the same site as it occurred in the diseased limb prior to amputation – suggest the possibility of a memory-like mechanism in pain.

5 *Spread.* The pains and trigger zones may spread to unrelated parts of the body where no pathology exists. This is further evidence that the central neural mechanisms involved in pain receive inputs from multiple sources. The organization of these mechanisms does not reflect the precise dermatomal (or segmental) innervation of the body by the somatic nerves. (This is immediately evident when Figures 6 and 7 on pp.77 and 81 are compared.) Instead, the mechanisms appear to be more widespread and receive inputs from all parts of the body.

6 *Resistance to surgical control.* The widespread distribution of the neural mechanisms associated with these pain states is also indicated by the frequent failure to abolish pain by surgical methods. Surgical lesions of the peripheral and central nervous systems have been singularly unsuccessful in abolishing these pains permanently, although the lesions have been made at almost every level from receptors to sensory cortex. Even after such operations, pain can often still be elicited by stimulation below the level of section and may be more severe than before the operation.

7 *Relief by modulation of the sensory input.* The most promising

method of treatment for these pains appears to be the modulation of the sensory input by either decreasing or increasing it. Phantom limb pain is sometimes relieved by successive local anaesthetic blocks of tender areas, peripheral nerves or sympathetic ganglia. It may also be relieved by vigorous vibration, transcutaneous electrical nerve stimulation, or by pain-producing injections of hypertonic saline into the stump or low-back interspinous tissues. Causalgia and the neuralgias can similarly be helped by anaesthetic blocks that temporarily decrease inputs from the affected areas, or by increased stimulation such as vigorous massage. These observations have given rise to new therapeutic methods that hold great promise for the relief of pain without producing irrevocable damage to the peripheral or central nervous systems.

These properties and their implications provide valuable clues towards an understanding of pain. They represent parts of a puzzle which, together with those obtained from psychology and physiology, will reveal the solution to a perplexing, urgent problem. Any satisfactory theory of pain must be able to explain the properties of these syndromes. If our theories do not lead eventually to effective treatment, they have failed, no matter how elegant or compelling they may seem. The clinical problems of pain, in other words, represent the ultimate test of our knowledge.

Part Two
The Physiology of Pain

'I was brought up in a medical generation in which . . . pain was [considered to be] a primary sensation dependent upon the stimulation of a specific sensory ending by a stimulus of a certain intensity, and conducted along a fixed pathway to ring a special bell in consciousness. Pain was as simple as that . . . The idea that anything might happen to sensory impulses within the central nervous system to alter their character, destination, or the sensation they registered in consciousness was utterly foreign to my concept. But in practice I found that it was incredibly difficult to make this concept consistent with clinical observations.'

William K. Livingston, 1943

5
The Physiology of Pain
Related to Injury

The psychological and clinical phenomena of pain provide a framework for the physiological problems we will now consider. Pain, as we have seen, is a highly personal, variable experience which is influenced by cultural learning, the meaning of the situation, attention, and other cognitive activities. How does the central nervous system function to permit such powerful cognitive control over the somatic sensory input? Pain, it is generally acknowledged, is primarily a signal that body tissues have been injured; yet pain may persist for years after tissues have healed and damaged nerves have regenerated. How can we account for neurophysiological processes that go on for such long durations? Similarly, pain and trigger zones sometimes spread to distant, unrelated parts of the body. Can we understand such phenomena in terms of the known connections among neurons in the nervous system? While present-day physiology has answers to some of these problems, it is not even close to explaining others. The physiological and anatomical data are no simpler than the psychological and clinical phenomena of pain.

Two terms are especially critical in our attempts to understand the physiology of pain: *specificity* and *specialization*. *Specificity* implies that a receptor, fibre, or other component of a sensory system subserves only a single specific modality (or quality) of experience; it assumes a rigid, fixed relationship between a neural structure and a psychological experience. *Specialization* implies that receptors, fibres, or other components of a sensory system are highly specialized so that particular types and ranges of physical energy evoke characteristic patterns of neural signals, and that these patterns can be modulated by other sensory imputs or by cognitive processes to produce more than one quality of experience or even none at all. It is the latter approach – specialization of function – that provides the conceptual framework for this chapter.

It is customary to describe the somatosensory system by proceeding from the peripheral receptors to the transmission routes that carry nerve impulses to areas in the brain. However, it is essential to remember that stimulation of receptors does not mark the beginning of the pain process. Rather, stimulation produces neural signals that enter an active nervous system that (in the adult organism) is already the substrate of past experience, culture, anticipation, anxiety and so forth. These brain processes actively participate in the selection, abstraction and synthesis of information from the total sensory input. Because sensory physiological processes are complex, a brief outline of the somatic sensory system will be provided first, and each step will then be examined in more detail. Only later, when we analyse the contemporary theories of pain, will we try to choose the data that seem most relevant and put them together in a way that is consistent with the psychological and clinical data.

Outline of somatic sensory mechanisms

We may ask at this point: what is the nature of the sensory nerve signals or messages that travel to the brain after injury? Let us say a person has burned a finger; what is the sequence of events that follows in the nervous system? To begin with, the intense heat energy is converted into a code of electrical nerve impulses. These energy conversions occur in nerve endings in the skin called receptors, of which there are many different types. It was once popular to identify one of these types as the specific 'pain receptors'. We now believe that receptor mechanisms are more complicated. There is general agreement that the receptors which respond to noxious stimulation are widely branching, bushy networks of fibres that penetrate the layers of the skin in such a way that their receptive fields overlap extensively with one another (Figure 9). Thus damage at any point on the skin will activate at least two or more of these networks and initiate the transmission of trains of nerve impulses along sensory nerve fibres that run from the finger into the spinal cord. What enters the spinal cord of the central nervous system is a coded pattern of nerve impulses, travelling along many fibres and moving at different speeds and with different frequencies.

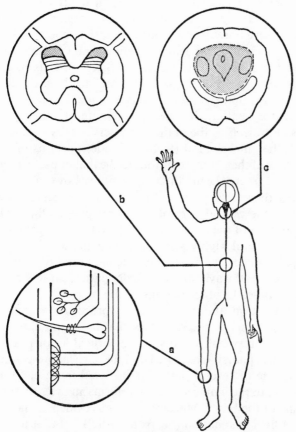

Figure 9. Schematic representation of the receptors and projection pathways of the somatic sensory system. A: The diagram of the skin shows widely branching free nerve endings (which produce overlapping receptive fields) as well as some specialized end-organs. The fibres project to the spinal cord. B: The cross section of the spinal cord shows the laminae (layers) of cells in the dorsal horns which receive sensory fibres and project their axons toward the brain. The crosshatched area represents the substantia gelatinosa (laminae 1 and 2). C: The brainstem (lower part of the brain) receives a large somatosensory input, and projects to higher as well as lower areas of the central nervous system. The crosshatched area represents the reticular formation. Below it on each side is the medial lemniscus. The spinothalamic projections – which are shown within the reticular formation – lie above the lemniscal tracts.

Before the nerve-impulse pattern can begin its ascent to the brain, a portion of it must first pass through a region of short, densely packed nerve fibres that are diffusely interconnected. This region, found throughout the length of the spinal cord on each side, is called the substantia gelatinosa (Figure 9). It is in the course of transmission from the sensory fibres to the ascending spinal cord neurons that the pattern may be modified.

Once the sensory pattern has been transmitted to the spinal cord neurons, it projects to the brain along nerve fibres – some of which occupy the anterolateral (front and side) portions of the spinal cord. Some of these fibres continue to the thalamus, forming the spinothalamic tract. The majority of the fibres, however, penetrate a tangled thicket of short, diffusely interconnected nerve fibres that form the central core of the lower part of the brain (Figure 9). This part of the brain is called the reticular formation, and it contains several highly specialized systems which play a key role in pain processes. From the reticular formation, there emerges a series of pathways, so that sensory patterns now stream along multiple routes to other regions of the brain.

Factual information about the afferent processes related to pain really ends at this point. We know that nerve impulses are projected to the cortex but, because large cortical lesions rarely diminish or abolish pain, it is assumed that the cortical projections represent only one of several pathways involved in pain. Other pathways project to the limbic system that forms an extensive and important part of the brain. Moreover, there is evidence that the cortex is not a final destination (or 'pain centre') but that it processes the information it receives and transmits it to deeper portions of the brain. In short, the afferent process from skin to cortex marks only the beginning of prolonged, interacting activities.

We are now ready to examine the somatic afferent processes in greater detail.

Receptor mechanisms

The traditional picture of skin sensitivity maintains that there are four kinds of receptors, each subserving one of four modalities of cutaneous sensation: pain, touch, warmth and cold. Each receptor is assumed to have a sensitive 'spot' at the skin above it, so that pain sensitivity at the skin, for example, is believed to take the form of discrete 'pain spots' subserved by 'pain receptors'. According to this concept, the free nerve endings are specific pain receptors while the more complex receptor organs (Figure 9) subserve the other modalities. This simple concept is the basis of the traditional *specificity theory of pain* which will be discussed later. For the present, it is sufficient to note that the free nerve endings can give rise to the full range of cutaneous sensory qualities. The pinna (outer part) of the ear contains only free nerve endings and the specialized endings around hair follicles. Yet we feel warmth, cold, touch, itch, tickle, pain, or erotic sensations when these areas are appropriately stimulated (Sinclair, 1967).

Histologists (anatomists who look at the fine structure of body tissues) have discovered a rich variety of receptor endings in skin and other tissues. The most common of all are the free nerve endings. Figure 9 shows how a sensory fibre branches out extensively so that its receptive field – the skin area innervated by all the branches of a single nerve fibre – covers a wide area of skin. The receptive fields of adjacent fibres overlap one another, so that stimulation of a spot of skin activates not one but several fields (Tower, 1943).

Intensive studies have been made of the types of receptor endings in skin and of the types of nerve fibre which lead from them (see Willis and Coggeshall, 1978). There are six anatomically recognized endings in hairy skin and in smooth skin. These connect to large myelinated sensory nerve fibres and respond in various ways to light mechanical stimulation (Table 2). As a nerve

	Adaptation rate		
	slow	*medium*	*fast*
Hairless skin	Merkel	Meissner	Pacinian
Hairy skin	Tactile disks	Hair follicle	Pacinian
	Ruffini		

Table 2. Adaptation rate of different types of specialized receptors.

is stimulated harder and harder, it generates more and more impulses per second. Some fibres only respond during the onset and offset of a stimulus and fail to generate nerve impulses if the stimulus is held steady; this is called fast adaptation. Other fibres generate a barrage of impulses which roughly matches the time course and intensity of the stimulus; this is called slow adaptation. In addition there are much larger numbers of free nerve endings that connect to all types of fibres and respond to all types of stimuli (Table 3). The sensory fibres are traditionally divided into three groups: A-beta or large myelinated, A-delta or small myelinated, and C or unmyelinated fibres. About sixty to seventy per cent of all the sensory afferents are in the C group.

	Myelinated		Unmyelinated
Fibre type	A-beta	A-delta	C
Diameter	5–15μm	1–5μm	0.25–1.5μm
Conduction velocity	30–100 m/sec	6–30 m/sec	1.0–2.5 m/sec
Receptor type	specialized & free	free	free
Respond to*	light pressure	1 light pressure	1 light pressure
		2 heavy pressure	2 heavy pressure
		3 heat (45°C +)	3 heat (45°C +)
		4 chemicals	4 chemicals
		5 cooling	5 warmth

*Each fibre in the A-delta and C group may respond to only one or to more than one of the types of stimuli; for example, there are C 'polymodal fibres' that respond to heavy pressure, heat and chemicals.

Table 3. Properties of different types of afferent fibres.

We must understand clearly exactly how physiologists have studied and classified these nerve fibres. They isolate single units and then search for the type of stimulus to which the fibre responds best: hair movement, skin indentation, skin crushing, warming, cooling, chemicals, and so on. Of course, not all fibres can be tested with all stimuli but it does appear that some fibres are exquisitely sensitive to specific stimuli. For example, Pacinian corpuscles respond briskly to tiny, fast skin indentations. Some A-delta fibres respond to cooling the skin by a fraction of a degree. It is tempting to label such fibres as vibration fibres or cold fibres. Furthermore it has been shown for some types of receptor-fibre units that the psychological sensation threshold for detecting vibration or cooling matches the ability of these fibres to detect the stimulus. For a just-detectable stimulus at psychological threshold intensity, it would seem highly reasonable that a particular class of receptors and fibres are uniquely responsible for carrying the message. However, the real world is full of intense stimuli, especially pain-producing stimuli. A good radio tuned perfectly to one station still gives a crackle if lightning strikes – and so it is with nerve fibre-receptor units. Any nerve fibre hit hard enough and fast enough gives off an injury discharge. That is what happens in our ulnar nerve when we hit our 'funny bone'. Similarly, if a needle is stabbed into tissue, it will fire all nerve fibres along its track. It will of course fire the low-threshold fibres and in addition it will recruit some high-threshold fibres which do not respond to low-level stimuli.

The crux of the issue we are discussing here is whether the pain is triggered only by those fibres which respond exclusively to intense stimuli or whether the nervous system responds to the total barrage and pain occurs when the barrage exceeds a critical level. The supporters of specificity theory propose that each class of fibres by itself evokes a specific class of sensation. In particular, pain would be evoked only by an afferent barrage in high-threshold afferents and the intensity of pain would depend on the frequency of nerve impulses in those afferents. We will see that this view is too simplistic and fails to fit the facts.

It is now possible, due to remarkable work initiated in Sweden by Vallbo and Hagbarth (1968), to record from single units with micro-electrodes gently inserted into human nerves in fully conscious volunteers. For our purposes, the most interesting types of sensory nerve fibres are the numerous 'polymodal nociceptors' which are the obvious candidates for the specificity theorists to label as 'pain fibres'. These unmyelinated fibres respond to all three of the commonly tested noxious stimuli: heat, pressure and chemicals. In this situation, there is the enormous advantage that it is not only possible to apply carefully controlled stimuli and then to record impulses in a single fibre on their way to the spinal cord, but also to ask the subject what he feels and thus to correlate input with sensation. We must be fully aware, however, that although only one fibre is being observed, many other types may be stimulated by the same stimulus. This fact is irrelevant to the true specificity enthusiasts who would predict that one dominant type of fibre would control the specific sensation which is reported – and how strong it feels.

Van Hees and Gybels (1972) have reported just such experiments in which they record from human fibres of the polymodal C type. The skin in the receptive field of a fibre is heated to a level where the subject reports pain, and the skin temperature and the frequency of nerve impulses are noted. Now we have a correlation between stimulus, afferent nerve impulses and verbal response. Specificity theory requires that if the same frequency of nerve impulses is evoked by another stimulus, pain should be felt. Pressure is now applied to the skin, nerve impulses appear in the fibre and at some level the subject declares that the stimulus is painful. The number of nerve impulses required to evoke pain by pressure is four to five times greater than that required by heat. This simple observation demolishes specificity theory. It can be explained by the fact that the pressure stimulus not only evokes impulses in the high-threshold afferents but also in low-threshold afferents which partially inhibit the effect of the high-threshold input (Wall and Cronly-Dillon, 1960). The heat stimulus does not evoke as many impulses in other fibres as does the pressure stimulus and, therefore, it is processed by spinal cord cells which have not been subject to the degree of inhibition produced by a pressure stimulus. The pattern of activity in different types of fibres is evidently one of the factors which controls the sensory outcome.

We now know that the transduction properties of any given receptor are a function of at least eight physiological variables: (1) threshold to mechanical distortion; (2) threshold to negative and positive temperature change; (3) peak sensitivity to temperature change; (4) threshold to chemical change; (5) stimulus strength–response curve; (6) rate of adaptation to stimulation; (7) size of receptive field; and (8) duration of after-discharge. It is suspected that many of these variables are interrelated. Since there is reason to believe that each of these variables has a continuous distribution, the specialization of any given receptor can be specified accurately in terms of its coordinates with respect to a number of the variables. Thus it is possible to define a particular receptor-fibre unit by saying, for example, that it has a low pressure threshold, a peak sensitivity at high temperature, a narrow receptive field, and a fast rate of adaptation. The specialization of each skin receptor would therefore be defined in terms of its position in a multidimensional space of physiological variables. If receptors are distributed throughout the space defined by these variables, the degree of specialization and number of different kinds of receptors must be very great indeed.

We propose that a receptor generates temporal patterns of nerve impulses rather than modality-specific impulses. These patterns would be determined by the effects of the physical stimulus within the limits set by the receptor's physiological properties such as its sensitivity range and rate of adaptation. Since many receptors respond to at least two different kinds of energy, they must be capable of generating more than one kind of temporal pattern.

Skin sensitivity and receptive fields

Recent studies of skin sensitivity provide a picture that is more consistent with the evidence of overlapping receptive fields than with the concept of a mosaic of sensitive spots. Maps of thermal sensitivity of large areas of skin (Figure 10) show highly sensitive areas surrounded by regions of decreasing sensitivity (Melzack, Rose and McGinty, 1962). These large sensitive areas, observed by psychological mapping techniques, undoubtedly reflect the activity of overlapping receptive fields that project to successive levels in the central nervous system.

Skin spots, then, appear to represent areas of peak sensitivity surrounded by valleys of lesser sensitivity. The fact that receptive fields overlap extensively makes it almost certain that even a pinprick will activate several receptor-fibre units. Thus, the evidence suggests that the 'skin spot', once believed to represent a single specific receptor lying beneath it, is the result of the ability

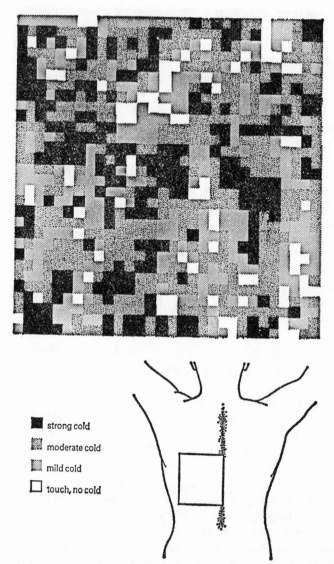

strong cold

moderate cold

mild cold

☐ touch, no cold

Figure 10. Distribution of cold sensitivity of approximately a quarter of the back. The position and size of the area tested is drawn in the lower right corner. The sensitivity distribution was mapped with a round stimulator tip 2.5mm in diameter, at a temperature of 10°C. The cold intensities reported by the subject are represented by different shades of stipple.
(from Melzack, Rose and McGinty, 1962, p.300)

of the central nervous system to integrate the impulses of many fibres having extensively overlapping receptive fields (Tower, 1943).

Even more remarkable are the observations of continuous shifts in skin sensitivity (Melzack, Rose and McGinty, 1962). Successive maps show that large sensitive fields may 'fragment' and 'coalesce', and thereby produce continually changing patterns of sensitivity distribution. It seems likely that these fluctuations represent changes in information transmission throughout the somatosensory projection system. They may be due to changes in activity in receptor-fibre units as well as at synapses throughout the transmission system.

Receptors in the skin, then, cannot be considered in isolation but can only be understood in terms of their relation to adjacent receptors and their projections to successive transmission levels in the central nervous system. Their sensitivity fluctuates, possibly because of blood flow or other changes in the skin, and the information they project through the central nervous system is also modified by messages descending from the brain. The brain receives impulses projected from many receptors, and these must be synthesized to produce the neural activities that are eventually felt as pain, touch, or any of the other cutaneous sensations.

The anatomy of a peripheral nerve

The major nerves, with names such as the sciatic nerve or the ulnar nerve, are large structures surrounded by their own sheath of connective tissue and special blood vessels (Figure 11). They are divided into bundles, surrounded by sheets of connective tissue, which are visible to the naked eye. The individual bundles are routinely dissected out by surgeons using low-power dissecting microscopes. Each bundle contains huge numbers of the real working units, the nerve fibres, each of which is comprised of a cell body, an axon and dendrites.

Each cell sends out a long cylindrical process called an axon (Figure 11). This is the basic structure which carries the nerve impulse and can also transport chemicals along its entire length. An adult human has tens of thousands of these to supply the foot

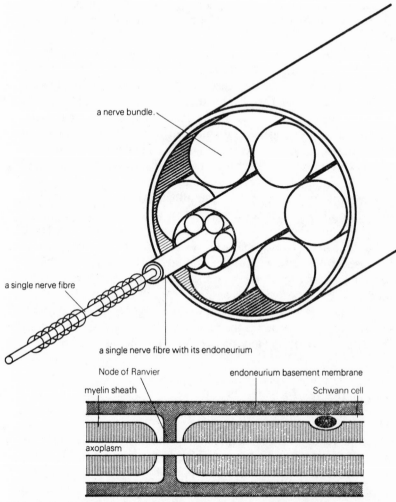

Figure 11. *Top:* drawing of the component parts of a peripheral nerve – with its sheath. *Bottom:* drawing of the detailed components of a single nerve fibre.

alone, and the tubular axons run all the way from the spinal cord to the foot – a distance of about one metre – without interruption. If the axon is more than 1 micron in diameter, it is covered by cuffs of myelin, a laminated fat-protein insulating material. The cuffs are one to two millimetres in length and there is a gap between them where they meet along the axon. The gaps are called 'nodes of Ranvier' and it is here that chemicals can pass in and out of the axon to generate the nerve impulses. The entire axon lies embedded within its own special type of cell, the Schwann cell, and, for the large axons, one such cell lies between each node of Ranvier. Many small fibres which do not have the myelin layer can nestle within one Schwann cell. Outside the Schwann cell there is a continuous tube of material, the basement membrane, and outside that, a connective tissue tube, the endoneurium. The axons therefore, in their entire distance from spinal cord to periphery, run in their own personal tubular channels. Each major nerve is a mixed nerve – that is, it contains three functional types of axons: (1) motor axons whose impulses cause muscle to contract; (2) sensory axons whose impulses deliver afferent signals to the spinal cord; (3) sympathetic axons whose impulses control such 'autonomic' activities as blood flow and sweating.

We are now in a position to consider, in detail, what happens when injury occurs at the skin.

A scratch: an injury in one dimension

We can learn a surprising amount from an injury as trivial as a scratch. Perhaps the best of all scientific traditions in matters of this kind is to be your own guinea pig. We propose that you – the reader – try one of the simplest experiments, one which was carried out long ago by Sir Thomas Lewis, who asked simple questions that led to profound answers. By doing such an experiment, you join a long scientific tradition of coming to a conclusion based on observation rather than preconceived notions. For example, Pliny, who witnessed the eruption of Vesuvius which destroyed Pompeii, tested the common belief of his time that goats breathed through their ears by putting wax plugs in a goat's ears and observing that it continued to breathe rather than die of asphyxiation. Harvey, who lived through the Great Plague and the Great Fire of London, was the first man to press a vein in his arm and to see that the blood must be moving towards his heart and not the other way as everyone said, and thereby made one of the greatest medical discoveries – the circulation of the blood. It had to wait for this century for Sir Thomas Lewis (1942) to be the first man to scratch himself and observe and think.

To repeat Lewis's experiment, bare your forearm, and rest it comfortably on a table or your lap. Then press the edge of your thumbnail hard into the skin near your wrist and drag it hard and fast in a line toward the elbow.

The first observation is that it does not hurt much. If you were to ask someone else to make an identical scratch on your arm, using the same pressure and speed which you can easily tolerate if you do it yourself, it will hurt a great deal more. Therefore, it is immediately apparent that the amount of pain felt depends not only on the injury but on other factors as well. With your self-inflicted scratch, the pain or discomfort, if any, coincides with the time and place of the scratch and then decreases. Now observe the scratch and it will be seen that it is a white line. Could this be because the blood has simply been squeezed out of the capillaries by the pressure and is taking time to return? This can easily be tested by pressing two fingertips together hard and then suddenly bringing them apart. It will be seen that, as the fingertips part, they are blanched but return to their normal colour in a second. Evidently the scratch must remain white for some additional reason. It is because the lining (endothelium) of the capillaries and the smooth muscle of the small arterioles and venules in the skin are directly sensitive to stretch and react by going into spasm. This is one of our mechanisms to prevent blood loss. While the damaged vessels are in spasm, substances are released which trigger the slower clotting mechanism, our second and much more powerful method of preventing blood loss. The effectiveness of this double mechanism is shown by the common observation that a small razor-blade cut may bleed quite profusely while a much more severe, blunt cut in the skin bleeds very little. The sharp razor blade exerts little pressure on the vessels while the blunt injury has triggered spasm and, by creating tissue damage, has released clotting agents.

Within a short time, the white line disappears as the spasm releases but the skin colour does not simply return to normal. It now becomes redder and redder until there is the clear red line of the scratch. Here, the blood vessels dilate (vasodilation) in the scratch region to a much wider diameter than normal. This will now remain for quite a long period of time and is produced by chemicals which leak from the damaged cells. Until repair processes have restored the cells to normal, the vasodilation will remain. It will be noticed that the line may feel sore or itchy. If you have scratched rather gently or if you have tough skin, this may be all that happens.

However, if the scratch has been more severe, two further reactions will occur. The skin over the red line begins to swell and becomes pale; this is the weal. You may have to look quite carefully for this swelling. Here the vessels are so dilated that fluid now leaks from the blood serum through the capillary walls into spaces between the tissue cells. Histological examination of such tissue shows that there are cell changes in progress. White blood cells (polymorphonuclear leucocytes) invade and destroy (phagocytose) broken cell debris. Soon special cells (fibroblasts) that form connective tissue begin to appear and there is evidence of growth of new tissue. At this stage, the line may ache or itch and feel sore if you move the arm. If you press gently on the line with a pencil tip, it will be clearly tender; that is, pressure which is felt as a light touch on normal skin is now sufficient to produce pain when it is applied to inflamed tissue.

So far, all reactions have been strictly limited to the area which received the scratch. However, it will soon be observed that an area of redness spreads on either side of the weal; this is the flare. Here, too, there is vasodilatation, little or no swelling but quite clear tenderness. This sequence of events – white line, weal and flare – was called 'the triple response' by Lewis.

Before your eyes, then, in slow motion, you have observed the development of inflammation. This classically has four cardinal signs: redness, heat, swelling and pain. The redness is caused by vasodilatation. The heat is produced locally by the presence of a large amount of hot blood close to the skin surface. The swelling, or oedema, is due to the leakage of fluids from blood vessels into the tissue. The cause of the pain is more complex. The pressure of the swelling contributes to the pain but that is not a sufficient explanation for it. If the swelling is removed or prevented, the pain is still present.

Why, then, is there pain and tenderness? All skin contains

nerve fibres (Figure 11). These nerve fibres are tuned to respond to particular events but an injury is such a massive event that at the moment of injury they all generate nerve impulses. Some of them will continue firing, giving the sting which rings on after even a minor injury. Those nerve impulses may be all that we need to know about to explain how the brain knows that an injury is occurring. But how are we to explain the long-lasting tenderness and, even more, how are we to explain the fact that the tenderness spreads into areas which were not injured? There are four explanations and they probably all play a part.

1 Primary changes in nerve terminals. First let us concentrate on changes which occur in the nerve endings as a direct consequence of the injury itself. The nerve ending is an extension of the sensory nerve cell and consists of a delicate bare membrane enclosing the end of the tubular axon. The diameter of these nerve endings is about one micron (one thousandth of a millimetre). It is no surprise that such endings will be destroyed in the injury. During their destruction, they generate a high-frequency burst of impulses which is transmitted to the brain. After that, they become insensitive and cannot fire again until they regenerate. Some larger endings or those a little further removed from the area of injury will be damaged but not put out of action. It is a property of a partially damaged nerve membrane that it becomes easier to excite. Therefore, we may expect that some nerve endings will be desensitized and others will be sensitized, and this is exactly what was observed by Campbell, Meyer and Lamotte (1979). In their experiments, using repeated heat pulses delivered by a laser beam on the hand, they found that the smallest fibres (C fibres) become inactivated while the slightly larger, myelinated fibres (A-delta fibres) became sensitized – so that while the initial stimulus had to be intense, the subsequent stimuli necessary to generate nerve impulses could be less and less intense until eventually the nerve fibre generated impulses even when there was no stimulus. Here we see one of the reasons why a sudden injury may be followed by immediate pain and then by tenderness: it is because the endings have become sensitized so that they now generate impulses continuously, which are presumably the basis of soreness and aching.

2 Pain-producing substances. We have seen that this primary effect cannot be the only explanation for pain and soreness because the tenderness spreads outside the immediate region of damage. We know that there are destroyed and damaged cells, as well as blood-vessel reactions, and new cells enter the region. All of this changes the environment surrounding the nerve endings. Nerve cells, like all cells, are affected by their external physical and chemical environment. Could it be that this new environment contains chemicals which fire or sensitize the nerve endings? Keele and Armstrong (1964) have done experiments on themselves and have shown that damaged tissue does in fact generate pain-producing substances. Their method was direct and simple. First, they produced a blister by applying an extract of Spanish Fly (cantharides) to the skin and then cut off the bulging skin to expose the blister base. As we all know, the skin of a blister is quite insensitive. The reason is that all the nerve ends in it have been ripped away from their parent nerve fibres. However, the exposed base is exquisitely sensitive to touch, to warmth, to washing, but does not hurt if left alone. They then placed various compounds known to be released from damaged tissue on the blister base and recorded their own pain.

The list is long and includes some well-known substances. Common substances present in all cells, such as potassium ions or adenosine triphosphate (ATP), are released from damaged cells and produce pain on a blister base. In addition, special pain-producing chemicals are released in inflamed tissue. These include histamine release, from specialized cells called mast cells, which is particularly characteristic of allergic reactions. Another intensely painful compound that is released is bradykinin, which is a molecule called a peptide, made up of a chain of amino-acids. Bradykinin produces intense excitation of many types of nerve ending and produces changes in blood vessels.

Compounds from outside the body can also produce pain and some are of considerable interest. Capsaicin is the substance in the Hungarian red pepper (paprika) which gives it its hot peppery taste. As any goulash fancier will know, a piece of paprika held on the tongue produces warmth, then heat, then pain if not washed down with some suitable fluid. Those who have managed this procedure with sufficient enthusiasm will know that a fairly impressive stomach-ache may follow as the compound begins to act on the gastric mucosa of the stomach. Jancso *et al.* (1967) showed that capsaicin produces intense firing of nerve fibres and later desensitizes them so that they become inactive for long periods of time. A single dose injected into anaesthetized new-born rats or mice will result in permanent destruction of the majority of small nerve fibres. Evidently this substance not only excites nerve fibres but is also a toxin to which some fibres are particularly sensitive. Capsaicin is described here not as a curiosity but because of the possibility of finding substances which might selectively destroy certain types of nerve fibres for therapeutic reasons.

A particularly interesting set of compounds produced in inflamed tissue is the prostaglandins. This is a family of compounds which all derive as breakdown products of the fatty acid known as arachidonic acid. The prostaglandins have many actions, one of which is to sensitize nerve endings. It is not certain if they ever rise to sufficient concentration to produce nerve impulses by themselves but it is clear that they sensitize nerve endings so that they are easily fired by other agents.

3 Action of nerves on nerves. The spread of sensitivity beyond the site of injury could be caused by the diffusion of pain-producing substances, but there is evidence for an additional factor involving the peripheral nerves themselves. The individual nerve fibres in skin spread out in many branches – the terminal arbor – to end like the branches of a tree. Injury to the tip of one of the branches will send impulses towards the nerve fibre ('the trunk of the tree') which conducts them to the spinal cord; however, as the impulse arrives at a branch point it not only proceeds up the fibre but also sends impulses backwards down the neighbouring branches to end in the terminal twigs. In this way, excitation of one part of the terminal arbor leads to invasion of all parts of the tree. Lewis called this the 'axon reflex' and he gave reasons to think that pain-producing substances are released from the nerve endings, which spread the effect of the injury. This contention is still controversial (Lynn, 1977). However, Fitzgerald (1978) has shown a fascinating additional effect. She recorded from single nerve fibres from skin and made a nearby injury which had no direct effect on the nerve fibres from which she was recording. After some time, the uninjured nerve fibres became more and more sensitive. Some effect was spreading from the injury. Was it produced by chemicals or were nerve impulses involved? She showed that if she injected a local anaesthetic into the injured area, which is believed to stop only the nerve impulses and not to affect the chemical changes, then there was no sensitization of the uninjured fibres. Because the area of the preparation was isolated from the central nervous system, the entire action had to be local. Taken at face value, the experiment seems to show that nerve impulses are involved locally in the spread of sensitivity from the damaged area to neighbouring intact tissue. Mechanisms such as these – both chemical and neural – are probably involved in cases of arthritis in which a single joint, such as a knuckle, is involved. The inflammation at the joint produces swelling, the release of chemical substances and the spread of pain to the whole finger and, sometimes, the adjacent fingers and hand.

4 Sensitization by way of the central nervous system. It is obvious that an injury more severe than a scratch would produce pain and tenderness over a wide area. This is apparent even at the moment of injury: when a person hits his thumb with a hammer, there is a flash of pain that is often felt in a wide area of the hand and wrist. With prolonged injury, such as an abcess, the tenderness spreads into areas so distant that it is impossible to propose that there are shared nerve endings between the distant and damaged area or that chemicals could spread or be transported to the distant tender areas. Here the explanation has to lie within the central nervous system, where the activity triggered by the primary lesion excites neighbouring areas in the central nervous system to produce heightened sensitivity. These conditions will be considered later.

A space-occupying lesion: injury in three dimensions

So far we have considered the simple incident of a scratch because it demonstrates the general principles which apply to the effects of an injury. Now we shall describe the additional factors that are involved in major injuries.

The sensitivity of different tissues

An opportunity to study the sensitivity of visceral tissue arose in the 1930s when a famous patient, Tom, drank burning-hot liquid that destroyed his oesophagus. Nowadays it is possible to replace the oesophagus by reconstructive plastic surgery, but this was not available at the time and the treatment was to make a permanent opening into the stomach through the abdominal wall (a gastrostomy). A liquid diet was then supplied by tube directly into the stomach. H. G. Wolff, one of the leading American pioneers of the study of pain, realized that Tom offered an unusual opportunity to study gastric function and sensitivity. Tom was a normal healthy man except for his gastrostomy, and Wolff arranged for him to be employed as janitor at a Medical School so that he could be observed. It was found that no sensation was evoked by touching, pinching or heating the stomach (Wolf and Wolff, 1943). This confirmed a great deal of evidence, obtained during abdominal surgery on lightly anaesthetized patients, that the gut does not evoke pain or spinal reflexes if it is manipulated, cut extensively, or even burned. However, pain is consistently evoked by stretching of the tissue by tugging, dilatation or spasm. This principle holds true for the stomach as well as the small and large intestine.

Nevertheless, Wolff discovered that if he artificially produced an area of intense vasodilatation and secretion in the stomach, the area became exquisitely sensitive to pressure. The same happened when Tom went through a period of anxiety, which raised the stomach secretion of acid and made the lining become inflamed, red and sensitive. Visceral tissue, then, is remarkably different from normal skin. It is totally insensitive to extremely damaging stimuli such as cutting or burning and is highly sensitive to distension or stretch. Clearly, pain is profoundly influenced by the properties of the tissue which is injured.

Viscera

It is evident, in considering deep structures, that we must consider at least three factors: (1) the degree of innervation and the location of nerve endings; (2) the type of stimulus which will fire the nerves; and (3) the state of the tissue. Normal gut, as we have seen, appears to evoke no sensation whatever unless it is stretched by tugging, dilatation or spasm. We have already discussed the special case of the ureter, an organ which normally does not produce sensation unless it is greatly stretched. The urinary bladder, as we all know, is able to evoke sensation. If a normal bladder is filled slowly through a urethral catheter, the patient is unable to guess the degree of filling until it is about half full. As filling continues, there is the feeling of increasing fullness until, at some stage, discomfort and then pain begin to accompany the urgency to urinate. However, as those readers who have had an attack of cystitis know all too well, inflammation dramatically changes the situation. What may appear in cystoscopic examination to be a minor infection of the lining of the bladder is associated with a marked lowering of the filling level at which pain and urgency are triggered, so that the frequency of the need to urinate rises to socially embarrassing levels.

The gall bladder appears to follow similar rules and never, in the normal person, reaches the threshold of awareness but becomes a dominating feature of the patient's life if dilated or inflamed. The uterus has a double innervation. The body of the uterus is supplied by nerves which originate from the upper lumbar segments of the spinal cord (Figure 12) and gives rise to pain only if extensively dilated or infected, or is in strong contraction as in menstruation (in some women) and in labour. In contrast, the cervix is supplied by sensory nerves from the sacral segments of the spinal cord (Figure 12) and in the normal state evokes excruciating pain if the opening of the cervix (the os) is suddenly dilated by a few millimetres.

Muscle

Muscles that move the limbs and torso (striated muscles) are heavily innervated by many types of sensory nerves but are rarely the source of pain – except in one special situation, in which muscle contraction occurs in the absence of an adequate blood supply (muscle ischaemia). Muscle cramps may occur during swimming in cold water when the muscles undergo strong contraction before an adequate blood supply can reach them. It is possible that some chemical substances may be released in this

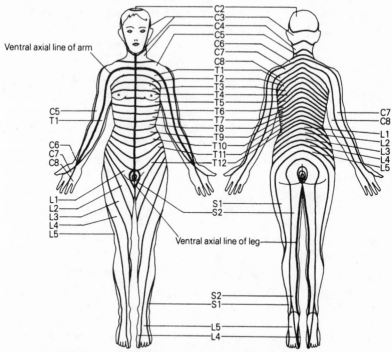

Figure 12. Distribution of dermatomes on the body surface. Each dermatome is the area of skin supplied by the dorsal roots of a given sensory nerve. The positions of the roots are labelled in terms of the level of the bones in the vertebral column. C: cervical; T: thoracic; L: lumbar; S: sacral. (from Keegan and Garrett, 1948)

condition, but none have yet been discovered. (Experimentally, muscle ischaemia can be induced by blocking blood flow to an arm by means of a pressure cuff and asking the person to open and close the hand.)

Smooth muscle of the viscera that contracts without adequate blood supply can also become ischaemic and a source of severe pain. Severe constriction of the arteries of the heart, for example, produces the pain of angina pectoris. Many patients with deteriorating blood flow through their coronary arteries begin to experience angina due to effort when the heart muscle must contract more strongly and the blood flow is inadequate to supply sufficient sugars and oxygen for energy. The same patients may suffer the equivalent condition – called intermittent claudication – at the same time in their leg muscles, when exercise triggers unbearable pain in the main muscles used. One of the limits of prolonged maximal activity by athletes, such as racing cyclists, is set by their threshold for triggering this kind of crippling pain which results in their instantly falling out of the race.

The sudden plugging of a main artery results in a major mismatch of muscle contraction and blood flow. This occurs in the classical heart attack, which is immensely painful until the contractions of the heart muscle which the artery supplies can decrease to a level that can be handled by the remaining blood flow – or until an alternative blood supply can open up. These mechanisms explain how it is possible to have 'silent' heart attacks – that is, major occlusions of blood vessels with such efficient shifting of the heart's contraction pattern and of its blood flow that the patient suffers no pain. Such attacks are noticed only by a general deterioration of the patient's physical ability or even by routine electrocardiograms which detect the marked change of contraction pattern.

Joints
Arthritis is one of the most common causes of pain. Although the causes of the changes at joints that occur in osteoarthritis and rheumatoid arthritis are poorly understood, the causes of the pain are less mysterious. Joints are diffusely innervated by many fine branches of nerves which are assumed to fire when their endings are activated by the mechanical pressure exerted by the swollen arthritic joints. General clinical evidence shows that, in the normal joint, pressure on tendons, on tendon sheaths, on periosteum and on joint capsules produces pain. It is suspected that the normal joint surface itself is not sensitive, but that the tissue destruction and the associated inflammation that occur in arthritis produce a drop in thresholds of the innervating fibres. As a result, minor changes of pressure produce great surges of pain.

The brain
Perhaps strangest of all the regions of our body which may be disturbed without producing pain is the brain. This astonishing

fact allowed the development of modern neurosurgery. In some types of brain operations, it is desirable to operate on the brain under local anaesthesia. It is still done where the verbal cooperation of the patient is needed to follow the effect of surgery in progress within his brain. The procedure is first to infiltrate large volumes of dilute local anaesthetic under the scalp of the patient. A line of fluid is injected in order to block all the nerves supplying the scalp to be incised. These nerves supply not only the skin but also the outer fibrous, vascular layer – the periosteum – of the skull. The surgeon may then proceed, without producing pain to the patient, to drill holes (trephination) through the skull and to saw between the holes in order to lift up a bone flap. This shows that the inner side of the skull is insensitive since no local anesthetic has reached this area. The surgeon now faces the dura mater – which resembles thick, flexible cellophane – that covers the brain. In man, the upper two-thirds of the dura is entirely without sensory innervation. The basal parts of the dura and the large blood vessels are innervated by branches of the fifth nerve. However, once the brain is exposed, the cerebral cortex itself may be cut into without the patient feeling any pain and, in most areas, without his feeling any sensation at all. Localized intense electrical stimulation in the depths of the brain has been frequently carried out in conscious man with no reports of pain unless the brainstem is entered.

The special case of cancer pain

Cancerous cells are made up of almost all the same chemical components as normal cells in the body. That is why cancer is so difficult to detect in its early stages, and also why the defence mechanisms of the body do not recognize it as foreign. Therefore, cancer does not induce the immune reactions which reject grafts. Furthermore, it does not even produce inflammation as a primary reaction. A crumb of bread accidentally breathed into the lungs sets off an immediate, painful violent coughing. A lung cancer may grow silently to the size of a grapefruit before any disorder is noticed. Yet cancer is rightly feared as a disease which is frequently painful in its last stages.

What, then, is the cause of pain if this silent enemy can infiltrate without disturbance? The answer is very largely mechanical and obeys the general principles we have already described. One of the commonest first signs of brain tumours is the appearance of severe, generalized headaches. Yet we have said that the brain itself is largely insensitive. The explanation is that the tumour has grown to sufficient size to begin to dam up the normal flow of cerebrospinal fluid which is generated in the ventricles of the brain. Since the fluid cannot escape, there is a rise of intracranial pressure so that brain tissue presses on innervated structures in the base of the skull and produces the headache. Any pharmacological or surgical manoeuvre which reduces this fluid pressure promptly relieves the headache although the cancer itself has in no way been changed.

Similarly, in abdominal cancer pains, by far the commonest cause is mechanical obstruction of one or another of the viscera, followed by dilatation above the block. The blocks may occur in intestine, bile ducts, ureters and the bladder, producing the sequence of dilatation and intense muscle contractions in the attempt to drive the contents of the structure past the blockade. Blood vessels and lymph ducts may become blocked in the same way. Since veins and lymph ducts contain fluid at a low pressure, they are easier to block than arteries and therefore swelling results from the build-up of pressure behind the block and may produce pain.

On occasion, the tumour may have directly painful effects by expanding and increasing the pressure on sensitive structures – such as a bone tumour which begins to involve the fibrous, vascular membrane that surrounds and nourishes the bone (the periosteum). However, tumours more commonly produce pain by the blocking effects of their mass. Tumours may send off secondary metastases which begin to grow in bone. Slowly the tumour grows at the expense of the bone which of course loses mechanical strength. Eventually the bone may collapse – a 'pathological' fracture. Tumours have a dominating, monopolizing character: they receive few blood vessels, push nerve fibres aside and are not themselves supplied by nerve fibres. Sometimes, therefore, these pathological fractures can be quite painless because all innervated tissue has been replaced by cancer. On other occasions, the long-range mechanical damage produced by the fracture involves normal tissue which is painful and undergoes normal inflammation.

A common target for secondary bony metastases are the bones of the vertebral column of the back. When such a bone collapses, it is certain that there will be serious problems because the sensory nerve roots are damaged in the collapse. The other serious consequence is the crushing of the spinal cord in the collapse, which produces paraplegia. Finally, cancer can directly invade nerves and produce a form of painful nerve injury.

The mislocation of pain from viscera: referred pain

When the skin is jabbed with a pin, the pain is accurately localized and the eyes and hands move exactly to the point of injury. This ability to localize pain in the region of injury is limited to skin and does not apply when the source of the pain is in deep tissue. Visceral pain is often felt in bizzare locations. Here the doctor needs to know these patterns of pain or he, like the patient, may be misled as to where to search for the seat of the trouble. Fortunately, these strange mislocations usually have regular rules which are found repeatedly in patient after patient.

Inflammation of the diaphragm, for example, produces pain which the patient insists is located in his shoulder. The explanation for this strange referral is as follows. The diaphragm which separates the chest (thorax) from the abdomen originates in the embryo from muscle tissue which forms in the fifth cervical segment. This muscle migrates from the neck to the chest to form the diaphragm. Here it develops into our main respiratory muscle. During its migration from neck to thorax, the muscle carries along its nerve supply which also originates from the fifth cervical segment. This is the phrenic nerve which runs down the lower neck and through the entire length of thorax to innervate the diaphragm. Apart from this special migration, the rest of the fifth cervical segment, like all other segments, forms local skin and muscle. The area of skin supplied by this segment, the dermatome, runs as a band from the midline of the back across the top of the shoulder blade and down the upper arm. As a result, pain triggered by nerve impulses arriving over the phrenic nerve is mistakenly interpreted as coming from the area of skin supplied by the rest of the spinal cord segment.

Appendicitis

The two commonest forms of referred pain are appendicitis and angina pectoris. The first signs of discomfort and pain from inflammation of the appendix seems to the patient to be located in the upper abdomen in the midline above the umbilicus. The appendix actually lies deep in the abdomen on the right side, nestled against the pelvis. In the embryo, the gut begins as a midline straight tube and then develops its coils and curves as the tube lengthens with growth. The overall pattern of sensory innervation is established early in embryonic life. The appendix grows at the junction of the small intestine as it enlarges to become the colon. Being a midline structure, it is innervated from both sides. The segments responsible for its nerve supply are in the lower thoracic part of the spinal cord which also develops into the lower ribs and upper abdominal wall. Thus, following the rule that the pain is referred to the segment of origin of the nerves, and since they come from both sides, the pain is first felt in the midline in the upper abdominal wall. As the appendicitis develops, the inflammation spreads and begins to involve the peritoneum – the membrane that covers the viscera – and the nearby abdominal wall. Now the rules change. When the abdominal wall is affected, it obeys rules like the skin, and the pain is correctly localized. Therefore, the classical course of events in appendicitis is a pain which is first felt in the midline above the navel, and which then shifts down to the right and is centred over the actual position of the appendix.

Angina pectoris

This condition is triggered, as we have noted above, by an inadequate blood supply to the heart. The word 'angina' means a yoke, the heavy collar put around farming animals. It feels to the patient as though a tight, broad belt is constricting his upper chest and then as the attack mounts, pains shoot down the left arm. The heart begins in the embryo as a midline structure innervated by the upper thoracic segments, so it is not surprising that the first pains should be felt in the upper chest wall. As the heart develops, the left side grows to a much greater mass since it is the left ventricle which does the major work of providing power for the entire arterial system except for the lung circulation.

Therefore the left side of the spinal cord has more tissue to innervate and it is reasonable that the pain should be referred to the left. The uppermost thoracic segments also play a part in the development of the arms, so that some spinal cells receive converging signals from the heart as well as the arm. This convergence appears to be the reason why pain is referred to the left arm.

There is more to referred pain than just a mislocation by the patient. If you touch the left arm of a patient during an angina attack, you find that it is tender, although the right arm is not. This even applies when he is on the verge of having the attack. This is strange because there is no disease in his left arm. It is clear, then, that in addition to mislocation there is a summation of impulses from both sources. The tenderness of the arm suggests that nerve impulses from the heart and from the region where the pain is referred must converge and summate and thereby increase the pain. There is a very simple way of testing that idea. By using local anaesthesia it is possible to eliminate one of the sources of nerve impulses. In the case of the arm, it is possible to infiltrate the brachial plexus, the massed bundle of nerves at the root of the upper arm. If this is done, the arm becomes numb and it is found that the patient suffering from angina can do more exercise than normal before he triggers his pain. This suggests that the pain is triggered by two sources of nerve impulses: a major one from the heart and a minor one from the arm. These two add together. If one source is removed, it becomes more difficult for the other to trigger the feeling of pain. This applies as a general rule to referred pains but even more universally it applies to all pains. It will be seen that summation – the excitatory effects of converging inputs – provides important clues to understanding the causes and treatment of these pains.

Toothache

Sufferers and their dentists often have problems in locating the origin of a toothache, which is usually evoked by bacterial infection in the pulp of a tooth. Patients sometimes report that they have an earache when, in fact, the problem is not the ear but decay of the back upper teeth. In the case of front teeth, the patient frequently points to the wrong tooth, missing by one or two on either side of the culprit. The dentist knows he must search carefully. He therefore examines, probes, X-rays and adds local stimuli to each tooth to detect where he can add a stimulus and enhance the pain.

In some cases, if the tooth infection is neglected, the pain increases as the pulpitis gets worse. Eventually the infection may leak out of the root of the tooth and begin to affect the gum. Now there is an instant and dramatic change: the patient accurately points to the exact area of trouble. The damage now involves superficial tissue with its ability to signal the true location of the injury. We have here, in a small area, a repetition of the changes in pain during appendicitis. In the initial stages, damage is limited to deep tissue and is incorrectly located. Later, superficial structures become involved and then the area in which the pain is felt coincides with the location of the damage.

6
Spinal Cord Mechanisms

The spinal cord has a strikingly similar appearance in all mammals. The cell bodies lie in the middle of the cord and form the grey matter with its characteristic butterfly shape (see Figure 9, p.101). Around this grey matter, the white matter consists of axons running up and down the cord bringing messages to and from the cord and the brain. The arriving afferent fibres from the body comprise the dorsal roots and terminate on cells in the dorsal horn. The output cells to the skeletal (or 'striped') muscle all lie in the ventral horn, and the output cells to the viscera, smooth muscle, sweat glands, and other structures under autonomic control tend to concentrate in the lateral horn. The trigeminal nerve which supplies the face has an equivalent central apparatus in the medulla with the same components as those seen in each spinal segment.

The cross-sectional size of the spinal cord varies in a quite predictable way (Figure 13). The nerves to the arms have grown out of the lower cervical and upper thoracic segments and so these segments are large, forming the cervical enlargement, which supplies a lot of sensitive skin as well as many muscles capable of fine control. Similarly, there is a lumbar enlargement for the legs. Since the body surface between the arms and legs consists of relatively insensitive skin and little muscle, the dorsal horns are quite small in these segments but there is a lot of white matter carrying ascending and descending information. The pelvis contains many visceral organs which need to be controlled, and so in the sacral segments one finds particularly large and elaborate visceral (autonomic) mechanisms. The overall plan is identical throughout the spinal cord, but each segment includes a self-contained mechanism for the reception and control of the particular structures which grew from that segment in embryo. While this is the basic pattern, all nervous system components are integrated and therefore the segments must coordinate with each other and must consult with the brain – which gains increasing control over the segmental circuits in higher animals.

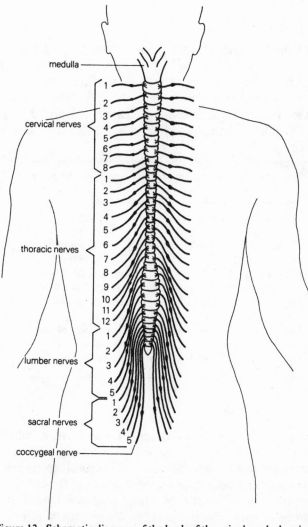

medulla

cervical nerves

1
2
3
4
5
6
7
8

thoracic nerves

1
2
3
4
5
6
7
8
9
10
11
12

lumber nerves

1
2
3
4
5

sacral nerves

1
2
3
4
5

coccygeal nerve

Figure 13. Schematic diagram of the back of the spinal cord, showing the entering sensory nerves, the enlarged ganglia that contain the cell bodies of the nerve fibres, and the roots at their level of entry into the cord. Cervical nerves 5 to 8 and thoracic 1 aggregate on each side to form the brachial plexus which innervates each arm. Similarly, lumbar and sacral nerves form the complex lumbosacral plexus which sends nerves to the pelvis and leg. Not shown are the vertebral bones which lie between each root or the chain of sympathetic ganglia that lie just outside the spinal cord on each side.

The components

The cells in the grey matter

Thanks to the Swedish anatomist, Bror Rexed (1952), we now recognize that the cells of the spinal cord are arranged in laminae (or layers) in a dorsal–ventral direction and that these laminae run the entire length of the spinal cord. The dorsal horn contains six laminae (Figure 14 and Table 4). Laminae 1 and 2 form a clear zone visible to the naked eye and are called the substantia gelatinosa Rolandi.

	Main cell size	Main sensory afferents	Commonest response
Lamina 1	Small and large	A-delta and C	Convergence of different inputs
2	Small	A-delta and C	Convergence of different inputs
3	Small and large	A-beta	Transitional between 2 and 4
4	Large	A-beta	Light cutaneous stimuli
5	Large	A-beta and delta	Convergence of different inputs
6	Large	Muscle afferents	Muscle stretch

Table 4. The dorsal horn laminae.

The ventral horn contains a further three laminae, numbers 7, 8 and 9, and finally there is an intriguing column of cells, lamina 10, clustered around the central canal. It is crucial to remember that this laminar anatomy refers to the location of the cell bodies, but these cells give off dendrites which always extend into the neighbouring or more distant laminae where they may contact axons from the periphery or from other cells.

The terminations of peripheral afferents

It is now possible to label single peripheral afferents by injecting the enzyme *horseradish peroxidase* which is transported to the

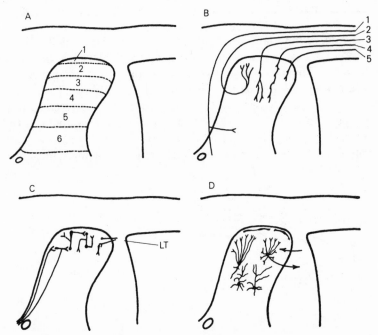

Figure 14. A cross section of lumbar dorsal quadrant of spinal cord.

A: The Rexed laminae into which cell bodies are divided. Laminae 1 and 2 are the substantia gelatinosa but lamina 3 contains similar small cells. Laminae 1, 4, 5 and 6 contain large cells.

B: The pattern of arriving peripheral nerve afferents: 1, represents the course of a large proprioceptive axon which terminates in lamina 6 and the ventral horn. 2, a hair follicle afferent with recurrent terminal arborizations in laminae 3 and 4; 3, a touch afferent; 4, a small delta myelinated afferent; 5, an unmeyelinated C afferent.

C: The small cells in substantia gelatinosa end on each other and perhaps on afferents and the dendrites of deeper cells. These send some axons into the Lissauer tract (LT) and back into substantia. They also send axons to the opposite substantia by way of the dorsal commissure.

D: Large cells in laminae 1, 4 and 5 and their dendrites. Descending fibres from the brainstem.

central terminals of the individual fibre. In this way, the detailed anatomy of the central terminals of particular fibre types can be observed. This careful work has been done particularly in

Edinburgh by Brown *et al.* (1978) and in North Carolina by Perl (1980). The general rule is that the thicker the fibre, the deeper it penetrates (Figure 15). The unmyelinated C fibres do not seem to penetrate beyond lamina 2. The small myelinated A-delta fibres terminate mainly in laminae 1 and 2, and some struggle down to lamina 5. The large myelinated cutaneous afferents penetrate more deeply, ending mainly in laminae 3, 4 and 5. The largest sensory afferents from the specialized muscle stretch afferents penetrate into lamina 6 and some even into the ventral horn where they terminate directly on motor neurons and form the basis of the monosynaptic reflexes such as the knee jerk.

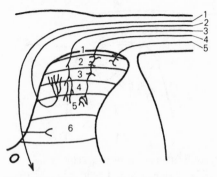

Figure 15. The course and destination of afferent fibres from dorsal root to dorsal horn containing six laminae. Afferent fibres: 1, muscle spindle afferent; 2, hair afferent; 3, touch corpuscle afferent; 4, δ afferent; 5, C afferent.

The origin and termination of control systems descending from the brain

The general rule is that nerve fibres descending in the white matter penetrate into the grey matter and innervate the cells nearest their tract in the white matter. The dorsolateral white matter is therefore well situated to send axons into the most dorsal laminae and does so. It contains fibres from the brainstem, particularly from the raphe nuclei, the locus coeruleus, the large cell region of the reticular formation and from the hypothalamus. Slightly more central, there is the pyramidal tract from the cortex and, although this is classically thought to be a motor system, it floods into the dorsal laminae as well and affects cell groups in laminae

3–6. More ventrally still, there are massive descending pathways from the vestibular system and the reticular formation which can directly or indirectly affect the firing of sensory cells. While we describe here only the direct input, the direct systems are, of course, themselves indirectly affected by all other parts of the brain.

The destination of fibres from cells in the dorsal horn

There are three general locations to which dorsal horn cells project: (1) cells in the same segment; (2) cells in other segments (the propriospinal system); and (3) cells in the brain (by way of the long running tracts). The local segmental circuits undoubtedly make up the bulk of the connections and, among other functions, form the reflex pathways by which arriving sensory signals produce motor outputs.

The small cells in substantia gelatinosa (Figure 16) seem to have predominantly intrasegmental effects; they project onto nearby laminae, although some of the axons project up and down the cord by way of a tiny tract on the surface of the cord named after Lissauer. There is convincing evidence (Gobel, 1979) of connections between a type of lamina 2 cell and a type of lamina 1 cell. But we still do not know the details of connections among cells in the other laminae, although several possibilities have been proposed (see Wall, 1980a). The short, intersegmental propriospinal fibres run in the grey matter and in white-matter bundles close to the grey matter, and end in nearby segments on both sides of the cord. It is obvious that these short connections could link with each other and eventually deliver messages to the brain.

However, attention has naturally focused on the large, long-running tracts which project directly to various brain structures. The furthest penetration into the brain is by way of a fibre system – the spinothalamic tract – which ends in the thalamus, and an inordinate amount of attention is paid to it in spite of the fact that, in man, it contains only about a thousand fibres. Adding to the fascination of the spinothalamic tract is the fact that it runs in the ventrolateral white matter which, if cut, leads to analgesia (see Fig. 6, p.77). In spite of the fact that the tract represents less than one per cent of the fibres that are cut, the operation is often

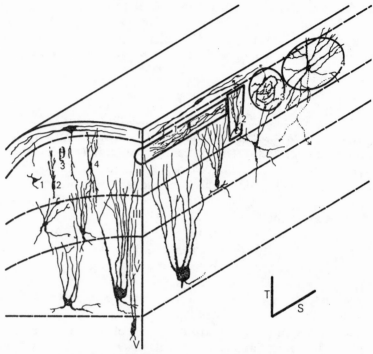

Figure 16. The arrangement of the various cell types found in the upper dorsal horn of the human spinal cord. The cell shapes are shown in the transverse plane T and in the sagittal plane S. The Rexed laminae I–IV are shown, see Figure 14 – A. The cell types in lamina II are: 1, islet cells; 2, filamentous cells; 3, stalk cells; 4, stellate cells. Axons of the cells are indicated by the dotted lines.

(from Schoenen, 1980)

called a spinothalamic tractotomy. Each of the six dorsal laminae, except for lamina 2, reports its state of activity to the brain. The destination of these fibres includes the reticular formation, the thalamus and the cerebellum, and are described in detail by Willis and Coggeshall (1978).

Finally, we must mention a special pathway – the dorsal columns – which contains primary afferent fibres. The large A-beta cutaneous afferents divide on entering the cord and send terminals into the nearby grey matter and a long branch which ends in the dorsal column nuclei at the entry point of the spinal cord into the skull. This pathway also contains fibres which come from the dorsal horn, particularly from lamina 5.

Chemistry
We have seen that the dorsal horn of the spinal cord contains three major neural components: (1) the afferent sensory fibres; (2) the cells in the grey matter; and (3) the descending controls. Each of these has its special chemistry. Astonishingly, there is no generally agreed chemical transmitter for the sensory afferents although there are a number of candidates. The terminals of the fine afferents which end in the substantia gelatinosa contain at least five active peptides (short chains of amino-acids). They are substance P, vasoactive intestinal peptide, somatostatin, angiotensin and cholecystokinin. Most work has so far been done on substance P, which is known to be released by arriving nerve impulses. In the substantia gelatinosa itself twelve more of these powerful agents are found: substance P, neurotensin, cholycystokinin, neurophysin, oxytocin, glucagon, somatostatin, vasopressin, angiotensin, motilin and bombesin (Gibson *et al.*, 1981). The greatest attention has been paid to the discovery of enkephalin and narcotic receptors in cells in the substantia gelatinosa, which has opened up the discussion of the local action of narcotics in the spinal cord to be discussed later. Also present are the well-known classical neurotransmitters, particularly gamma-aminobutyric acid (GABA), a powerful inhibitory transmitter. The descending axons contain the well-known compounds serotonin and noradrenalin and some of the peptides. We see here an alchemist's laboratory of many powerful stimulators and inhibitors of nerve cells, but we know almost nothing in detail of when and where they act. They offer an exciting future not only for exploration but also as potential agents for pharmacological control of sensory transmission.

Responses of cells
The immediate response of the cells to single stimuli
For the best of reasons – simplicity of experiment – investigators began by recording from single spinal cord cells and by applying

single stimuli to the skin, looking for excitation of the cells. The same procedure used for peripheral nerve fibres was also used to study spinal cord cells and, of course, the bias of the experimenters is evident in the experimental design. Those who were convinced that the specialization at the periphery is continued into the brain – the basis of the specificity theory – looked for 'best' stimuli or for cells monopólized by one type of stimulus, and tended to neglect cells which did not fit the expected specificity pattern. Those who were impressed by the functional aspects of control and convergence used several stimuli and stressed the multiplicity of effective stimuli. An unbiased survey of the thousands of dorsal horn cells reported by various workers shows a small minority, about 10%, which responds only to intense stimulation by pressure, heat or chemicals. About 20% respond only to light mechanical stimuli of the skin. The great majority – over 70% – respond to mixtures of different types of peripheral stimuli.

As might be expected, there is specialization of function in the laminae of the dorsal horns. In 1967, Wall showed that laminae 4, 5 and 6 were clearly differentiated by their most common type of cell. In lamina 4, the cells have small receptive fields and many respond only to low-threshold A-beta mechanoreceptors. In lamina 5, the receptive fields are larger and much more complex, and the cells respond to both low- and high-threshold afferents and to heat and chemicals. In a search for cells that respond to visceral inputs, Pomeranz, Wall and Weber (1968) found them in lamina 5 and, interestingly, found no cells which did not also respond to a cutaneous input. Here then, we see, at the first central cells, an explanation for referred visceral pain at the skin surface and for the convergences which are know to occur between deep and surface inputs (see p.124). Recent physiological evidence shows that cells that respond directly (monosynaptically) to unmyelinated afferents are found in laminae 1 and 2, although many cells in laminae 5 and 6 also respond massively, but perhaps indirectly, to these afferents (Fitzgerald and Wall, 1980).

As techniques improved, it became possible to examine the firing of small cells as well as large ones in laminae 1, 2 and 3. The results and discussions of the various experimenters are described in detail elsewhere (Wall, 1980a and b). Perl and his associates concentrated on a search for cells that respond specifically to noxious stimuli and identified them particularly in lamina 1. Other teams also found such cells, but rarely; most cells which were studied received several types of convergent input. Wall, Merrill and Yaksh (1979) carried out a special study of the small cells in the substantia gelatinosa and found a mixture of specialized and generalized cells. Since we are here discussing injury and pain, we will now concentrate on those cells which receive the incoming messages from the high-threshold afferents. The large transmitting cells are concentrated in laminae 1 and 5, and the small cells with short axons are found most commonly in laminae 1 and 2.

The interactions of convergent inputs

The specificity enthusiast has to dismiss cells with convergent inputs as irrelevant to the specific pain pathway which he believes must exist. We, on the other hand, consider them to be important because they can still signal highly specialized information and, furthermore, are likely to provide mechanisms which could explain the summations, convergences and controls which are observed in the real world, especially in the clinic. Hillman and Wall (1969) started with a study of lamina 5 cells and first restricted themselves to very light stimuli, hair movement and gentle skin indentation. They found cells which respond to a brief stimulus applied to an area of skin by a brief burst of impulses, followed by a silent period of inhibition. Surrounding this excitatory area, there is a large area of skin in which gentle stimuli produce only inhibition of the cell's activity. This is a common pattern of receptive fields in all sensory systems, in which an excitatory receptive field has an inhibitory surround. This pattern of receptive field has many advantages as a signalling system because, as a stimulus moves out of the centre, it does not just fade away but actually produces the opposite effect. When Hillman and Wall used intense stimuli, such as pinching, they found that there is a much larger area from which the cell could be excited; but beyond this large area there is an even larger area in which intense stimuli produce inhibition of the lamina 5 cell. This enormous inhibitory surround has now been given a special name of DNIC or 'diffuse noxious inhibitory control' (Le Bars, Dickenson and Besson, 1979a and b).

It is clear, then, that we have evidence for two superimposed receptive fields – one for gentle stimuli, and one for intense stimuli, each with different spatial organizations. Now we can understand the curious fact that has been known for years: that stimulation of large, low-threshold afferents tends to inhibit the response of cells to small, high-threshold afferents. The large afferents are connected to both excitatory and inhibitory mechanisms but, on the whole, the inhibition wins. The practical development of transcutaneous electrical nerve stimulation, in which gentle stimuli are given to inhibit pain (Wall and Sweet, 1967), appears to depend on tricking a delicately balanced, spatial mechanism which controls receptive fields. Furthermore, the older folk methods of fighting pain with distant pain – such as acupuncture or cupping (which we will discuss in Chapter 14) – may be explained at the spinal cord level in terms of activation of a large inhibitory surround. It appears that these properties are not unique to lamina 5 cells but apply also to lamina 1 cells. Even more surprising, the cells in both laminae which are dominated by the excitatory input from high-threshold afferents are inhibited by the simultaneous activation of low-threshold afferents.

In summary, many cells are excited by injury-detecting afferents and the majority of these are also excited by gentle stimulation of a small area of skin. In addition, the activation of low-threshold afferents partially inhibits the responses of all types of cells to injury-detecting afferents. We do not know if both lamina 1 and 5 cells contribute to trigger pain in man, but an analysis by Mayer *et al.* (1975) opts for lamina 5 cells as the dominant input.

The effects of descending controls

Electrical stimulation of particular brainstem structures inhibits activity in many single dorsal horn cells. The decerebrate animal (in which the brainstem is sectioned completely at the midbrain level) is fixed in a frozen 'posture' of both the sensory and motor systems, and many structures in the pons and medulla steadily bombard the spinal cord with descending streams of nerve impulses. It is possible to interrupt these descending messages reversibly by cooling a segment of the thoracic cord, and this allows single cells to be examined repeatedly with and without the brainstem control (Wall, 1967; Hillman and Wall, 1969). It appears that the descending control generally inhibits the response of cells to cutaneous afferents and particularly to noxious stimuli. This effect is so powerful that the injection of the pain-producing compound bradykinin into a leg fails to excite cells in the decerebrate animal, but produces massive firing if the descending control is blocked. The most striking functional change is seen in lamina 6 cells which are dominated by muscle input in the decerebrate animal and by a cutaneous input if the descending control is blocked. Here we see that the control not only influences the intensity of response but also the type of response.

More details of these controls have been revealed. Fetz (1968) showed that the pyramidal tract inhibits lamina 4 cells, has mixed effects in lamina 5 and tends to excite lamina 6 cells. Later it became apparent that drugs and electrical stimulation of parts of the brain which produce behavioural analgesia and inhibition of the responses of spinal cord cells to noxious stimuli act through these descending pathways. Basbaum *et al.* (1977) showed that the dorsolateral white matter is particularly crucial for carrying these impulses, and Basbaum and Fields (1979) have shown that the origin of some of these pathways is in the raphe nuclei and in the reticular formation.

The role of the substantia gelatinosa
We have so far discussed the short-term responses of dorsal horn cells which project to the brain, and have shown that they are subject to excitatory and inhibitory convergences from the periphery and to descending control. Some of these controls undoubtedly act directly on the surface of the transmitting cells. But, in addition, it is possible that the short-axon small cells in the substantia gelatinosa (SG) may also play an important role in modulation of the sensory input. The fact that they are anatomically well placed to control the transmission of impulses from the

incoming afferents to the spinal transmitting cells is the basis of the gate-control theory which we will discuss in Chapter 10.

The evidence for the role of SG cells in the modulation of transmission is reviewed in detail elsewhere (Wall, 1980a and b) and can be summarized here. Some cells may be excitatory links. There is good evidence that a type of lamina 2 cell excites a type of lamina 1 cell (Gobel, 1979). It is also certain that lamina 5 cells respond to activity in unmyelinated C afferents, and lamina 2 cells may connect the C fibres to these cells. In a recent experiment (see Wall, 1980b), stimulation of the small axons from SG in the Lissauer tract excited twenty-nine per cent of nearby cells in laminae 4 and 5. Turning now to the possible inhibitory role of these cells, we so far know of seven examples where a change of excitability of SG cells is associated with a change of excitability in the opposite direction in cells of laminae 4 and 5. These reciprocal changes are produced by: (1) stimulation of the raphe nuclei; (2) stimulation of the dorsal columns; (3) stimulation of the nucleus magnocellularis of the reticular formation; (4) stimulation of the dorsolateral white matter; (5) application of naloxone; (6) stimulation of the Lissauer tract (which inhibits forty-eight per cent of nearby lamina 5 cells); and (7) selective blockade of A afferents (which abolishes the responses of SG cells to A afferents, does not affect their response to C afferents but greatly enhances the response of lamina 5 cells to C afferents). A striking example of these effects is the discovery (Fitzgerald and Woolf, 1980) that naloxone inhibits the activity of SG cells (implying that they are activated by opioid compounds) but excites cells in laminae 4 and 5 (suggesting that they are influenced by the SG cells).

All of these facts add up to a strong argument that the small SG cells may modulate input signals by increasing or decreasing their effect on the large spinal transmission cells which send their messages to distant structures. The fact that there are at least four different shapes of small SG cells and a large number of different chemistries suggests that the substantia gelatinosa is not simple and uniform but capable of many different types of control.

Long-term actions

For the same reason of simplicity which led neurophysiologists to use single, brief stimuli to examine single fibres and single cells, it seemed reasonable to examine only a brief period, perhaps 50 milliseconds (msec.), after the arrival of the volley, since this period contained the large, obvious surge of activity. Everyone knew that most stimuli in the real world are slow and prolonged, and it was generally accepted that there must be slow changes in the nervous system but their study was put off until the brief, initial responses were understood. The fastest reaction time of a person who detects and responds to a stimulus is more than 150 msec. If the person is required to respond to discrete stimuli presented in a series, the reaction times range from 230 to 500msec. It is evident, therefore, that we must consider the state of the sensory pathways for some time even after a sudden, brief stimulus.

No matter how brief and isolated, a stimulus does not activate a quiescent nervous system which is a blank register (or 'tabula rasa'). The nervous system in which the sensory signal flows has a short- and long-term history. Is the animal alert or asleep, oriented to the stimulus or going about some other business, prepared for an expected, learned signal or receiving it for the first time? All of these aspects of immediate history influence the set of the nervous system, including the receiving cells in the spinal cord. Furthermore, no stimulus really occurs in isolation. There is always a background or platform on which the stimulus occurs. Even a subject in an experimental psychology experiment who is in a dark, soundproof room and is asked to report on the presence of a stimulus is not really isolated. He knows which way is up, he feels his body, he is bored or alert, in a good or bad mood, under control or free. In other words, even under the most controlled experimental conditions, a stimulus is never genuinely isolated. In the real world, a pain-provoking stimulus is necessarily presented against a background of events such as pressure on the tissue, local blood flow, the motion of the limbs, the situation of the body, and the state of attention. Just as the body has a posture from which any movement starts, so the sensory system has a setting from which it receives and analyses a novel event.

This setting or control is produced by steady or slowly acting mechanisms in all parts of the nervous system. We will now consider some candidates in the spinal cord.

The control of sensory afferent terminals

If there is a sudden, gentle, brief stimulus, the afferent fibres carry a brief input volley and the spinal cord cells with long-running axons emit a short burst of impulses which outlasts the input by several tens of milliseconds. However, in the dorsal horn, a prolonged shift in voltage – the dorsal root potential – accompanies the brief input–output sequence and can last for hundreds of milliseconds. Wall (1958) showed that this potential was a sign of a change of membrane potential in the terminals of the afferent fibres. He went on to show that it was likely that the change – primary afferent depolarization – was produced by action involving the small cells of substantia gelatinosa (reviewed in Wall, 1980a). The significance of the change is that it is associated with a change in the effectiveness of the terminals in their ability to produce firing of the cells deep in the dorsal horns. This so-called presynaptic inhibition works either by blocking the impulses or by controlling the amount of neurotransmitter released by the terminals.

A mechanism thus exists which is able to control sensory inputs. The same mechanism may also exert a postsynaptic influence on the cells on which the sensory fibres end. This slow, long-lasting mechnism may well be steadily active, continually controlling the impulses which affect particular cells. It can be brought into a new state of activity not only by impulses arriving from the periphery but also by impulses descending from the head. It may act to increase as well as decrease the effectiveness of arriving sensory signals and represents one of the controls which make up the 'gate' through which entering impulses must pass. It must be realized that since we think of this control as being in continuous action, it can be modified to a more open or a more closed position either by inputs from the periphery or by volleys descending from the brain.

So far we have spoken only of the transient and steady control of the terminals of afferent fibres, but we now have two examples of long-term control which are highly relevant to pain problems.

If a peripheral nerve is cut in a rat or a cat, the ability of that nerve to modulate the excitability of its own central terminals and those of its neighbours disappears in a few days (Wall and Devor, 1981). This observation may be an example of a homeostatic mechanism, whereby the spinal cord reacts to the partial loss of sensory input by removing an inhibitory control and thereby exaggerating the central effects of any arriving impulses.

There is convincing evidence, which we will describe later, that the section of nerves is frequently followed by gross exaggerations of the central effects of inputs from adjacent intact nerves. We believe that the unmyelinated fibres are responsible for these abnormal central effects.

The reason for this assumption is that animals injected with the compound capsaicin at birth have a very large loss of their unmyelinated C fibres but the myelinated A fibres seem to remain intact. In these animals, brief (phasic) inputs are unable to generate a depolarization of their afferent terminals (Wall, 1980b), indicating that an important control has been lost. We can go further and ask what it is about the C fibres which exerts the necessary influence for the control to work. Curiously enough, it is not the nerve impulses since the control remains if the nerve is crushed rather than cut, yet we know that these two procedures have the same effect on nerve impulses. If it is not the nerve impulses, what is left? Nerve fibres have a double function: first, to transmit nerve impulses, and second, to transport chemical substances. We know that whenever presynaptic control has been abolished, there is an interference with the transport of substances. We are not certain what these substances are, but we suspect that the peptides are involved, and, in this particular case, that substance P is a crucial compound which is needed for the control to work. This slow action could be one of the functions of the peptides in gradually setting the relative excitabilities of connections. It is apparent that we have moved from the initial period of interaction which lasts for a period of less than a hundred milliseconds to considering longer and longer periods lasting up to days.

Responses of spinal cord cells

In an anaesthetized animal, the action of spinal cord circuits seems relatively fixed, rigid and abrupt. However, it is possible to examine these same cells in an animal without anaesthesia after the forebrain has been removed (the decerebrate preparation) under a general anaesthetic. We know from studies of people and animals that such preparations can be considered to cause no feeling and suffering. They allow the study of the state of the spinal cord, medulla, pons and lower midbrain without influence from thalamus and cortex, and without the dampening effects of anaesthetics. In these preparations, a far more lively picture emerges which tells us more of what such cells would be capable of doing if they were in an intact, freely moving animal. First, one observes, in some transmitting cells, long-term facilitations which last over one second so that repeated identical stimuli build up a longer and longer discharge. This phenomenon, called the 'wind-up' effect, occurs especially if the inhibitory controls have been abolished, and is reminiscent of the temporal summation of pain which is so characteristic of some nerve injuries (p.91).

While the wind-up can be seen in the large transmitting cells of lamina 5, a much more striking form of prolonged firing can be seen in about twenty per cent of the small cells of the substantia gelatinosa, where some respond for minutes to a single stimulus (Wall, Merrill and Yaksh, 1979). Some cells show the opposite effect where repeated stimuli produce a smaller and smaller effect (habituation). This is particularly striking in the substantia gelatinosa, where a cell may respond well to a single brush stroke of hairs but then fail completely if the cell's receptive field is again stimulated in the next minute or so. Such cells have been called 'novelty cells' and they too have their counterparts in overall behaviour.

In a paraplegic man, a strong stimulus evokes a strong flexion of the limb but on repetition the response gradually fades. Dimitrijevic and Nathan (1970) have shown that this turn-off can last as long as a day. We have all experienced the huge startle response which even a light, unexpected touch can evoke, and yet, if the stimulus is repeated, the response rapidly declines or disappears. These are examples of the brain's ability to impose an inhibition or censorship on incoming messages.

Among the neurons in the spinal cord, the cells of the substantia gelatinosa are the best candidates so far discovered as mediators of these long-term facilitations and inhibitions. In addition to their interesting reactions to peripheral stimuli, these small cells are strongly excited for long periods after brief stimuli to the various descending pathways (Dubuisson and Wall, 1980).

Receptive fields

Each peripheral or spinal cell transmits information from a definite area of tissue, the receptive field. We have noted that spinal cells can collect inputs from widely separated areas – as in the case of cells which receive inputs from the viscera as well as the skin. We have also seen that cells with convergent inputs have complex receptive fields with both excitatory and inhibitory components. To understand pain, it is important to know if these receptive fields remain stable or if they change in the presence of disease; an answer is necessary in order to explain the expansion of the painful areas beyond the region of disease, and the unpleasant feelings evoked in normal tissue after injury in a distant part of the body.

The basis of all receptive fields must depend on anatomy, since nerve fibres must run directly or indirectly from the periphery to affect the observed central cell. The basic anatomy is undoubtedly fully formed in the embryo, or at least during the first few weeks after birth. However, while there is strong anatomical evidence that the incoming sensory nerve fibres and their central connections are spread over a very wide area, the normal animal shows a very discrete, highly localized distribution of *physiological* responses to stimulation. In other words, there is a mismatch between an excess of anatomical connection and the observed precise localization of physiological responses. The reason, we believe, is that many of the anatomical connections are normally kept suppressed but may be released when there is damage to the central or peripheral nervous systems (Wall and Devor, 1981). We are able to make these statements because, in the intact brain and spinal cord, the receptive fields form an overlapping mosaic to produce maps within the brain of the body surface. Each cell has its receptive field, and its neighbour has a slightly shifted field, so that by putting them all together a somatotopic map is formed which shows that the cells and their inputs are arranged in an orderly manner to serve the entire body surface. For example, if cells in the lumbar enlargement are examined one by one from the medial edge to the lateral edge of the dorsal horn, one finds that the most medial cells receive inputs from the toes, the most lateral cells serve the upper leg, and in between there is a predictable strip of skin, the dermatome, connecting the two extremes. The existence of these maps allows a reliable prediction of which area a particular cell will serve in the normal state. These maps allow one to observe deviations from the normal in diseases.

Most of the pathways that transmit sensory information from the body to the brain have relays in the spinal cord. However, one system sends axons directly from the periphery up the dorsal columns of the spinal cord (see Figure 6) to end in the dorsal column nuclei which lie at the beginning of the medulla. Cells in these nuclei send their axons across the midline to form a large tract, the medial lemniscus. This projects to the thalamus, which in turn projects to the cortex. At each stage of the dorsal column–medial lemniscus system there is a detailed map of the body surface (Figure 17). Dostrovsky, Millar and Wall (1976) wondered what would happen to this map if the input from the hind legs was eliminated by a cord block. The prediction was that a hole should develop in the map since cells have lost their input. Indeed, they found that this is what happens to most cells in the leg area. However, they also observed that a minority of cells promptly begin to respond to a new input (Figure 18). Thus a cell which normally responds to toes suddenly begins to respond to abdomen. When the block is removed they revert immediately to their normal input.

A similar phenomenon was seen in cells at the next stage in the thalamus (Nakahama *et al.*, 1966). The receptive field of a cell was determined and then that area of skin was locally anaesthetized. Some cells promptly responded to a new receptive field. Recently, the most spectacular example of this immediate

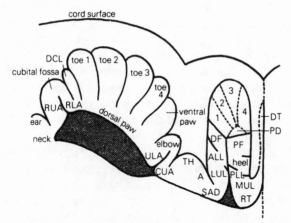

Figure 17. A 'felinculus' of the body surface representation within the gracile and cuneate nuclei. Abbreviations from left to right: R U A, rostral upper arm; R L A, rostral lower arm; D C L, dew claw; U L A, ulnar lower arm; C U A, caudal upper arm; T H, thorax; A, abdomen; S A D, saddle and lumbar back; L U L, lateral upper leg; A L L, anterior lower leg; D F, dorsal foot; P D, foot pad; P F, plantar foot; P L L, posterior lower leg; M U L, medial upper leg; R T, root of tail; D T, distal tail. Cross-hatching indicates areas where deep pressure is necessary to fire the cells.
(from Millar and Basbaum, 1976)

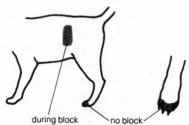

Figure 18. An example of how the input to some cells can change as soon as the normal input is blocked. Here a single cell was being studied in the foot area of the gracile nucleus (see Figure 17). It responded only to pressure on the toes – 'no block'. Then all input from the leg was blocked by cooling the lumbar spinal cord. As soon as the leg input was blocked, the cell began to respond to touch on an area of the flank – 'during block'. When the block was removed by rewarming the lumbar cord, the receptive field of the cell returned to the foot and the responsive area on the flank disappeared.
(from Dostrovsky, Millar and Wall, 1976)

switching has been seen in the sensory cortex of freely moving cats (Metzler and Marks, 1979). Once a cell's receptive field on the hind leg was located, the hind leg was locally anaesthetized with an indwelling epidural catheter and new receptive fields appeared. Evidently, in this system, the arriving nerve impulses to some cells are under constant fast control so that abolition of one input unmasks another. If the afferent nerve is cut rather than blocked, there are slow changes in addition to the fast ones so that over periods of many days novel receptive fields appear in more and more cells (Dostrovsky *et al.*, 1976). A possible explanation for these slow changes is that new nerve fibres sprout from intact afferent neurons and invade the area which has lost its input. An additional possibility is that many remaining intact fibres are unmasked by slow processes, but the evidence for this depends largely on spinal cord experiments to which we will now turn.

In the spinal cord, unlike the areas we have just discussed, there is no evidence for rapid, major changes of receptive fields when a particular input is lost (Devor and Wall, 1981a and b). The cells in lamina 4 have remarkably rigid receptive fields, although their excitability can be varied over a wide range. The cells of lamina 5 have complex receptive fields which can expand and contract under variations of the controls we have discussed, but the dramatic, sudden shifts seen in the lemniscal projection system are not observed. However, peripheral nerve lesions lead to substantial changes of spinal receptive fields over a period of days (Devor and Wall, 1978). If the nerves to a rat's foot are cut, there is the expected gap in the spinal cord map for three days after loss of the input. Then, during the period of four to ten days after the nerve lesion, some forty per cent of the cells which have been functionally deafferented begin to respond to the nearest intact nerves. The central parts of the axons which have been cut in the periphery remain intact and can still be made to excite the cell if they are electrically stimulated. In spite of this, the cells respond to a new input and we attribute this to the slow decay of inhibitory mechanisms, including the disappearance of control of the membrane potential of the primary afferent terminals. Of all the different types of axons damaged, we suspect the unmyelinated afferents as being most important because animals that have lost these fibres at birth from capsaicin poisoning do not show the customary organization of the normal receptive fields and maps. It seems that the unmyelinated afferents may control the organization of spinal cord connections, rapidly by way of nerve impulses and slowly by way of transported substances. Whatever the mechanism may be, it is apparent that the origin of the inputs which dominate cells is under control, and even the adult nervous system is capable of substantial plasticity of connection and response, especially after nerve injury.

The special example of narcotic analgesia

The pain-killing effect of morphine and the other narcotics is produced in the central nervous system. But where and how does this action occur? The modern story begins with the discovery of stimulation-produced analgesia which will be discussed in the next chapter. Recently, narcotic-like substances which are produced by the body were discovered in the central nervous system. These come in two types: large molecules called the endorphins and small peptides containing five amino-acids called the enkephalins. Enkephalins and narcotic receptors are highly concentrated in an area of the midbrain called the periaqueductal grey, which produces analgesia when it is electrically stimulated. The question immediately arose, how could this area produce analgesia?

Basbaum *et al.* (1977) showed that if the dorsolateral white matter in the thoracic spinal cord was cut, both electrical stimulation and narcotics failed to produce the expected analgesia in the hind legs but did so in the arms and face. This experiment showed that the midbrain area generated impulses that descended into the spinal cord. These impulses prevented pain signals from being sent from the cord to the brain. This descending control relay system seems to use serotonin (5-hydroxytryptamine) as one of its neurotransmitters.

The presence of these narcotic-induced descending controls naturally shifted attention to the spinal cord and particularly to the most dorsal laminae where they terminated. Here, it turns out, the story is repeated. Laminae 1 and 2 contain high concentrations of enkephalins and there are morphine receptors present in these laminae, particularly on the terminals of fine afferent fibres. As in the midbrain, local injections of a small amount of narcotic into the substantia gelatinosa produce a striking inhibition of the response of lamina 5 cells to afferent signals from an injured area (Duggan *et al.*, 1976). Yaksh and Rudy (1976) applied morphine to the surface of lumbar cord and produced local analgesia, and this has evolved into the injection of narcotics locally onto the surface of the spinal cord in man, with the result that minute doses produce a long-lasting analgesia in the segments that absorb the compound. Thus far, the results seem convincing: that there are two sites – one in the midbrain and one in the cord – where narcotics produce their action, and that they do so by imitating an existing system which uses enkephalins.

Jessell and Iversen (1977) recently produced a chemically labelled version of the gate-control system, which we will describe later, in which large fibres stimulated small cells in the substantia gelatinosa; these released enkephalin which acted on the opiate receptors on the fine afferent fibres and reduced the release of substance P, a peptide present in these fibres. Sjolund *et al.* (1979) showed that transcutaneous electrical stimulation in man relieved pain, released endorphins locally and was reversed by naloxone which is a specific narcotic antagonist. There remain many problems with this grand scheme, particularly in its details (Wall and Woolf, 1980), but the greatest mystery is that we do not know the natural circumstances under which this internal pain control comes into operation. This problem will be considered further in the next chapter on brain mechanisms.

7
Brain Mechanisms

Studies of the organization of the spinal cord, described in Chapter 6, show clearly that pain signals are transmitted to the brain by multiple pathways and that the information processed in the dorsal horns is controlled by descending systems. Brain processes related to pain are even more complex; the old concept of a 'pain centre' is obviously nonsense. Many areas of the brain are involved in pain processes and they interact extensively. We will first outline the basic anatomical organization of the brain and then look at the mechanisms related to pain.

Basic organization of the brain

The spinal cord begins to enlarge and change shape as it enters the skull. This marks the transition from the spinal cord to the brainstem. In the lowest part of the brainstem, some nuclei (groups of cell bodies) receive fibres from the dorsal columns and spinocervical tract. This area also contains the nerve cells which receive fibres from the trigeminal nucleus, which is the sensory nerve of the face. As we move rostrally (toward the top of the head), the brainstem becomes larger until it terminates in the large group of nuclei that form the thalamus. On the basis of anatomical landmarks, portions of the brainstem up to the thalamus are designated as the medulla, the pons, and the midbrain (Figure 19). The pons – an enlarged portion of the brainstem – is the level of origin of the cerebellum, which carries out complex functions related to movement. The midbrain lies between the pons and the thalamus, which is the major relay station of the forebrain (or cerebrum).

The structure of the brainstem is basically the same in all

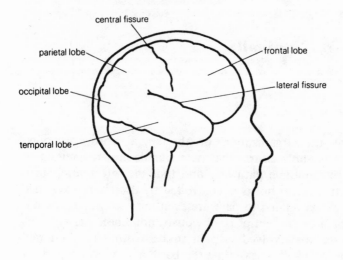

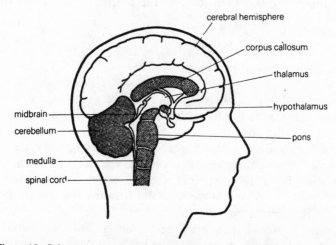

Figure 19. Schematic diagrams of the brain. *Top:* the major lobes and fissures. *Bottom:* a cross-section through the centre of the brain revealing the major components of the brainstem and other structures.

vertebrate species. Knowledge of the groundplan in one species allows relatively easy identification of comparable (homologous) structures in other species. (However, although structurally similar, their functions are not necessarily the same in all species.) If a cross-section of the medulla or midbrain of the rat, for example, is compared to a homologous cross-section in the human brain, the similarities are striking. The naked eye can easily see the medial lemniscus on each side, which consists of a large bundle of myelinated fibres that project to the posterior (back) part of the thalamus. These posterior nuclei send most of their axons to the somatosensory cortex. Between the medial lemnisci in the midbrain lies a wide area of small, densely packed cells and fibres which comprise the reticular formation. The reticular formation is not homogeneous, and, examined under a microscope, consists of distinct structures, some easily identified, others not. The periaqueductal grey, for example, is highly visible, but specialized areas within it and below it can be distinguished only on the basis of microscopic differences. The reticular formation is a particularly fascinating structure because it is superbly organized to integrate information from diverse sources and exerts a profound influence on sensory, motor and autonomic activity. Many of its fibres project back down to the spinal cord while others extend directly or indirectly to virtually all the areas of the cerebrum.

A 'ring' of structures – often called the 'limbic system' – surrounds the thalamus on each side of the brain. These structures, which play a major role in pain as well as virtually every other kind of behaviour, include the hypothalamus, hippocampus, amygdala, septum and cingulum. Lying on top of all of these structures – and enveloping them like a thick, intricately folded 'mantle' – is the cerebral cortex, which becomes larger in more highly evolved animals.

The major function of the brain is to receive and integrate sensory inputs, relate the inputs to past experience, and to bring about purposeful behaviour that is optimally adapted to the survival of the animal or person in its particular environment. Pain in man comprises two components – behaviour and conscious experience – which can both be measured with appropriate tools. Pain in animals, however, can only be measured by examining overt behaviour. The experience of pain is often inferred from the behaviour of mammals, and it is also reasonable to attribute pain experience to birds, amphibia and fish.

Ascending systems

Embryological and anatomical studies of fish, amphibians, and reptiles reveal that, even in the lowest vertebrates, reflexes are created by internuncial cells (the 'neuropil') that link the sensory input to the motor output. During embryological development in these species, behaviour becomes increasingly a function of earlier sensory inputs as a result of the memory traces they have etched into the neural connections. Behaviour, then, is not merely the expression of a response to a stimulus, but a dynamic process comprising multiple interacting factors. Coghill (1929) was first to propound this principle, based on his brilliant neuro-embryological-behavioural studies of salamanders, which has been substantially confirmed by later investigators. Given this fundamental principle – that organisms are not passive receivers manipulated by environmental inputs but act dynamically on those inputs so that behaviour becomes variable, unique and creative – the remainder of evolution becomes comprehensible as a gradual development of mechanisms that make each new species increasingly independent of the push-and-pull of environmental circumstances.

One of the most striking discoveries in the 1950s was the fact that injury signals are transmitted to the brain by multiple ascending pathways, each with distinctive conduction velocities and terminations in the brain (Kerr, Haugen and Melzack, 1955; Bowsher and Albe-Fessard, 1965). On the basis of the evolution of the pathways and their anatomical distribution in the brainstem, it is possible to distinguish between two major systems: (a) the phylogenetically old pathways – the spinoreticular, paleo-spinothalamic, and propriospinal systems – which course medially through the brainstem (Figure 20), and (b) the newer pathways which maintain a lateral course in the brainstem and project ultimately to areas in the thalamus and thence to the cortex – the neospinothalamic, spinocervical, and dorsal-column postsynaptic pathways (Figure 21). The fact that most of these pathways, including the phylogenetically old ones, are still continuing to evolve (Noback and Schriver, 1969) suggests that each has distinctive functions.

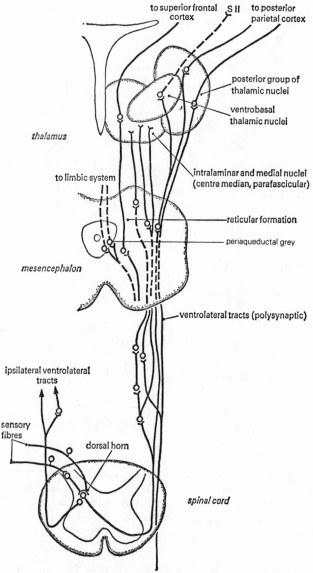

Figure 20. The slowly conducting somatosensory projection pathways.
The breaks in the projection lines represent multi-synaptic connections.
The propriospinal fibres are not shown, but consist of short fibres which are
distributed throughout the cord.
(adapted from Milner, 1970)

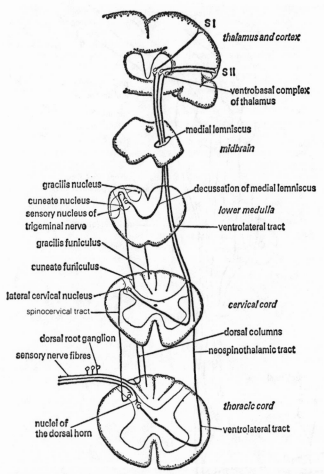

Figure 21. The rapidly conducting somatosensory projection pathways. The three main projection pathways are the dorsal column–medial lemniscal pathway, the dorsolateral tract (of Morin), and the neospinothalamic tract. The lower sections are shown on a larger scale than the upper sections. (from Milner, 1970)

The medial systems

The *spinoreticular system* (Figure 20) consists of short, multi-synaptic chains of fibres that ascend in the ventrolateral spinal cord and, beginning at the medulla, course medially into the brainstem reticular formation and terminate mostly on reticular cells on the same (ipsilateral) side – although some penetrate to the opposite (contralateral) side (Kerr and Lippman, 1974). Some of the fibres carry information exclusively about light touch or intense (noxious) tactile or thermal stimuli, but the majority are multimodal – that is, they carry information evoked by several kinds of stimuli, and respond with higher frequencies of firing as the stimulus intensity increases (see Dennis and Melzack, 1977). Generally, reticular cells have large receptive fields and exhibit a gross somatotopic organization. Moreover, they receive inputs from other sensory modalities as well as from adjacent reticular cells and a variety of more distant brain structures.

The *paleospinothalamic tract* is a relatively small pathway which projects directly to the medial and intralaminar nuclei of the thalamus. This tract has many of the properties of the spino-reticular pathway – its fibres have large receptive fields and most of them carry multimodal information, with noxious input predominating.

The *propriospinal system* consists of chains of small fibres that ascend throughout the spinal cord, particularly in the grey matter, in contrast to the ventrolateral tracts we have just discussed, which lie primarily in the white matter. Although these proprio-spinal fibres have long been assumed to play an important role in pain (Noordenbos, 1959), they are elusive and difficult to study. Nevertheless, an ingenious study has shown that they are indeed involved in pain. Basbaum (1973) attempted to section all the long-fibre tracts in rats and thereby to isolate the short-fibre system. He did this by cutting one half of the thoracic spinal cord on one side and later, at a slightly lower level, cutting half the spinal cord on the other side. In this way, only the chains of small fibres that carry signals through the spinal grey matter could carry information about pain. Basbaum showed that this opera-tion did not abolish a learned response in which a painful electric shock made the rat turn its head to stop the shock. Even more remarkable was Basbaum's ability to train a rat to learn this response *after* the two hemisections of the cord. Of course, when the cord was totally cut through at a single level, the learned response was abolished. The evidence, then, suggests that a portion of the signals about pain are carried by short fibres that ascend diffusely through the cord, although their destination and other properties are unknown.

The lateral systems

In contrast to the medially projecting systems, the pathways that comprise the lateral group (Figure 21) are rapidly conducting and somatotopically highly organized. Although the three pathways – the spinocervical and neospinothalamic tracts and the dorsal column system – share many properties in common, there are also important differences among them.

The *spinocervical tract* ascends in the dorsolateral spinal cord. Many of the neurons in the tract respond to noxious mechanical and thermal stimuli and some show the 'wind-up' effect characteristic of injury-signalling systems. Of the cells that respond to light touch, a substantial proportion (forty-four per cent) show increased discharge to intense pressure. Although this tract has been found in all higher species, it is sometimes difficult to identify in humans. About 75% of the fibres terminate in the lateral cervical nucleus, and the remainder appear to go to the rostral part of the dorsal column nuclei. The majority of fibres from the lateral cervical nucleus cross the midline in the upper cervical cord and lower medulla and ascend in the medial lemniscus to an area in the lateral, posterior thalamus which is known as the ventrobasal complex (Figure 21). However, there is a small but definite projection to the rostral reticular formation (zona incerta), and to the posterior group and medial nuclei of the thalamus.

The *neospinothalamic tract* ascends to the thalamus from the ventral and ventrolateral regions of the spinal cord. Its cells respond to a wide range of stimuli (Price and Mayer, 1974); some respond exclusively to tactile or noxious stimuli, but the majority respond to both, with higher discharge rates to more intense stimulus levels. Although the neospinothalamic tract is more easily observed in monkeys than in cats, its existence in the cat, though less pronounced, is no longer in doubt, and the system clearly carries nociceptive information in both species (see Dennis and Melzack, 1977). In monkeys, the neospinothalamic tract is the most rapidly conducting somatic pathway. The majority of fibres of the neospinothalamic tract terminate in the ventrobasal thalamus. However, there are also substantial terminations in the rostral reticular formation and in the medial and intralaminar group of nuclei in the thalamus.

The *dorsal column postsynaptic system* was discovered as recently as 1968. Traditionally, the dorsal columns were believed to carry only fibres activated by innocuous touch and proprioception. However, Uddenberg (1968) discovered postsynaptic fibres in the dorsal columns which are activated by small to medium-sized receptive fields, and which produce a sustained, high-frequency discharge to noxious pinch. Later, Angaut-Petit (1975a) confirmed the existence of these neurons, and reported that they comprise about 10% of dorsal column fibres and that most of them (77%) respond differentially to both gentle and noxious levels of stimulation. About 7% respond only to noxious stimuli, and the remainder only to light tactile stimuli. Cells with similar properties are also found in the rostral portions of the dorsal column nuclei (Angaut-Petit, 1975b). There is evidence, which we will review shortly, to suggest that such a system may exist in man and that it may play a role in pain. It is important to note that the dorsal column nuclei project not only to the ventrobasal thalamus but also to the posterior group of nuclei in the thalamus (Figure 20) and the midbrain reticular formation (see Dennis and Melzack, 1977).

Similarities and differences among the systems

It seems remarkable that there should be three rapidly conducting, somatotopically organized systems from the spinal cord to the ventrobasal thalamus. Why should all three have evolved? It is true that one of them (the spinocervical tract) appears to diminish in size in the evolution of primates. It is possible to discount the tract as being 'vestigial', like an appendix, but this may be misleading and we may lose valuable clues on the functional organization of pain-signalling systems.

The similarities among the three systems are clear. Each carries nociceptive, thermal and light tactile information, and each is rapidly conducting, has relatively few synapses, and contains fibres with small to medium-sized receptive fields. However, the systems differ in two respects. First, their pattern of termination in the brain is different. The dorsal column postsynaptic system may terminate in the dorsal column nuclei although there is the possibility of a more rostral projection (see Dennis and Melzack, 1977). The neospinothalamic tract and spinocervical tract project to the same general area of the thalamus, but the terminations of each are concentrated in different though adjacent areas (Boivie, 1971). The second – and more striking – difference among the systems is the kind of inhibitory control exerted on each. In the spinocervical tract system, the inhibitory control from higher brain structures is exerted primarily on nociceptive signals while light tactile responses are relatively unaffected (Brown, 1971); in contrast, the inhibitory control exerted on neospinothalamic tract units is predominantly on light tactile rather than nociceptive inputs (Coulter *et al.*, 1974). (Although there is evidence of descending control of the dorsal column postsynaptic fibres, no studies have examined the effects on different inputs.) The available evidence on the lateral systems, then, suggests that they are not simply redundant but may each play a distinct role in the transmission of information related to pain (Dennis and Melzack, 1977).

Behavioural evidence

The behavioural evidence shows clearly that there are functional differences between the medial and lateral systems and even among the component pathways of each. Electrical stimulation of the ventrolateral spinal cord in people undergoing neurosurgery often, but not always, produces reports of sharp, burning pain. Electrical stimulation of the dorsal columns does not produce such reports, but mechanical stimulation often does (White and Sweet, 1969). Furthermore, Sourek (1969) found that insertion of a fine needle into the medial part of the dorsal columns produces pain sensations felt in the lower part of the body, while insertion of the needle into the more lateral portion produces pain sensations at higher levels. These sensations are felt on the same side as the needle insertion; when the midline is crossed, the pain shifts to the other side of the body. The data suggest that dorsal column postsynaptic fibres exist in man and that they play a role in pain perception and behaviour. At the midbrain level, electrical stimulation of the neospinothalamic tract in man produces pain described as bright and sharp. Surprisingly, stimulation of the medial lemniscus at high frequencies is described as hot and painful (Nashold *et al.*, 1969). In the rat, stimulation of the medial lemniscus produces clear signs of pain: cringing, writhing, running, jumping and some vocalizing, and the animals rapidly learn to press a lever to turn off the stimulation, indicating that it is highly aversive. In fact, there even appear to be two distinctly different aversive populations of fibres in the medial lemniscus of the rat (Dennis *et al.*, 1976).

Studies which produce lesions to reveal the functions of the ascending systems suggest that the pathways of the lateral systems are involved in pain. In man, attempts have been made to relieve phantom limb pain by sectioning the dorsal columns on the same side as the stump. Although cramping pain was relieved in some of the patients, the pain usually returned after several months (Browder and Gallagher, 1948). In monkeys, unilateral ablation of the dorsal columns briefly reduced reactivity to electric shocks of the legs on the same side (Vierck *et al.*, 1971). In cats, section of the dorsolateral cord (which included the spino-cervical tract) temporarily impaired pain responses, and the effect lasted longer when a lesion was made of the whole dorsal half of the cord (Levitt and Levitt, 1968). These and other studies (see Dennis and Melzack, 1977) suggest that spinocervical and dorsal column lesions have at least temporary effects on some aspects of pain. The data of these studies, however, like those of all studies that involve lesions, must be treated with caution because the lesion often destroys adjacent structures as well as descending pathways. Nevertheless, the data, taken together, suggest that all six pathways of the medial and lateral projection systems play a role in pain processes. The possible roles they play and the implications of multiple systems with similar (though not identical) properties will be discussed in Chapter 11.

Brain systems

Not long ago, when pain was still considered to be a simple projection system, there was a hypothetical pain centre in the brain. Precisely where this pain centre was to be found was the source of considerable controversy. The favourite site of centres of all sensation was the cortex, but no such centre could be located. Wilder Penfield, the great neurosurgeon, electrically stimulated the exposed cortex thousands of times in hundreds of patients in the course of neurosurgical operations for epilepsy or tumours. On a few rare occasions, the patients reported feeling pain, but this happened so infrequently that few writers were willing to place the 'pain centre' in the cortex. Special attempts were made to place phantom limb pain in the somatosensory projection areas of the cortex, and these areas were excised in many patients. Nevertheless, the phantom limb pain usually returned, and the painless phantom itself was rarely altered, so that cortical ablations for phantom limb pain were soon given up.

If the 'pain centre' is not in the cortex, where is it? The next obvious site is the sensory thalamus which receives input from the major pain-signalling pathways that originate in the spinal cord. Head (1920) long ago proposed that the 'pain centre' resides in the thalamus and that the cortex exerts an inhibitory control over it. The thalamic syndrome, he suggested, could be due to vascular or other lesions that destroy cortico-thalamic fibres so that all inputs to the thalamus are unmodulated and cause excruciating pain. It was natural, then, that neurosurgeons would destroy thalamic nuclei in the attempt to abolish pain. The operation at first appeared successful but later turned out to be a failure (Spiegel and Wycis, 1966). The pain usually returned, even after extensive lesions, and was often worse than before. Nevertheless, we now know that electrical stimulation of the somatosensory thalamus (Hosobuchi *et al.*, 1973; Turnbull *et al.*, 1980) or the fibres that fan out from it and project via the internal capsule to the cortex (Mazars *et al.*, 1976) can sometimes relieve chronic pain. These observations indicate that the sensory thalamus is involved in pain, but is not the pain centre.

It is now becoming increasingly evident that virtually all of the brain plays a role in pain. Even seemingly unrelated brain activities such as seeing, hearing and thinking are important. Seeing the source of injury, hearing the sounds that accompany a rifle shot or a falling beam, and thinking about the consequences of an injury all contribute to pain. Any satisfactory understanding of pain must include all of these processes which interact with inputs from the injured area or from deafferented neurons that produce pain signals when injury is absent.

Reticular formation
It is now well established that the reticular formation is involved in aversive drive and similar pain-related behaviour. Stimulation of nucleus gigantocellularis in the medulla (Casey, 1971a), and the central grey and adjacent areas in the midbrain (Spiegel, Kletzkin and Szekeley, 1954; Delgado, 1955) produces strong aversive drive and behaviour typical of responses to naturally occurring painful stimuli. In contrast, lesions of the central grey produce marked decreases in responsiveness to noxious stimuli (Melzack, Stotler and Livingston, 1958). Similarly, at the thalamic level, 'fear-like' responses associated with escape behaviour have been elicited by stimulation in the medial and adjacent intralaminar nuclei of the thalamus (Roberts, 1962). In the human, lesions in the medial thalamus (parafascicular and centromedian complex) and intralaminar nuclei have provided temporary relief from intractable pain (Mark, Ervin and Yakovlev, 1963; White and Sweet, 1969).

Although these reticular areas are clearly involved in pain, they may also play a role in other somatosensory processes. Casey (1971a) found that sixteen out of twenty cells in nucleus gigantocellularis responded to tapping or moderate pressure on the skin. The response pattern of the cells, moreover, was a function of the intensity of stimulation; the cells responded with a more intense and prolonged discharge to stimuli (pinch, pinprick) that elicited withdrawal of the tested limb. Similarly, Becker, Gluck, Nulsen and Jane (1969) found that many cells in the midbrain central grey and tegmentum responded to electrical stimulation of large, low-threshold fibres. An increase in the stimulus level in order to fire the small, high-threshold fibres produced distinctively patterned responses showing high discharge rates, prolonged afterdischarges for several seconds, and the 'wind-up' effect (increasing neural response to repeated intense stimuli).

The role of the reticular formation in pain is especially clear in an elegant series of experiments by Casey (1971a and b; Casey, Keene and Morrow, 1974). He demonstrated a correlation between pain-related behaviour and single neuron activity in cells of the nucleus gigantocellularis of the medullary reticular formation. Cats with electrodes placed in this area were trained to cross a barrier to escape repeated single shocks to a cutaneous nerve. Weak shocks that did not elicit escape behaviour produced low-level discharge in the reticular neurons. However, the neural response increased when shock intensity was increased, and became maximal only when the shock elicited escape. Strong pinching was the only natural stimulus that excited some of these cells. Casey also found that direct electrical stimulation through the recording microelectrode was an effective escape-producing stimulus when delivered in or near the region of the responding cells. In a single set of experiments, then, Casey demonstrated a correlation between intense inputs that produce escape, a particular pattern of neural activity in reticular cells, and escape behaviour when the cells were directly stimulated.

Casey (1980) has recently proposed that reticular neurons are especially well suited to carry out integrated functions in the brain that are related to pain. A substantial number of reticular neurons have bifurcating axons that project caudally to the spinal cord and rostrally to the thalamus and hypothalamus. Stimulation of the reticular formation often elicits well-coordinated motor responses in animals deprived of forebrain function, and also produces marked changes in autonomic activity. In addition to being a major receiving station for pain signals and inputs from other sensory systems, it also exerts control over virtually all the sensory systems. Because noxious stimulation is so effective in influencing the discharge of these neurons, the reticular formation appears to be organized to play a major integrating role in pain experience and behaviour.

Limbic system

The reciprocal interconnection between the reticular formation and the limbic system is of particular importance in pain processes (Melzack and Casey, 1968). The midbrain central grey, which is traditionally part of the reticular formation, is also a major gateway to the limbic system (Figure 22). It is part of the 'limbic midbrain area' (Nauta, 1958) that projects to the medial thalamus and hypothalamus which in turn project to limbic forebrain structures. Many of these areas also interact with portions of the frontal cortex that are sometimes functionally designated as part of the limbic system. Thus the phylogenetically old medial ascending systems, which are separate from but in parallel with the newer neospinothalamic projection system, gain access to the complex circuitry of the limbic system.

It is now firmly established that the limbic system plays an important role in pain processes. Electrical stimulation of the hippocampus, amygdala, or other limbic structures may evoke escape or other attempts to stop stimulation (Delgado, Rosvold and Looney, 1956). After ablation of the amygdala and overlying cortex, cats show marked changes in affective behaviour, including decreased responsiveness to noxious stimuli (Schreiner and Kling, 1953). Surgical section of the cingulum bundle, which connects the frontal cortex to the hippocampus, also produces a loss of 'negative affect' associated with intractable pain in human subjects (Foltz and White, 1962). This evidence indicates that limbic structures, although they play a role in many other functions, provide a neural basis for the aversive drive and affect that comprise the motivational dimension of pain.

Intimately related to the brain areas involved in aversive drive,

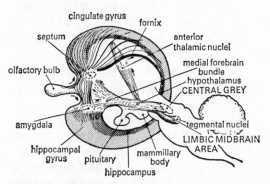

Figure 22. Schematic drawing of the limbic system, which is known to play an important role in emotional and motivational processes. The arrows indicate the direction of flow of nerve impulses through the system.
(adapted from MacLean, 1958, p. 1723)

and sometimes overlapping with them, are hypothalamic and limbic structures that are involved in approach responses and other behaviour aimed at maintaining and prolonging stimulation ('self-stimulation'; Olds and Olds, 1963). Electrical stimulation of these structures often yields behaviour in which the animal presses one bar to receive stimulation and another to stop it. These effects, which may be due to overlap of 'aversive' and 'reward' structures, are sometimes a function simply of intensity of stimulation, so that low-level stimulation elicits approach and intense stimulation evokes avoidance. Complex interactions among these areas (Olds and Olds, 1962) may explain why aversive drive to noxious stimuli can be blocked by stimulation of reward areas in the lateral hypothalamus (Cox and Valenstein, 1965) or septum (Abbott and Melzack, 1978). In fact, in the lateral central grey, there is a strong correlation between current thresholds of brain stimulation to block pain and those for self-stimulation (Dennis, Choinière and Melzack, 1980).

The role of limbic system structures is subtle and complex. Injury, in higher animals, occurs in a spatial and social context that often requires complex responses. Thus, the hippocampus appears to provide a 'cognitive map' in which spatial relations among objects in the environment are important in responses such as escape or hiding from dangerous predators or social rivals (O'Keefe and Nadel, 1978). The amygdala seems to provide an 'affective bias' as a result of matching incoming information against past experience, so that animals and people can respond adaptively to familiar or unfamiliar stimuli (Gloor, 1978). After ablation of the amygdala, monkeys unhesitatingly ingest hot, sharp, or otherwise injurious objects that normally, on the basis of past experience, elicit caution or avoidance.

Ventrobasal thalamus and its cortical projection
The medial pathways that project to the reticular formation and limbic system are not organized to carry precise somatotopic information about the location, nature, extent and duration of an injury. Yet an injury, initially at least, is usually precisely localized. A burn on a finger by a hot cinder from a pipe is immediately located and examined. A jab in the buttock by a sharp object similarly elicits a sudden movement of the hand to

rub the precise point. If the reticular formation and limbic system are not organized to transmit precise information rapidly to the brain, it is reasonable to assume that the laterally projecting pathways are involved (Melzack and Casey, 1968; Dennis and Melzack, 1977). Indeed, recent studies suggest that the sensory-discriminative dimension of pain is subserved, at least in part, by the neospinothalamic projection to the ventrobasal thalamus and somatosensory cortex (Figure 21).

Neurons in the ventrobasal thalamus, which receive a large portion of their afferent input from the neospinothalamic projection system, show discrete somatotopic organization even after dorsal column section. Studies in human patients and in animals (see Wall, 1970) have shown that surgical section of the dorsal columns, long presumed to subserve virtually all of the discriminative capacity of the skin sensory system, produces little or no loss in fine tactile discrimination and localization. Furthermore, Semmes and Mishkin (1965) found marked deficits in tactile discriminations that are attributable to injury of the cortical projection of the neospinothalamic system. These data suggest that the neospinothalamic projection system has the capacity to process information about the spatial, temporal, and magnitude properties of the input.

Cortical functions
We have already seen that cognitive activities such as memories of past experience, attention and suggestion all have a profound effect of pain experience. In addition, there is evidence that the sensory input is localized, identified in terms of its physical properties, evaluated in terms of past experience, and modified *before* it activates the discriminative or motivational systems. Men wounded in battle may feel little or no pain from the wound but may complain bitterly about an inept vein puncture (Beecher, 1959). Dogs that repeatedly receive food immediately after the skin is shocked or cut soon respond to these stimuli as signals for food and salivate, without showing any signs of pain, yet howl as normal dogs would when the stimuli are applied to other sites on the body (Pavlov, 1927, 1928).

The neural system that performs these complex functions of identification, evaluation, and selective modulation must conduct rapidly to the cortex so that somatosensory information has the opportunity to undergo further analysis, interact with other sensory inputs, and activate memory stores and pre-set response strategies. It must then be able to act selectively on the sensory and motivational systems in order to influence their response to the information being transmitted over more slowly conducting pathways. We have proposed (Melzack and Wall, 1965) that the dorsal column and spinocervical projection pathways act as the 'feed-forward' limb of this loop. The dorsal column pathway, in particular, has grown apace with the cerebral cortex (Bishop, 1959), carries precise information about the nature and location of the stimulus, adapts quickly to give precedence to phasic stimulus changes rather than prolonged tonic activity, and conducts rapidly to the cortex so that its impulses may begin activation of central control processes.

The powerful descending inhibitory influences exerted on dorsal-horn cells in the spinal cord (Hagbarth and Kerr, 1954; Hillman and Wall, 1969) can modulate the input before it is transmitted to the discriminative and motivational systems. Indeed, direct corticospinal neurons that project to lamina 5 cells have properties that suggest that they could act like a rapid switching mechanism, changing the role of the spinal neurons from a tactile to a nociceptive one (Fetz, 1968; Coulter *et al.*, 1976). These rapidly conducting ascending and descending systems can thus account for the fact that psychological processes play a powerful role in determining the quality and intensity of pain.

The frontal cortex may play a particularly significant role in mediating between cognitive activities and the motivational-affective features of pain (Melzack and Casey, 1968). It receives information via intracortical fibre systems from virtually all sensory and associational cortical areas and projects strongly to reticular and limbic structures. Patients who have undergone a frontal lobotomy (which severs the connections between the prefrontal lobes and the thalamus) rarely complain about severe clinical pain or ask for medication (Freeman and Watts, 1950). Typically, these patients report after the operation that they still have pain but it does not bother them. When they are questioned more closely, they frequently say that they still have the 'little' pain, but the 'big' pain, the suffering, the anguish are gone. It is certain that the sensory component of pain is still present because these patients may complain vociferously about pinprick and mild burn. Indeed, pain perception thresholds may be lowered (King, Clausen and Scarff, 1950). The predominant effect of lobotomy appears to be on the motivational-affective dimension of the whole pain experience. The aversive quality of the pain and the drive to seek pain relief both appear to be diminished.

Similarly, patients who exhibit 'pain asymbolia' (Rubins and Friedman, 1948) after lesions of portions of the parietal lobe or the frontal cortex are able to appreciate the spatial and temporal properties of noxious stimuli (for example, they recognize pinpricks as sharp) but fail to withdraw or complain about them. The sensory input never evokes the strong aversive drive and negative affect characteristic of pain experience and response.

The data on the brain systems described so far suggest that there are specialized, interacting neural substrates for three major psychological dimensions of pain: sensory-discriminative, motivational-affective, and cognitive-evaluative (Melzack and Casey, 1968). An essential element in all of these interactions is descending inhibitory control mechanisms. Like every other aspect of pain, they are highly complex.

Descending systems

If the 1950s was the decade of discovery of multiple ascending pathways related to pain, then the 1970s was the decade that revealed the power of descending control systems. It was the exhilarating decade of the discovery of endorphins and enkephalins and, as a result, a better understanding of the mechanisms of analgesia than anyone would have dreamed possible at the beginning of the decade.

The story of the 1970s really begins in 1956, when Hagbarth (of Sweden) and Kerr (of Australia) worked together with Magoun (in the United States) to explore the recently discovered descending control functions of the reticular formation. Hagbarth and Kerr (1954) found that the responses evoked in the ventrolateral spinal cord could virtually be abolished by stimulation of a variety of brain structures including the reticular formation, cerebellum, and cerebral cortex. The implications were clear: the brain must exert an inhibitory control over transmission in the dorsal horns. In 1958, Melzack, Stotler and Livingston discovered, totally unexpectedly, that lesions of a small area of the reticular formation (the central tegmental tract adjacent to the lateral periaqueductal grey) produced hyperalgesia and hyperaesthesia in cats. That is, the cats over-responded to pinpricks and often cried and shook their paws as though in pain. The observers concluded that fibres in this area exert a tonic (or continuous) inhibitory control over pain signals; removal of the inhibition allows pain signals to flow unchecked to the brain, and even permits the summation of non-noxious signals to produce spontaneous pain.

These conclusions led David Reynolds, a young psychologist at the University of Windsor, Ontario, to test the hypothesis that the tonic inhibition from the central tegmental-lateral periaqueductal grey area could be enhanced by electrical stimulation, and might produce analgesia. In 1969, he reported that the stimulation did indeed produce a profound analgesia – sufficient to carry out surgery on awake rats without any chemical anaesthetic, and in 1970 he reported a replication of these results in higher species. Reynolds' observations met with scepticism and were generally ignored. In 1971, Mayer, Liebeskind and their colleagues, unaware of Reynolds' discovery, independently found the same phenomenon, which has come to be known as 'stimulation produced analgesia'. A series of brilliant experiments by Mayer, Liebeskind, Akil, Besson, Fields, Basbaum and their colleagues (see Liebeskind and Paul, 1977; Mayer and Watkins, 1981) led rapidly to reports that (1) electrical stimulation of the lateral periaqueductal grey and adjacent areas produces strong analgesia in awake animals; (2) the analgesia often outlasts stimulation by many seconds or minutes; (3) stimulation of the area inhibits lamina 5 cells in the dorsal horns, and acts selectively on noxious rather than tactile inputs; (4) the system seems to involve serotonin as a transmitting agent; and (5) the effects of stimulation are partially diminished by administration of naloxone, a morphine antagonist.

New discoveries followed in rapid succession. One set of studies showed that the injection of small amounts of morphine directly into the periaqueductal grey area produces analgesia (see Herz *et al.*, 1970; Mayer and Watkins, 1981), indicating that a major action of morphine is to activate descending inhibitory neurons in the brainstem. It was also found that the area that elicits analgesia has a broad somatotopic organization (Balagura and Ralph, 1973; Soper, 1979). Moreover, there is evidence that stimulation of the area for several minutes before a painful stimulus is administered produces an enhanced analgesic effect, suggesting that some pharmacological substance is released into the area (Melzack and Melinkoff, 1974). It was also discovered that the brainstem inhibitory fibres descend through a distinct pathway in the dorsolateral spinal cord, that opiate analgesia and stimulation-produced analgesia are abolished or reduced by section of this pathway (Basbaum, Marley, O'Keefe and Clanton, 1977), and that serotonin is the pathway's major transmitter (Basbaum and Fields, 1978). The picture that emerged is a relatively simple one despite the complexity of connections (Figure 23): the periaqueductal grey neurons, which are rich in enkephalin receptors and surrounding enkephalins, activate cells in the nucleus raphe magnus which, in turn, send fibres to the dorsal horns and inhibit dorsal horn cells by the release of serotonin.

During this period, the stage was set for a remarkable breakthrough in the whole field of analgesia and pain. Several biochemists and pharmacologists in the United States were convinced that the reason why morphine was a powerful analgesic was because there were specialized chemical receptacles – opiate receptors – on nerve cells, whose structure was such that a morphine molecule fit into them like a key into a lock. After much research these opiate receptors were finally discovered (see Snyder, 1980). The next question was obvious: why would such opiate receptors evolve when the probability of a person or animal ingesting morphine is negligible? The answer, to Terenius (1978), Hughes and Kosterlitz (1977), and others (see Terenius, 1979; Snyder, 1980) was that the body manufactured its own opioid substances – chemicals similar in structure to morphine. And, indeed, when these investigators searched for such molecules, they found them, and called them endorphins (endogenous morphine-like substances) and enkephalins (opioid substances 'in the brain'). Soon, it was discovered that a large pituitary molecule –

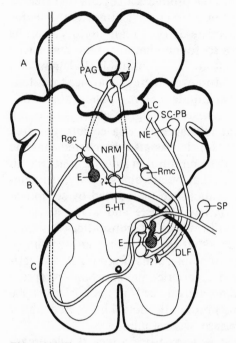

Figure 23. The endogenous pain control system as proposed by Basbaum and Fields (1978).

A: Midbrain level. The periaqueductal grey (PAG), an important locus for stimulation-produced analgesia, is rich in enkephalins (E) and opiate receptor, though the anatomical details of the enkephalinergic connections are not known. Microinjection of small amounts of opiates into PAG also produces analgesia.

B: Medullary level. Serotonin (5HT)-containing cells of the nucleus raphe magnus (NRM) and the adjacent nucleus reticularis magnocellularis (Rmc) receive excitatory input from PAG and, in turn, send efferent fibres to the spinal cord.

C: Spinal level. Efferent fibres from the NRM and Rmc travel in the dorsolateral funiculus (DLF) to terminate among pain-transmission cells concentrated in laminae 1 and 5 of the dorsal horn. The NRM and Rmc exert an inhibitory effect specifically on pain-transmission neurons. The pain-transmission neurons, which are activated by substance P (SP) containing small-diameter primary afferents, project to supraspinal sites and indirectly, via the nucleus reticularis gigantocellularis (Rgc), contact the cells of the descending analgesia system in the PAG and NRM, thus establishing a negative-feedback loop.

beta-lipotropin – splits up to produce ACTH (adrenocortico-trophic hormone) and endorphin. Furthermore, the enkephalin molecule has the same structure as a part of the larger endorphin molecule. Presently, several endorphin molecules have been discovered, their chemical structure has been determined, and some of them can be synthesized in the laboratory. They have been found to be extremely powerful analgesics.

Still further revelations appeared to strengthen the role of enkephalins and endorphins in pain and analgesia. They were found to be distributed in precisely those areas that would involve them in this role: in the substantia gelatinosa of the dorsal horns, in the periaqueductal grey, and in many areas of the limbic system (see Snyder, 1980). Furthermore, the morphine antagonist naloxone, which was assumed to antagonize all opiate-like compounds, including the endorphins and enkephalins, was used to determine whether the opioid compounds played a role in pain and analgesia (see Mayer and Watkins, 1981). Consequently, evidence soon appeared which showed that the injection of naloxone in patients suffering dental pain produced increases in their pain, suggesting that opioids exert a continual inhibitory control over pain. Naloxone was also found to diminish or abolish the analgesic effects of periaqueductal stimulation, acupuncture, and transcutaneous electrical stimulation, suggesting that these effects are mediated through pathways containing opioid transmitters. Even the placebo effect was attributed to the release of endorphins because naloxone appeared to diminish the effect. In general, then, the story that unfolded seemed to point to a solution, at last, of the entire problem of pain and analgesia.

Multiple descending systems
Even while this elegant picture was emerging, experimenters began to report evidence at variance with it. For every experiment that reported that naloxone had the predicted effect on pain, another soon appeared that failed to confirm it: naloxone did not

Catecholamine-containing neurons of the locus ceruleus (LC) in rat and subceruleus-parabrachialis (SC-PB) in cat may also contribute to pain-modulating systems in the DLF. (NE = norepinephrine.)
(from Basbaum and Fields, 1978)

modify either spontaneous pain or heat pain thresholds in patients suffering chronic pain (Lindblom and Tegner, 1979); it did not alter stimulation-produced analgesia in rats suffering moderate pain after subcutaneous injection of formalin (Dennis, Choinière and Melzack, 1980); it did not affect the formalin-produced pain itself (North, 1978); it failed to modify the placebo effect (Mihic and Binkert, 1978); it failed to reverse acupuncture analgesia in a study of dental pain (Chapman *et al.*, 1980).

It soon became apparent that there is not one but several descending control systems, and that some are sensitive to naloxone and others are not. Furthermore, a host of non-opioid transmitters – such as noradrenalin, acetylcholine and dopamine – are also involved in analgesia.

The story at present is extremely complicated and it would be premature to attempt a summary of a field of research that is in such a state of flux. Rather, we will examine two trends in research. First, after the exciting period of discovery of endogenous opioid compounds, we are now entering a new period in which they are being critically evaluated. There is increasing research on non-opioid and non-naloxone-sensitive pathways, and on their interactions with one another. The role of endorphins and enkephalins – despite their undoubted existence – is becoming more hazy. They play a role in pain and analgesia, but the nature of that role is poorly understood. It is possible that they are involved in sudden stress or sudden injury to prevent the animal or person from being overwhelmed by pain, but there is little evidence that they play a role beyond that. Moreover, morphine, which was assumed to exert so much of its effect on systems that have downstream inhibitory effects, is now known to also act directly at spinal levels (Yaksh, 1978; Bromage *et al.*, 1980) and may affect fibres that project to higher levels of the brain (see Abbott, 1980; Beecher, 1959).

Part of the reason for questioning the earlier data derives from the second trend in recent research: to consider carefully the conditions in which pain is tested. The traditional methods for examining pain in animals in the laboratory involve brief pains at threshold level. The tail-flick and hot-plate tests are the favourite methods. In the former, a rat's tail is stimulated by hot water (45°C.) or radiant heat, and pain is inferred when the rat flicks the tail aside. In the latter, the rat is placed on a hot plate until it licks its paws or jumps up, which signals that it is in pain. But these kinds of momentary, threshold-level pains are utterly different from the intense, long-lasting pains that concern us most, such as a burned finger, a broken bone, a migraine headache or phantom limb pain. Recently, a test has been developed in which it is possible to administer pain to a rat that is moderate in intensity and lasts for about two hours. The test consists of injecting a small amount of dilute formalin under the skin of a paw and recording a distinct set of responses which can be given numerical values (Figure 24; O'Keefe, 1964; Dubuisson and Dennis, 1977). In man, the pain feels like a bee sting – definitely painful, but moderate, tolerable, and of reasonable duration.

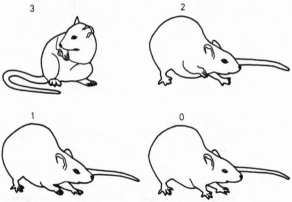

Figure 24. Typical responses used for rating pain intensity in rats. The animal's right forepaw has been injected with a dilute solution of formalin. Numerical values assigned to these responses are shown: 3, the rat licks the injected paw; 2, the paw is raised without touching the floor; 1, the paw is kept gingerly on the floor without full pressure; 0, the paw bears full normal weight as the rat ambulates in the cage.
(from Dubuisson and Dennis, 1977)

A series of recent experiments has shown that the formalin, tail-flick and hot-plate tests each reveal different components of the mechanisms of pain and analgesia. For example, when the periaqueductal grey is stimulated, much less electrical current is necessary to produce analgesia in the formalin test than in the other tests (Dennis, Choinière and Melzack, 1980). This is astonishing, because the pain in the formalin test is more intense and prolonged. Furthermore, each test reveals a unique profile of effects when drugs are administered which are agonists or antagonists of major transmitters such as serotonin, noradrenalin, dopamine, and acetylcholine (Dennis and Melzack, 1980; Dennis *et al.*, 1980). The formalin test is more sensitive to the effects of some drugs, while the tail-flick or hot-plate test is more sensitive to others. It is not that one test is 'good' and another is 'bad'. Rather, each test appears to reveal different aspects of complex neural and pharmacological mechanisms which involve multiple ascending systems, descending controls, and their interactions. It is now certain, for example, that cells of the nucleus raphe magnus are excited by fibres from the periaqueductal grey (Figure 23) but are inhibited by noradrenergic fibres from other, as yet unknown, origins (Hammond *et al.*, 1980). The descending inhibitory effect of nucleus raphe magnus, then, depends on a balance of facilitatory and inhibitory influences, and it is possible that one or the other may predominate, depending on the nature of the noxious stimulation and the type of response pattern that is involved in each test.

By utilizing different tests, it has also been possible to shed light on the conflicting evidence concerning tolerance to morphine. Studies of people who take morphine for months or years to control cancer pain show little evidence of tolerance to the morphine. The same dose maintains its effectiveness for the entire period and, in fact, may be lowered when the pain diminishes due to spontaneous or therapy-induced remission (Twycross, 1974, 1978; Mount *et al.*, 1976). Experimental studies of morphine in humans and animals, on the other hand, show striking tolerance, so that the morphine dose, to maintain effectiveness, has to be continually raised (Goodman and Gilman, 1980). Abbott (1980) investigated morphine tolerance in rats, using the formalin and tail-flick tests, and found rapid tolerance to morphine in the tail-flick test (confirming earlier studies) but little or no tolerance in the formalin test. Evidently, when morphine is given for moderate, continuous pain, there is virtually no tolerance, but when it is given for brief, just-perceptible pain, there is rapid tolerance. The results with the formalin test are clearly like those observed in people suffering chronic severe pain.

These data indicate that the combination of ascending and descending neural mechanisms and the pharmacological substrates of each may differ in each kind of pain test. Moreover, pain sensitivity appears to be modulated by a diurnal rhythm (McGivern and Berntson, 1980) and by a host of other factors such as environmental and social variables and prior stress (Dennis *et al.*, 1980). Careful, patient research is necessary to unravel these influences, but by recognizing multiple interacting factors we at least appear to be pointed in the right direction.

Summary

The physiological evidence shows that the receptors, fibres, and central nervous system pathways involved in pain are specialized to generate and transmit patterned information rather than modality-specific impulses. Injurious stimuli activate multiple fibre systems which converge and diverge a number of times so that the patterning can undergo change at every synaptic level. Nerve impulses in large and small fibres that converge onto the cells of the dorsal horns are subjected to modulation by the activity of the substantia gelatinosa. Similarly, the convergence of fibres onto cells in the reticular formation permits a high degree of summation and interaction of inputs from spatially distant body areas. Divergence also occurs: fibres fan out from the dorsal horns and the reticular formation, and project to different parts of the nervous system that have specialized functions. One of these functions is the ability to select and abstract particular kinds of information from the temporal patterns that are conveyed by the incoming fibres. Central cells, it is now also apparent, monitor the input for long periods of time. The after-discharges, and other prolonged neural activity produced by intense stimuli, may persist long after cessation of stimulation, and may play a particularly important role in pain processes.

This convergence and divergence, summation and pattern discrimination all go on in a dynamically changing nervous system. Stimuli impinge on sensory fields at the skin that show continuous shifts in sensitivity. Furthermore, fibres that descend from the brain continually modulate the input, facilitating the flow of some input patterns and inhibiting others. The widespread influences of the substantia gelatinosa and the reticular formation, which receive inputs from virtually all of the body, can modify information transmission at almost every synaptic level of the somatosensory projection systems. These ascending and descending interactions present a picture of dynamic, modifiable processes in which inputs impinge on a continually active nervous system that is already the repository of the individual's past history, expectations and value systems. This concept has important implications: it means that the input patterns evoked by injury can be modulated by other sensory inputs or by descending influences, which may thereby determine the quality and intensity of the eventual experience.

The somaesthetic system is a unitary, integrated system comprised of specialized component parts. Several parallel systems analyse the input simultaneously to bring about the richness and complexity of pain experience and response. Some areas are specialized to select sensory-discriminative information while others play specialized roles in the motivational-affective dimension of pain. These parallel information-processing systems interact with each other, and must also interact with cortical activities which underlie past experience, attention, and other cognitive determinants of pain. These interacting processes produce the myriad patterns of activity that subserve the varieties of pain experience.

8
Pain after Injuries of the Nervous System

Some of the most terrible forms of pain result from direct injury of the peripheral and central nervous systems. We have already seen, in Chapter 4, that lesions of peripheral nerves are associated with such dreaded pain syndromes as phantom limb pain, post-herpetic neuralgia, and causalgia. Terrible, persistent pain is also often the consequence of some forms of damage of the spinal cord and brain. The primary aim of this chapter is to look at the possible neural mechanisms that underlie pain related to injury of peripheral nerves, the spinal cord, and the brain.

Peripheral nerve injury

Peripheral nerves are the target of metabolic disorders, poisons, infections and injury, all of which produce pathological changes in nerve fibres. Some of these neurological states result in intense pain. This large variety of disorders, which includes a number of genetic diseases, has been studied by sampling the structure of the damaged nerve (see Wall, 1978). The results reveal that the loss of any combination of large and small fibres may occur in the disease without any obvious correlation of fibre size with pain. Dyck, Lambert and O'Brien (1976) have suggested that the cause of pain may be the presence of actively degenerating and regenerating nerve fibres, but even this correlation is not a strong one. The majority of their cases with pain and acute degeneration had only a slight degree of pain that was not a chief complaint and analgesics were not used. It is reasonable to conclude that fibre diameter alone is not enough or may be completely irrelevant to explain the origin of pain in the neuropathies.

The anatomical effect of damage

The cell bodies of sensory fibres lie in the dorsal root ganglia (see Figure 6, p.77). Two such ganglia exist for each segment – one on each side – and they lie just outside the spinal cord. If a nerve fibre is transected, the distal part, which is physically isolated from its cell body, degenerates completely. The surrounding endoneurial tube, including the Schwann cells, remains intact except at the point of injury (see Figure 11, p.110). The debris of the degenerating fibre is absorbed by specialized nearby cells. While this process is going on, the end of the fibre nearest to the spine has sealed over and, within a day, begins to send out fine sprouts. This is the beginning of regeneration.

In the case of a simple crush injury of a nerve, the endoneurial tubes have remained intact, and so the new sprouts are likely to find adjacent Schwann cells and grow into the tubes with ease. Here we can expect an orderly regeneration at a rate of about one to three millimetres per day in which, eventually, the nerves will grow back to their original destinations. However, a different picture emerges when a nerve is completely transected and the central end (which is in continuity with the dorsal root ganglion) is tightly ligated with a suture, thereby closing the surrounding nerve sheath around the end of the nerve. The degeneration process in the distal part of the fibre is identical to that just described, but the cut ends of the central fibres send sprouts out into an entirely different kind of tissue from that encountered by the sprouts in a crush injury. They enter a region of severe injury with all the tissue breakdown and repair reactions associated with inflammation. They find themselves among invading blood vessels and fibroblasts instead of their familiar tubes. Furthermore, they collide with the thick connective tissue sheath around the nerve through which they cannot penetrate. At first each axon emits multiple sprouts which probe the surrounding tissue for about a week and then most of them give up. The long-term result is called a neuroma, which is the cut end of a nerve after regeneration has failed. It is filled with a jumble of scar tissue and very fine nerve sprouts still attempting to escape from their trap.

Finally, let us take the practical situation of an accident where a nerve has been transected and the surgeon now rejoins the cut ends of the nerve. As we have seen, nothing prevents the total degeneration of the distal part of the nerve, but the surgeon aims to produce the best possible conditions for regeneration. If the length of nerve which is damaged is very short – for example, where broken glass has cut cleanly across a nerve – the two jagged ends of the nerve can be cut carefully and sutured end to end. Surgeons now do this with great dexterity, using extremely fine filaments as suture material. They join the nerve, bundle by bundle, so that the two faces match gently and accurately. Unfortunately, the matching of the cut ends of the tubes cannot be perfect and, at a microscopic level, the damage seems vast. Under ideal conditions in nerves in the rat, the most careful suturing of cut nerves is followed by no better than seventy-five per cent of the nerves crossing the gap successfully. Those sprouts which fail remain on the central side of the injury and form a partial neuroma.

In cases where the original injury has torn a large gap in the nerve, much ingenuity has been used to find suitable material to allow the regenerating fibres to bridge the gap. The most successful technique has been to remove a section from a healthy nerve which will regenerate normally, such as the long fine sural nerve from the leg, and 'splice' it into the gap by carefully suturing multiple strands across the gap. Most of the tubes in the graft survive and provide a track along which fibres may grow. Since the graft comes from the patient himself, it does not trigger immune reactions and so the graft is not rejected. The results are better than they used to be but are still not perfect because of failure by many fibres to cross the gap or to find the right destination.

The physiology of regenerating sprouts
If you – the reader – feel behind the inner flange of your elbow, you will be able to palpate a thick strand that runs from the upper arm to lower arm. That is your ulnar nerve and you can roll it under your fingers and press on it quite hard without feeling anything unusual. This test shows you that normal nerve is not particularly sensitive to pressure. If you accidentally bang your elbow (hitting the 'funny bone'), a strange and very unpleasant feeling shoots down your forearm into the little and ring

fingers. Here, by violence, you have artificially generated nerve impulses in the middle of the ulnar nerve and the brain interprets this as a kind of blow delivered to the area supplied by the nerve. The brain cannot detect that the messages have an unusual source. It reacts as though they came from the normal ends of the nerve which in this case supply the medial forearm, the palm, and the two medial fingers.

Mechanical sensitivity. The physiology of regenerating sprouts or of sprouts in a neuroma has recently been investigated (Wall and Gutnick, 1974). The first obvious new property of these sprouts is that, unlike the parent fibre which is emitting them, they are highly sensitive to pressure. A very small displacement makes them generate nerve impulses. This is the basis of a common test used by neurologists when they search for signs of nerve damage and regeneration. It is called the Tinel sign and consists of gently tapping over the course of a nerve. As you have seen on yourself, nothing happens if you do this quite strongly to a normal nerve. If you tap over a neuroma or over sprouts reaching out towards their destination, the patient reports a mild 'electric shock feeling' in the area of skin supplied by the nerve. If motor fibres are damaged or regenerating and are in contact with a muscle, a tap over the nerve will produce a muscle contraction because the pressure has produced impulses which arrived at the muscle and caused it to contract.

Ongoing activity. The second unusual property of nerve sprouts is that many of them show spontaneous activity. Most normal sensory nerve fibres are silent unless there is some special event taking place at their endings. Many of the sprouts begin to generate impulses spontaneously when no obvious stimulus is applied. The time-course of this new property and the others mentioned is the following: firing starts up within a few hours to a day after the injury, and then increases for the first two weeks; after that, there is usually a decline of spontaneous firing activity to a fairly low level by about one month.

Sensitivity of sprouts to adrenalin. The most surprising new property of nerve sprouts is that they are extraordinarily sensitive to small amounts of adrenalin or noradrenalin applied either locally or by injection into the blood vessels supplying the neuroma. The importance of this finding is twofold. Noradrenalin is the chemical transmitter released by sympathetic nerve fibres. Because a mixed nerve inevitably contains sympathetic nerve fibres, these grow out into the neuroma along with all the other nerve fibres. A second source of sympathetic fibres derives from those that run along with regenerating blood vessels which invade the region of damage as part of the inflammatory reaction. Adrenalin circulates in the blood and is released from the adrenal gland under conditions when the sympathetic system is active, such as during the states of alertness, arousal, stress, 'fight, fright and flight'. Gentler and more specific actions of the sympathetic system occur during cooling and movement. Normal nerves are little affected by actions of the sympathetic system. Now that we know that a damaged nerve becomes highly sensitive to adrenalin we can begin to understand why it is that certain pains are intimately connected with the sympathetic system.

Crosstalk between fibres: ephaptic transmission. In the normal nerve, the myelin sheath and Schwann cells we described earlier (p.110) provide a perfect insulation between parallel nerve fibres so that they do not excite each other. This is the expected property of a signalling system whose independent lines are kept private. With the growth of sprouts which no longer run in their special tubular sheaths, there is a hint that, after about a month, a small number of nerve fibres begin to excite each other. It can be seen that this would have serious sensory consequences if motor impulses on their way out jumped across to sensory fibres and came back to the spinal cord to be interpreted as incoming signals.

Consequences of peripheral nerve injury in animals

If a nerve is transected or crushed, the area supplied by the nerve becomes completely anaesthetic, since this zone cannot send impulses to the spinal cord. In the case of a crush injury, as we have seen, the sprouts grow out into their original tubes and undergo relatively minor physiological changes limited to the first week or so. Animals with crush injuries show no abnormal behaviour other than the temporary anaesthesia and paralysis which lasts until the fibres regenerate back to their original targets

(Wall, Scadding and Tomkiewicz, 1979; Wall *et al.*, 1979). In sharp contrast, animals with neuroma injuries begin to act very strangely in the second and third weeks after the nerve has been cut. They behave as though the anaesthetic region is disturbing them and they begin to lick it vigorously and even attack the area by biting it. Realizing that this period coincides with the peak of abnormal sensitivity of the neuroma sprouts, and knowing that the sprouts are sensitive to noradrenalin, an attempt was made to see if the abnormal behaviour could be stopped by blocking the sympathetic nervous system during the sensitive period. Fortunately, a large number of different types of sympathetic blocking drugs have been developed, particularly for the control of high blood pressure (Goodman and Gilman, 1980). Several of these drugs were tried and it was found that they completely abolished the self-attack behaviour in the rats and at the same time reduced the major phase of sensitivity of the nerve ends.

Effects of sympathetic–blocking agents in man

The fact that sympathectomy is so effective in abolishing causalgia and that one or more blocks of the sympathetic ganglia can often cure a variety of neuralgic pain states (such as the neuralgias and reflex sympathetic dystrophies) leads to questions about the mechanisms involved. Is it genuinely a sympathetic effect or could it be due to section or block of somatic afferent fibres?

Hannington-Kiff (1974) has introduced a new technique which shows with certainty that the effect of sympathectomy is truly dependent on blocking of the sympathetic efferents. He places a blood-pressure cuff around the upper part of the painful limb, inflates the cuff so that the blood can no longer circulate, and gives an intravenous injection of the drug guanethidine. Guanethidine is one of a large number of chemicals which effectively block the ability of the sympathetic efferent fibres to release noradrenalin and has a long-lasting action. The guanethidine permeates from the veins into the surrounding tissues. It is allowed to act for about fifteen minutes and then the circulation is released. The drug has been 'fixed' in the nerve endings by this time and any excess drug is swept away in highly diluted form so that it has no effect on the rest of the body. This simple treatment thereby produces a sympathetic block of the entire limb. Sensory fibres are not blocked by the drug, but the pain often disappears for long periods of time.

The practical importance of this procedure is that it saves the patient the misery and danger of a direct approach to his sympathetic ganglia from which the sympathetic efferent fibres emerge. The basic importance is that it solves an old controversy in which it was thought possible that sympathectomy acted by cutting not only the sympathetic nerves but also the sensory nerves which pass through the ganglia on their way to the spinal cord. Guanethidine blocks *only* the ability of the sympathetic nerves to emit noradrenalin and seems not to affect sensory fibres directly. In the untreated limb, a positive feedback is set up since sympathetic efferent activity – especially noradrenalin output – generates impulses in sensory afferents which reflexly trigger even more sympathetic output so that the area is not only painful but glossy and wet.

Unfortunately for some patients, there is more to the story than the abnormal sympathetic efferent-sensory afferent interactions. Some patients respond only temporarily to sympathetic denervation. Noordenbos and Wall (1981) examined seven such patients. They all showed an intractable causalgia-like syndrome and it was decided to make a large excision of the damaged nerve and to replace it with a graft from the sural nerve. This, of course, resulted in a temporary denervation of the painful region and, in each case, the area was eventually reinnervated from the grafted nerve end. Unfortunately, all seven reported a return to their previous condition, including pain, dysaesthesia, radiation and summation. Considering the fact that causalgia is a rare consequence of nerve injury, and that the surgical resection and grafting constituted an entirely different type of injury from the original one, the recurrence of the condition suggests that the primary site of the problem may have shifted from the location of the injury to some more central region which was set into a new mode that handled arriving signals in a highly abnormal fashion.

Effects of peripheral nerve injury on central processes

Immediate effects. Pain following a peripheral nerve injury often develops fully within a few hours after injury. From that time on, the pain persists. This cannot be explained by the presence of an injury discharge in the cut nerves since the discharge dies down within minutes of the injury (Wall, Waxman and Basbaum, 1974). Furthermore, it cannot be explained by the sensitivity of the sprouts from the cut nerves since that activity builds up over the first two weeks after injury. Other mechanisms must explain the rapid onset and persistence of pain. Noordenbos (1959) proposed that the brain normally receives a delicate balance of inputs, some of which excite and others which inhibit. In the gate-control theory, which we will describe later, we extended this idea and added central controlling factors. It is apparent that the presence of an excitatory input, or the absence of an inhibitory input, or central readjustment could promptly tilt the sensory systems into a pain-producing mode. If that is the case, it should be possible to readjust the balance.

Chronic anatomical changes. Turmoil can be seen by electron microscopy in the central (spinal) terminals of the fine fibres within six days of cutting the sciatic nerve in the rat (Csillik and Knyihar, 1978). The conduction velocity of impulses begins to drop by four days. The sensory nerve of the face seems particularly sensitive to peripheral damage, and degenerating fibres are seen in the brain within a few weeks. Section of the main nerve to the leg produces central degeneration within months. Evidently, even though the stump of an amputated limb remains innervated, its anatomical connections to the spinal cord begin to change soon after injury.

Chronic chemical changes. The cell bodies of sensory nerves, which comprise the dorsal root ganglia, synthesize chemicals which are transported to the central terminals of the sensory nerves. One of these is an enzyme – a special acid phosphatase – and it disappears from the central ends of the sensory fibres by four days after peripheral nerve injury (Devor and Claman, 1980). One of the peptide family, substance P, whose molecule is made up of a chain of eleven amino-acids, exists in the terminals of fine nerve fibres and affects the excitability of nerve cells. It begins to disappear by five days after nerve section (Barbut *et al.*, 1981). This compound does not disappear if the nerve is crushed but does if it is cut.

Chronic physiological changes. When excitatory impulses arrive at the spinal cord, they also activate inhibitory processes, one of which is presynaptic and acts on the terminals of the sensory fibres which are carrying the input. This inhibitory feedback to the terminals fails to occur by seven days after section of the sciatic nerve in the rat but is not affected by a crush injury (Wall and Devor, 1981). Coincident with the disappearance of substance P and the feedback on the terminals, the spinal nerve cells which are cut off from the periphery now begin to respond to new inputs from adjacent and distant body areas (Devor and Wall, 1978).

Dorsal root lesions

If the sensory fibres are cut in the dorsal root central to the dorsal root ganglion – a rhizotomy (Figure 7) – this is followed by degeneration of all the fibres and a rapid rise of the excitability of the central cells on which they end. These denervated cells become so excitable that they begin to fire spontaneously. The consistent and persistent pain of patients with brachial plexus avulsions may well be produced by just this spontaneous ongoing activity. No wonder, then, that cutting dorsal roots has a very poor record in relieving phantom limb pain (White and Sweet, 1969). It is adding insult to injury.

Spinal cord lesions and pain

Several forms of pathology of the spinal cord are associated with pain. Spinal blood vessels, for example, may rupture, producing a local haemorrhage with consequent damage to spinal tissue. Not only are there sensory and motor losses, but terrible pain may occur. Sometimes the pain abates, but more often it persists in spite of any measures that are taken. So far, no effective treatment has been found for such pain.

Infections of the spinal cord may also produce pain. Syphilis, if left untreated, may selectively affect the dorsal half of the spinal cord, producing *tabes dorsalis*, a syndrome characterized by abnormally intense pain after stimulation of the skin, and the pain typically occurs after long delays. There are many other forms of spinal pathology, some of which are associated with pain. Syringomyelia, in which there is degeneration of the fibres that cross the central core of the cord, was long thought to be 'painless', but there are now ample reports that syringomyelia may be a painful disease in some cases. More commonly known is the fact that multiple sclerosis – a demyelinating disease – is sometimes accompanied by pain, producing even more misery in people already afflicted with a frightening disease.

A variety of spinal lesions may cause pain. Gunshot wounds and knife wounds that penetrate the back may sometimes slice through a portion of the spinal cord, leaving a substantial portion intact, yet producing a state of terrible pain in the part of the body that is denervated (or 'deafferented'). Surgical lesions of the spinal cord that were intended to relieve pain may not only fail to do so, but sometimes increase the earlier pains. At other times, parts of the body that had never been in pain now suddenly become a source of pain. This phenomenon is known as 'unmasking', as though the new pain were always there, but was not felt because it was 'masked' or dominated in consciousness by the old pain. But this is unlikely. It is more reasonable to suspect that the surgical lesion destroyed fibres that are part of an inhibitory system. The removal of inhibition leads to heightened excitation in spinal cells that now send nerve impulses to the brain that produce pain.

Very little is known about the pain-causing mechanisms of these pain states or, unfortunately, how to treat them. More is known about pain states which are due to peripheral nerve damage which has clearly extended into the spinal cord. We have shown earlier that cutting peripheral nerves sets off a sequence of changes starting in the periphery and quite clearly extending into the spinal cord. If they have occurred this far, it is possible that they may spread further and trigger a central chain of events. Curiously, the troubles may originate from the nervous system's attempt to counteract the consequences of the injury. The outgrowing sprouts are an attempt to reconstruct the lost nerve but they are highly sensitive. The changes in the spinal cord may be seen as homeostatic mechanisms in which structures, cut off from their normal source of information, open the floodgates. In such a state, small inputs add up to produce devastating effects, such as hyperpathia and summation. The raised excitability eventually results in ongoing activity and spontaneous pain. Furthermore, the loss of inhibitory mechanisms allows normally discrete messages to spill out of the normal channels – 'radiation' – and affect neighbouring neurons.

The 'opening of the floodgates' after loss of input via sensory roots may also explain the back pain that occurs after a disc protrudes and presses against the sensory roots. The usual explanation is that the roots are irritated by the disc and send volleys of nerve impulses to the brain. But, astonishingly, prolonged pressure against roots has the opposite effect – it may produce a cessation of activity (Wall, Waxman and Basbaum, 1974). As a result of the *loss* of activity, an abnormal hyperexcitability of spinal cord cells may occur, so that the hyperactive cells fire spontaneously and persistently, thereby producing chronic low back pain. The fact that removal of the disc sometimes does not produce relief of pain suggests that a prolonged – possibly permanent – abnormal state has now been initiated by the initial pathology and persists in the absence of input.

Pain in paraplegic patients, which we discussed in Chapter 4, is particularly puzzling, but may be explained in terms of similar mechanisms. How is it that even after a total section of the spinal cord – especially after a neurosurgeon has removed a whole segment of the cord (cordectomy) – paraplegic patients continue to feel pain in specific parts of the body well below the level of the section? The most likely answer (Melzack and Loeser, 1978) is that the massive loss of sensory input, after a total break of the spinal cord, produces a huge number of uncontrolled, spontaneously firing cells that send abnormal volleys to those parts of the brain that subserve pain experience.

Loeser and Ward (1967) showed that cutting several dorsal roots in the cat produces abnormal bursts of firing in dorsal horn cells that persist for as long as 180 days after the root section. Furthermore, single shock pulses to adjacent intact roots produce prolonged firing that persists for hundreds of milliseconds. These abnormal patterns are commonly seen after deafferentation. Since total section of the spinal cord produces a massive deafferentation, it is not surprising that recordings of spinal cells above the level of the cord transection in man show highly abnormal bursting activity which resembles that seen after chronic deafferentation in the cat spinal cord (Loeser, Ward and White, 1968). These abnormal, hyperactive neuron pools may act as 'pattern generating mechanisms' which produce the terrible pains that are sometimes observed in paraplegic patients (Melzack and Loeser, 1978).

Pain after brain injury

In the previous chapter, we saw that some areas of the brain, particularly the brainstem reticular formation and the cortex, exert a powerful inhibitory control over the transmission of pain signals. We also noted that limbic system structures are involved in the total pain experience, especially its emotional and motivational aspects. It is abundantly clear that there is no 'pain centre'; rather there is a complex interaction among multiple structures involving most of the brain.

Damage to the central areas of the brain is often the cause of severe, intractable pain. Unfortunate people who suffer a stroke – rupture or blockage of a major blood vessel of the brain – usually exhibit a variety of signs, such as loss of speech, movement, or some kinds of sensation, depending on the location of the damage. If the central core of the brain, especially the thalamus, is damaged, however, they often suffer terrible pain. The syndrome is commonly known as the 'thalamic pain syndrome' but the pathology usually encroaches into surrounding areas, including portions of the limbic system, the hypothalamus and fibre areas just below the cortex. From all that is known, lesions at any level of the somatic projection system from the spinal cord up to the cortex may be accompanied by severe, intractable pain.

These 'central pains' are especially dreaded by physicians who have to treat them because they are so intractable. No drug, no operation, no technique yet invented seems to be able to control these pains. Even the cause of these pains, such as the 'thalamic pain syndrome', is unknown. In fact, there may be three possible causes and, conceivably, all three may play a role. The pain may be due to irritation of brain tissue by the necrotic tissue damaged by the stroke, or it may be due to the loss or disruption of a neural system that normally exerts an inhibitory control over lower levels of the pain-signalling pathways. A potential treatment to overcome the loss of inhibition is reported by Adams *et al.* (1974), who have stimulated the nerve tracts close to the thalamus and relieved thalamic-syndrome pain in some patients. The third possible mechanism is that the brain lesion triggers a cascade of changes which spreads to involve distant areas. The reason for considering this rather pessimistic possibility comes from the work of Loh *et al.* (1980). They showed that the hyperaesthetic aspect of the patient's pain is associated with effects by the sympathetic nerves on the sensory nerves, as in causalgia. This finding implies that although the original lesion is undoubtedly in the brain, it has changed the properties of nerve cells in the distant periphery. We have shown that a peripheral lesion produces changes in the spinal cord and perhaps higher in the brainstem. Here is a hint that brain lesions may induce changes in lower levels of the nervous system, perhaps even as far away as the peripheral nerves themselves. This possibility is supported by the remarkable discovery (Loh *et al.*, 1981) that pains caused by a lesion of the spinal cord or brain may be reduced or abolished by blocks of the sympathetic supply to the periphery. Though the relief is usually temporary, repeated blocks sometimes produce long-lasting effects.

All of this, of course, is highly speculative. But speculation and theory lie at the heart of science. They are the launching pad, as it were, of experiments and concepts that produce giant steps in science. The field of pain, like every other scientific field, is rich in theory and speculation, and the next several chapters examine the history of pain theories.

Part Three
Theories of Pain

'The "real world" is a construct, and some of the peculiarities of scientific thought become more intelligible when this fact is recognized . . . Einstein himself in 1926 told Heisenberg it was nonsense to found a theory on observable facts alone: "In reality the very opposite happens. It is theory which decides what we can observe."'

D. O. Hebb, 1975

9
The Evolution of Pain Theories

So far, we have been concerned primarily with experimental and clinical observations related to pain. Some of the data, as we have seen, are still surrounded by controversy, and the scientist often has to sift the genuine facts from those 'clues' which may only lead into blind alleys. But facts alone, scientists have discovered over the centuries, usually fall short of providing a complete understanding of difficult problems. Books have been written which bring together all the known facts about pain, yet the puzzle persists. There are still too many fundamental questions for which we have no answers. Nevertheless we grope towards understanding and, for that reason, invent theories that bring us closer to it.

Although the notion of a scientific theory sounds formidable, a theory is primarily an attempted solution to a puzzle or problem – not unlike a guess made by a detective presented with an array of clues in a mystery. Several clues may lead to a theory or guess on the nature of the solution. The theory, in turn, may lead to a search for further clues that were previously not evident.

A theory alone, however, may not be enough to convince (or convict). New facts are tested against the theory to see whether or not they fit. If they support the theory, all the clues may fit together to make a coherent picture. Sometimes they demand alterations of the theory. At other times they are so much at odds with the theory that it must be rejected. In this chapter we will examine and evaluate the theories of pain that have evolved during the past century.

Specificity theory

The traditional theory of pain is known as 'specificity theory'. It is described in virtually every textbook on neurophysiology, neurology and neurosurgery, and is so deeply entrenched in medical school teaching (until recently, at least) that it is often taught as fact rather than theory. It is presented as though we already have the major answers to pain problems, and all that remain are a few minor questions that deal with therapy. It also proved to be a very powerful theory during the first half of this century, giving rise to excellent research and to some effective forms of treatment. It has several basic flaws, however, and new, more powerful theories have recently been proposed.

Specificity theory proposes that a specific pain system carries messages from pain receptors in the skin to a pain centre in the brain. To understand the theory, we must first consider its origins, The best classical description of the theory was provided by Descartes in 1664, who conceived of the pain system as a straight-through channel from the skin to the brain. He suggested that the system is like the bell-ringing mechanism in a church: a man pulls the rope at the bottom of the tower, and the bell rings in the belfry. So too, he proposed (Figure 25), a flame sets particles in the foot into activity and the motion is transmitted up the leg and back and into the head where, presumably, something like an alarm system is set off. The person then feels pain and responds to it. Despite its apparent simplicity, the theory involves several major assumptions, which we will examine shortly. First, however, we will see how Descartes' theory has evolved in the last three centuries.

The theory underwent little change until the nineteenth century, when physiology emerged as an experimental science. A major problem faced by sensory physiologists in the nineteenth century was this: how can we account for the different qualities of sensation? Our visual and auditory sensations are qualitatively different from each other, just as our skin sensations are obviously different from those of taste or smell. What is the basis of these different sensory qualities? As a result of studies by early anatomists and physiologists, it became apparent that the brain is aware of the outside world only by means of messages conveyed to it by the sensory nerves. The qualities of experience, therefore, are somehow associated with the properties of sensory nerves. It was Johannes Müller who first stated this proposition in scientific

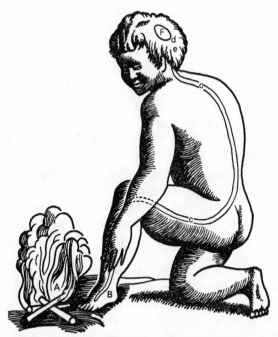

Figure 25. Descartes' (1664) concept of the pain pathway. He writes: 'If for example fire (A) comes near the foot (B), the minute particles of this fire, which as you know move with great velocity, have the power to set in motion the spot of the skin of the foot which they touch, and by this means pulling upon the delicate thread (cc) which is attached to the spot of the skin, they open up at the same instant the pore (d e) against which the delicate thread ends, just as by pulling at one end of a rope one makes to strike at the same instant a bell which hangs at the other end.'

form, and his statement has become known as the 'doctrine of specific nerve energies'.

Müller's doctrine of specific nerve energies
Müller's monumental contribution (1842) to our understanding of sensory processes lies in his formal statement that the brain receives information about external objects only by way of the sensory nerves. Activity in nerves, then, represents coded or symbolic data concerning the stimulus object. It is essential to note that Müller recognized only the five classical senses, the sense of

touch incorporating for him all the qualities of experience that we derive from stimulation of the body. He wrote:

Sensation is a property common to all the senses; but the kind of sensation is different in each: thus, we have the sensations of light, of sound, of taste, of smell, and of feeling or touch. By feeling and touch we understand the peculiar kind of sensation of which the ordinary sensitive nerves generally, as the trigeminal, vagus, glossopharyngeal, and spinal nerves, are susceptible; the sensations of itching, or pleasure and pain, of heat and cold, and those excited by the act of touch in its more limited sense, are varieties of this mode of sensation.

For Müller, then, the somaesthetic sensations are a function of a unitary sensory system. The various qualities of somatic sensory experience provide no difficulty for the theory; no more, that is, than the different qualities of form, depth and colour perception provide difficulty for anyone regarding the visual system as a single integrated system.

Müller was uncertain, at that time, whether the quality of sensation is due to some specific energy inherent in each of the sensory nerves themselves, or whether it is due to some special properties of the brain areas at which the nerves terminate. By the late nineteenth and early twentieth centuries, however, it was apparent that nerve impulses are essentially the same in all sensory nerves, and it was concluded that the quality of sensation is given by the termination of the nerves in the brain. The impact of all this was a search for a terminal centre in the brain for each of the sensory nerves.

Müller's concept, then, was that of a straight-through system from the sensory organ to the brain centre responsible for the sensation. Since the cortex is seemingly at the 'top' of the nervous system, a search was made for cortical centres. Visual and auditory projections to cortex were found very early, and it was assumed that these cortical areas were the seat of seeing and hearing. The physiologists of the day were so convinced of the truth of this doctrine that DuBois-Reymond (see Boring, 1942) proposed that if the auditory nerve could be connected to the visual cortex, and the visual nerve to the auditory cortex, then we would see thunder and hear lightning!

It was at this time that Max von Frey, a physician, first began to contemplate these problems and between 1894 and 1895 he published a series of articles in which he proposed a theory of the cutaneous senses. This theory was expanded during the next fifty years, and is the basis of modern-day specificity theory.

Von Frey's theory

The way von Frey developed his theory (Boring, 1942) makes a fascinating story in the history of science. He had three kinds of information that he put together to form it. The first was Müller's doctrine of specific nerve energies. It was apparent to him, as it was to others, that Müller's notion of a single sense of touch or 'feeling' was inadequate. The great physicist and physiologist Helmholtz proposed that there must be thousands of different specific auditory fibres, one kind for each discriminably different sound. Volkmann had similarly proposed that there must be several kinds of specific nerve fibres from the skin, one for each quality of cutaneous sensation. It was reasonable, then, for von Frey to expand Müller's concept to four major cutaneous modalities: touch, warmth, cold, and pain, each presumably with its own special projection system to a brain centre responsible for the appropriate sensation.

The second kind of information von Frey had was the spot-like distribution of warmth and cold sensitivity at the skin. He made two simple devices that are still used in neurological tests. He put a pin on a spring, and could gauge the pressure on the pin necessary to produce prick-pain, thus finding pain spots. He also put two-inch snippets of horse-tail hairs on pieces of wood and made 'von Frey hairs' to map out distributions of touch spots. Thus he believed that the skin comprises a mosaic of four types of sensory spots: touch, cold, warmth, and pain.

The third kind of information used by von Frey derived from the development, during the nineteenth century, of chemical techniques to study the fine structure of body tissues. Anatomists used particular chemicals to stain thin slices of tissue from all parts of the body, and then observed the tissues through a microscope. When they examined the skin in this way, they found a variety of specialized structures. To achieve immortality of sorts, some of the anatomists named the specialized structures after themselves. Thus, we still know these structures as Meissner corpuscles, Ruffini end-organs, Krause end-bulbs, Pacinian corpuscles and so forth. Two types of structure were so common that no one dared attach his name to them: the free nerve endings that branch out into the upper layers of the skin, and the nerve fibres that are wrapped around hair follicles.

The way von Frey utilized these three kinds of information is a remarkable example of scientific deduction. He reasoned as follows: since the free nerve endings are the most commonly found, and pain spots are found almost everywhere, the free nerve endings are pain receptors. Furthermore, since Meissner corpuscles are frequently found at the fingers and palm of the hand where touch spots are most abundant and most sensitive, they (in addition to the fibres surrounding hair follicles) are the touch receptors. The next association was an imaginative deduction: he noted that the conjunctivum of the eye and the tip of the penis are both sensitive to cold, but the conjunctivum is not sensitive to warmth and the penis is not sensitive to pressure; moreover, Krause end-bulbs are found in both locations; therefore, he concluded, Krause end-bulbs are cold receptors. Finally, he had one major sensation – warmth – left over, and one major receptor – Ruffini end-organs – so he proposed that Ruffini end-organs are warmth receptors.

Von Frey's theory dealt only with receptors. Others carried on, however, and sought specific fibres from the receptors to the spinal cord, then specific pathways in the spinal cord itself.

Extensions of von Frey's theory. Following von Frey's postulation of four modalities of cutaneous sensation, each having its own type of specific nerve ending, the separation of modality was extended to peripheral nerve fibres (see Chapter 5). Ingenious experiments (reviewed by Bishop, 1946; Rose and Mountcastle, 1959; Sinclair, 1967) were carried out to show that there is a one-to-one relationship between receptor type, fibre size, and quality of experience. The concept of modality separation in peripheral nerve fibres represents the most literal interpretation of Müller's doctrine of specific nerve energies. Since fibre-diameter groups are held to be modality specific, the theory imparts 'specific nerve energy' on the basis of fibre size, so that specificity theorists speak of A-delta-fibre pain and C-fibre pain, of touch fibres and cold fibres as though each fibre group had a straight-through transmission path to a specific brain centre.

Finally, a search was made for the 'pain pathway' in the spinal cord (Keele, 1957). Studies and operations on humans and animals suggested that the anterolateral quadrant of the spinal cord was critically important for pain sensation (see p.77, on cordotomy). As a consequence, the spinothalamic tract which ascends in the anterolateral cord has come to be known as 'the pain pathway'.

The location of the 'pain centre' is still a source of debate among specificity theorists. Head (1920) proposed that it is located in the thalamus because cortical lesions or excisions rarely abolish pain. Indeed, they may make it worse. Thus, the thalamus is held by some to contain the pain centre, and the cortex is assumed to exert inhibitory control over it.

Analysis of specificity theory

Von Frey's designation of the free nerve endings as pain receptors is the basis of specificity theory. Its solution to the puzzle of pain is simple: specific pain receptors in body tissue project via pain fibres and a pain pathway to a pain centre in the brain. Despite its apparent simplicity, the theory has three facets, each representing a major assumption. The first of these, that receptors are specialized, is physiological in nature and has achieved the proportions of a genuine biological law. The remaining two assumptions, anatomical and psychological in nature, are not supported by the facts.

The physiological assumption. Von Frey's assumption that skin receptors are differentiated to respond to particular stimulus dimensions represents a major extension of Müller's concept of the 'specific irritability' of receptors. The assumption is that each of the four types of receptors has one form of energy to which it is especially sensitive. This concept of physiological specialization of skin receptors provides the power of von Frey's theory and appears to be the main reason for its survival through the decades. Sherrington (1900, p.995) stated it in a manner that is acceptable to all students of sensory processes:

The sensorial end-organ is an apparatus by which an afferent nerve fibre is rendered distinctively amenable to some particular physical agent, and at the same time rendered less amenable to, i.e. is shielded from, other excitants. It lowers the value of the limen of one particular kind of stimulus, it heightens the value of the limen of stimuli of other kinds.

The beauty of Sherrington's definition of receptor specificity in terms of the lowest limen (or threshold) for a particular stimulus is that it makes no assumptions concerning the eventual psychological experience. This concept of the 'adequate stimulus' (Sherrington, 1906) is so generally accepted that it is rightfully considered to be a biological principle or law.

The anatomical assumption. It is von Frey's anatomical assumption that is the most specific, the most obviously incorrect and the least relevant aspect of the theory. Von Frey assumed that a single morphologically specific receptor lay beneath each sensory spot on the skin and he assigned a definite receptor type to each of the four modalities. He postulated his correlations on the basis of logical deduction rather than experimental evidence and he was fully aware of their defects and weaknesses. Regarding the correlation between cold and Krause's end-organs, von Frey (1895; see Dallenbach, 1927) notes that 'out of this supposition arises an obviously serious difficulty, because the ability to feel cold appears not only at the spots but also at the surrounding skin'. He also acknowledges that 'whether the number of end-organs in the skin is sufficient to account for all the cold spots is a question that has yet to be decided'.

The crucial experiment of making a histological examination of the skin under carefully mapped temperature spots has been performed at least a dozen times (see Melzack and Wall, 1962), without a single investigator finding any support for von Frey's anatomical correlations. Indeed Donaldson's (1885) and Goldscheider's (1886) earlier demonstrations of only free nerve-endings beneath temperature spots have been confirmed repeatedly. Even Ruffini (1905), from the viewpoint of the histologist, noted that there are not four but a numberless variety of receptor types and considered the correlations to be nonsense. Weddell and Sinclair, during the 1950s, again destroyed every conceivable aspect of von Frey's anatomical assumption. Yet the theory has held its ground without a single counterattack. The reason, it appears, is that the anatomical assumption usually attacked lies at the periphery of von Frey's concept. The assumption that skin receptors have specialized physiological properties remains valid regardless of the correctness or incorrectness of the particular anatomical correlations suggested by von Frey. Free nerve-endings may all look alike yet each may have highly specialized properties (see Chapter 5).

The psychological assumption. It is the assumption that each psychological dimension of somaesthetic experience bears a one-to-one relation to a single stimulus dimension and to a given type of skin receptor that is the most questionable part of von Frey's theory (Melzack and Wall, 1962). Like all psychological theories, von Frey's theory has an implicit conceptual nervous system; and the model is that of a fixed, direct-line communication system from the skin to the brain – of distinct nerves and pathways of four different qualities (analogous to the differently coloured wires of an electrical circuit) running from four specific kinds of stimulus transducers in the skin to four specific receivers in the brain. Figure 26 illustrates the modern-day specificity conception of the pain projection system. Despite its obvious sophistication, showing free nerve endings, anterolateral pathway, and so forth, it is essentially similar to Descartes' concept of pain (Figure 25, p.197) which was proposed three hundred years earlier. It depicts a fixed, straight-through conceptual nervous system. It is precisely this facet of the specificity concept, which imputes a direct, invariant relationship between a psychological sensory dimension and a physical stimulus dimension, that has led to attempts at repudiation of the doctrine of specificity in its entirety.

Consider the proposition that the skin contains 'pain receptors'. To say that a receptor responds only to intense, noxious stimulation of the skin is a physiological statement of fact; it says that the receptor is specialized to respond to a particular kind of stimulus. To call a receptor a 'pain receptor', however, is a psychological assumption: it implies a direct connection from the receptor to a brain centre where pain is felt, so that stimulation of the receptor must always elicit pain and only the sensation of pain. It further implies that the abstraction or selection of information concerning the stimulus occurs entirely at the receptor level and that this information is transmitted faithfully to the brain. The crux of the revolt against specificity, then, is against

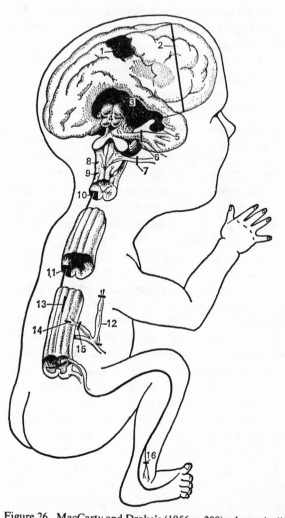

Figure 26. MacCarty and Drake's (1956, p.208) schematic diagram illustrating various surgical procedures designed to alleviate pain: 1, gyrectomy; 2, prefrontal lobotomy; 3, thalamotomy; 4, mesencephalic tractotomy; 5, hypophysectomy; 6, fifth-nerve rhizotomy; 7, ninth-nerve neurectomy; 8, medullary tractotomy; 9, trigeminal tractotomy; 10, cervical cordotomy; 11, thoracic cordotomy; 12, sympathectomy; 13, myelotomy; 14, Lissauer tractotomy; 15, posterior rhizotomy; 16, neurectomy.

psychological specificity. This distinction between physiological specialization and psychological assumption also applies to peripheral fibres and central projection systems.

The facts of physiological specialization provide the power of specificity theory. Its psychological assumption is its weakness. This assumption will now be examined in the light of the psychological, clinical, and physiological evidence concerning pain (Melzack and Wall, 1962, 1965).

Psychological evidence. The psychological evidence on pain described in Chapter 2 fails to support the assumption of a one-to-one relationship between pain perception and intensity of the stimulus. Instead, the evidence suggests that the amount and quality of perceived pain are determined by many psychological variables in addition to the sensory input. For example, American soldiers wounded at the Anzio beach-head 'entirely denied pain from their extensive wounds or had so little that they did not want any medication to relieve it' (Beecher, 1959, p.165). If the men had felt pain, even pain sensation devoid of negative affect, they would, it is reasonable to assume, have reported it, just as lobotomized patients report that they still have pain but it does not bother them. Instead, these men 'entirely denied pain'. Similarly, Pavlov's dogs that received electric shocks, burns, or cuts, followed consistently by the presentation of food, eventually responded to these stimuli as signals for food and failed to show 'even the tiniest and most subtle' (Pavlov, 1927, p.30) signs of pain. If these dogs felt pain sensation, then it must have been nonpainful pain (Nafe, 1934) or the dogs were out to fool Pavlov and simply refused to reveal that they were feeling pain. Both possibilities, of course, are absurd. The inescapable conclusion from these observations is that intense noxious stimulation can be prevented from producing pain, or may be modified to provide the signal for eating behaviour.

The concept of four rigid modalities of cutaneous experience has been criticized by Head (1920), Nafe (1934), Livingston (1943), Hebb (1949), Weddell (1955), Sinclair (1955) and many others. The dimensions of somaesthetic perceptions have never been experimentally determined, so that psychologists are unable to agree on the number of distinctly different sensory qualities produced by skin stimulation (Titchener, 1920). The number chosen by von Frey is based purely on conjecture. To say, for example, that itch is produced by a particular pattern of stimulation of 'pain receptors' (Bishop, 1946) indicates only that the patterning of the input is more important in determining the different qualities of experience than any modality label we might arbitrarily attach to the receptor (Nafe, 1934). The four modalities of von Frey represent broad categories of different perceptual experiences that have been labelled in terms of those perceptions which are most easily named.

Clinical evidence. Phantom limb pain, causalgia, and the neuralgias provide a dramatic refutation of the concept of a fixed, direct-line nervous system. We have already noted in Chapter 4 that:

1 Surgical lesions of the peripheral and central nervous system have been singularly unsuccessful in abolishing these pains permanently.

2 Gentle touch, vibration, and other non-noxious stimuli can trigger excruciating pain, and sometimes pain occurs spontaneously for long periods without any apparent stimulus.

3 The pains and new 'trigger zones' may spread unpredictably to unrelated parts of the body where no pathology exists.

4 Pain from hyperalgesic skin areas often occurs after long delays and continues long after removal of the stimulus, which implies a remarkable temporal and spatial summation of inputs in the production of these pain states.

These clinical facts defy explanation in terms of a rigid, straight-through specific pain system.

Physiological evidence. There is convincing physiological evidence (see Chapter 5) that specialization exists within the somaesthetic system, but none to show that stimulation of one type of receptor, fibre, or spinal pathway elicits sensations in only a single psychological modality. Specialized fibres exist that respond only to intense stimulation, but this does not mean that they are 'pain fibres' – that they must always produce pain, and only pain, when they are stimulated. Similarly, central cells that respond exclusively or maximally to noxious stimuli are not 'pain cells'. There is no evidence to suggest that they are more important for pain perception and response than all the remaining somaesthetic cells that signal characteristic firing patterns about multiple properties of the stimulus, including noxious intensity. The view that only the cells that respond exclusively to noxious stimuli subserve pain and that the outputs of all other cells are no more than background noise is purely a psychological assumption and has no physiological basis. Physiological specialization is a fact that can be retained without acceptance of the psychological assumption that pain is determined entirely by impulses in a straight-through transmission system from the skin to a pain centre in the brain.

In Müller's formulation of the doctrine of specific nerve energies, the varieties of cutaneous experience are subserved by a single integrated system. Von Frey's postulation of four modalities is able to account for at least four different qualities of somaesthetic experience, but it necessarily divides the somaesthetic system into four separate subsystems, each having a direct-line transmission route to a specific termination in the brain. Müller's integrated, unspecialized conceptual nervous system was thus replaced by four specialized, unintegrated subsystems.

We can have the advantages of an integrated somaesthetic system comprised of specialized component parts if we relinquish the concept that the various sensory qualities are determined by the terminations of the ascending fibres in the brain. There is no evidence for discrete thalamic or cortical 'centres' for any dimensions of somaesthetic experience. We must assume, therefore, that the dimensions of somaesthetic perception are subserved by different patterns of excitation evoked in the brain by different sensory stimuli. The arrival of sensory messages at the thalamus and cortex appears to mark only the beginning of a web of activity travelling in all directions to widespread areas of the central nervous system. In view of all this the idea of 'terminations' in the brain becomes a difficult concept: where does a pattern of excitation terminate? Surely not in the thalamus and cortex which appear to act as the hub of changing, constantly on-going processes.

If somaesthetic sensory qualities are not determined by specific terminal centres but by particular nerve impulse patterns coursing through widespread portions of the brain, there is no longer the theoretical necessity for postulating a separate system for each sensory quality. Pathways do indeed diverge, and there is no question of the specialization of central pathways for particular functions. But if we maintain the distinction between physiological specialization for information transmission and the perception and response that eventually occur, we are left free to take cognizance of any degree of specialization the data call for without encountering the difficulties of separate modality transmission routes.

Pattern theory

As a reaction against the psychological assumption in specificity theory, other theories have been proposed which can be grouped under the general heading of 'pattern theory'. Goldscheider (1894), initially one of the champions of von Frey's theory, was the first to propose that stimulus intensity and central summation are the critical determinants of pain.

Goldscheider was profoundly influenced by studies of pathological pain, especially those by Naunyn (1889) on *tabes dorsalis*, which occurs in patients suffering the late stages of syphilis. *Tabes* is characterized by degeneration in the dorsal spinal cord and dorsal roots, and one of its major symptoms is the temporal and spatial summation of somatic input in producing pain (Noordenbos, 1959). Successive, brief applications of a warm test-tube to the skin of a tabetic patient are at first felt only as warm, but then feel increasingly hot until the patient cries out in pain as though his skin is being burned. Such summation never occurs in the normal person, who simply reports successive applications of warmth. Similarly, a single pinprick, which produces a momentary, sharp pain in normal subjects, evokes a diffuse, prolonged, burning pain in tabetic patients.

Not only are the intensity and duration of pain out of proportion to the stimulus, but there is often a remarkable delay in the onset of pain. A pin prick may not be felt until many seconds later – usually a few seconds but sometimes as long as forty-five seconds (Noordenbos, 1959). Observations such as these had a powerful impact on Goldscheider, who was compelled to conclude that mechanisms of central summation, probably in the dorsal horns of the spinal cord, were essential for any understanding of pain mechanisms.

Goldscheider's pattern, or summation, theory proposes that the particular patterns of nerve impulses that evoke pain are produced by the summation of the skin sensory input at the dorsal horn cells. According to this concept, pain results when the total output of the cells exceeds a critical level as a result of either excessive stimulation of receptors that are normally fired by non-noxious thermal or tactile stimuli, or pathological conditions that enhance the summation of impulses produced by normally non-noxious stimuli. The long delays and persistent pain observed in pathological pain states, Goldscheider assumed, are due to abnormally long time-periods of summation. He proposed, moreover, that the spinal 'summation path' that transmits the pain signals to the brain consists of slowly conducting, multi-synaptic fibre chains. The large fibres that project up the dorsal column pathways were presumed to carry specific information about the tactile discriminative properties of cutaneous sensation.

Several theories have emerged from Goldscheider's concept. All of them recognize the concept of patterning of the input, which is essential for any adequate theory of pain. But some ignore the facts of physiological specialization, while others utilize them in proposing mechanisms of central summation.

Peripheral pattern theory
The simplest form of pattern theory deals primarily with peripheral rather than central patterning. That is, pain is considered to be due to excessive peripheral stimulation that produces a pattern of nerve impulses which is interpreted centrally as pain. The pattern theory of Weddell (1955) and Sinclair (1955) is based on the earlier suggestion by Nafe (1934) that all cutaneous qualities are produced by spatial and temporal patterns of nerve impulses rather than by separate modality-specific transmission routes. The theory proposes that all fibre endings (apart from those that innervate hair cells) are alike, so that the pattern for

pain is produced by intense stimulation of nonspecific receptors.

The physiological evidence, however, reveals a high degree of receptor-fibre specialization. The pattern theory proposed by Weddell and Sinclair, then, fails as a satisfactory theory of pain because it ignores the facts of physiological specialization. We have already noted in Chapter 5 that it is more reasonable to assume that the specialized physiological properties of each receptor-fibre unit (such as thresholds to different stimuli, adaptation rates, and size of receptive field) play an important role in determining the characteristics of the temporal patterns that are generated when a stimulus is applied to the skin.

Central summation theory

The analysis of phantom limb pain, causalgia and the neuralgias in Chapter 4 indicates that part, at least, of their underlying mechanisms must be sought in the central nervous system. Livingston (1943) was the first to suggest specific central neural mechanisms to account for the remarkable summation phenomena in these pain syndromes. He proposed that pathological stimulation of sensory nerves (such as occurs after peripheral nerve damage) initiates activity in reverberatory circuits (closed, self-exciting loops of neurons) in the grey matter of the spinal cord. This abnormal activity can then be triggered by normally non-noxious inputs and generate volleys of nerve impulses that are interpreted centrally as pain.

Livingston's theory is especially powerful in explaining phantom limb pain. He proposed that the initial damage to the limb, or the trauma associated with its removal, initiates abnormal firing patterns in reverberatory circuits in the dorsal horns of the spinal cord, which send volleys of nerve impulses to the brain that give rise to pain. Moreover, the reverberatory activity may spread to adjacent neurons in the lateral and ventral horns and produce autonomic and muscular manifestations in the limb, such as sweating and jerking movements of the stump. These, in turn, produce further sensory input, creating a 'vicious circle' between central and peripheral processes that maintains the abnormal spinal cord activity (Figure 27). Even minor irritations of the skin or nerves near the site of the operation can then feed into these active pools of neurons and keep them in an abnormal,

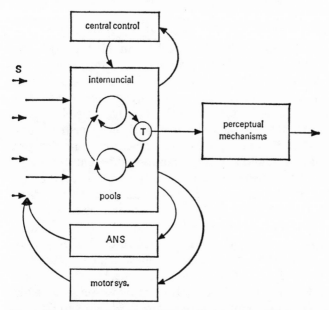

Figure 27. Schematic diagram of W. K. Livingston's (1943) theory of pathological pain states. The intense stimulation (S) resulting from nerve and tissue damage activates fibres that project to internuncial neuron pools in the spinal cord, creating abnormal reverberatory activity in closed self-exciting neuron loops. This prolonged, abnormal activity bombards the spinal cord transmission (T) cells which project to brain mechanisms that underlie pain perception. The abnormal internuncial activity also spreads to lateral and ventral horn cells in the spinal cord, activating the autonomic nervous system (ANS) and motor system, producing sweating, jactitations, and other manifestations. These, in turn, produce further abnormal input, thereby creating a 'vicious circle'. Brain activities such as fear and anxiety evoked by pain also feed into and maintain the abnormal internuncial pool activity.

disturbed state over periods of years. Impulse patterns that would normally be interpreted as touch may now trigger these neuron pools into greater activity, thereby sending volleys of impulses to the brain to produce pain. In addition, emotional disturbance may evoke neural activity that feeds into the abnormal neuron pools. Once the abnormal cord activity has become self-sustaining, surgical removal of the peripheral sources of input may not stop it. Rather, clinical procedures that modulate the sensory input, such as local anaesthetic injections or physiotherapy, may again reinstate normal cord activity.

Gerard (1951) has suggested a theory that is similar in concept, although different in hypothetical mechanism. He proposed that a peripheral nerve lesion may bring about a temporary loss of sensory control of firing in spinal cord neurons. These may then begin to fire in synchrony, just as isolated bits of nerve tissue in an appropriate solution fire synchronously, possibly due to spread of electrical fields. Such synchronously firing neuron pools 'could recruit additional units, could move along in the grey matter, could be maintained by impulses different from and feebler than those needed to initiate it, could discharge excessive and abnormally patterned volleys to the higher centres'.

Although Livingston's and Gerard's concepts have considerable power in explaining phantom limb pain, they fail to account for the fact that surgical lesions of the spinal cord often do not abolish the pain. Instead, the neurosurgical evidence points to mechanisms in the brain itself. If the crucial mechanism lay in the spinal cord dorsal horns, then cutting the major sensory routes through which spinal activity projects to the brain should stop the pain. Yet it is now generally recognized that, once the pain syndrome is well established, attempts to relieve it by surgery of spinal cord pathways are often ineffective. White and Sweet (1969) report the return of phantom limb pain after cordotomy in seven out of eighteen lower limb and three out of four upper limb cases. Even bilateral cordotomy may fail. Efforts have been made to find 'the leak' in the pain projection system, and the multi-synaptic propriospinal fibre chain has been proposed as one possibility (Noordenbos, 1959). But if there is a leak, and impulses ascending the cord determine pain without further elaboration, it is hard to imagine that so small an input (after the extensive surgical cuts) can produce such massive pain. Surgeons have therefore turned to the dorsal columns, the traditional 'touch-proprioception pathway' in the spinal cord, particularly for cramping pains in the phantom limb. Yet here too the operation is usually ineffective in producing a permanent cure (White and Sweet, 1969).

This emphasis on spinal cord activity is avoided by Hebb (1949), who suggests that synchronized firing in thalamocortical neural circuits provides the signal for pain. Hebb is particularly explicit in his concept that pain is determined by central summation mechanisms. He notes that pain frequently occurs after lesions at any level of the somaesthetic pathway. The loss of sensory control of patterned thalamocortical activities, he proposes, would produce excessive, synchronous firing in brain cells, which would disrupt the patterned activities that normally subserve perceptual and cognitive processes. The disruption itself, he suggests, *is* pain.

Sensory interaction theory

Related to theories of central summation is the theory that a specialized input-controlling system normally prevents summation from occurring, and that destruction of this system leads to pathological pain states. This theory derives from Goldscheider's original concept, and proposes the existence of a rapidly conducting fibre system which inhibits synaptic transmission in a more slowly conducting system that carries the signals for pain. Historically (see Melzack and Wall, 1965), these two systems are identified as the epicritic and protopathic (Head, 1920), fast and slow (Bishop, 1946), phylogenetically new and old (Bishop, 1959), and myelinated and unmyelinated (Noordenbos, 1959) fibre systems. Under pathological conditions, the fast system loses its dominance over the slow one, and the result is protopathic sensation (Head, 1920), slow pain (Bishop, 1946), diffuse burning pain (Bishop, 1959), or hyperalgesia (Noordenbos, 1959).

Noordenbos' theory (Figure 28) represents an especially important contribution to sensory-interaction concepts. The small fibres are conceived as carrying the nerve impulse patterns that produce pain, while the large fibres inhibit transmission. A shift in the ratio of large-to-small fibres in favour of the small fibres would result in increased neural transmission, summation, and excessive pathological pain. Just as important as the input control by the large fibres, in Noordenbos' concept, is the idea of a multisynaptic afferent system in the spinal cord. It stands in marked contrast to the idea of a straight-through system, and has the power to explain why spinothalamic cordotomy may fail to abolish pain. The diffuse, extensive connections within the ascending multi-synaptic afferent system, he proposes, can rarely (if ever) be totally abolished (unless the whole spinal cord is cut), so that there is always a 'leak' for impulses to ascend to the brain to produce pain.

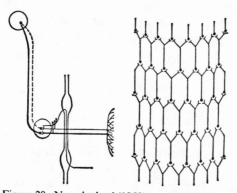

Figure 28. Noordenbos' (1959) concept of pain mechanisms. *Left:* small-diameter, slowly conducting somatic afferents and small visceral afferents (which travel through the sympathetic ganglia) project onto cells in the dorsal horn of the spinal cord. The summation of inputs from the small fibres produces the neural patterns that are transmitted to the brain to produce pain. The large-diameter fibres inhibit transmission of impulses from the small fibres and prevent summation from occurring. A selective loss of large fibres brings about a loss of inhibition and thereby increases the probability of summation and abnormal pain phenomena. The small fibre projection system – drawn as a dashed line – is indicated to be multi-synaptic. *Right:* Noordenbos' representation of the 'Multi-synaptic Afferent System' in the spinal cord. The diffuse, widespread conduction through the system, Noordenbos suggests, is the basis of 'the leak' of nerve signals that evoke pain even after extensive surgical section of the anterolateral pathways.

Noordenbos' theory has considerable power in explaining many of the pathological pain states described in Chapter 3. The concept of a shift in the fibre-diameter groups in favour of the small fibres is consistent with the observed relative loss of large fibres after peripheral nerve injury, and is able to explain the delays, temporal and spatial summation, and many other properties of pathological pain. The development of 'girdle pains' after cordotomy, he proposes, may similarly be due to the relative loss of the large fibres in the anterolateral pathways which still leaves the small diffusely conducting fibres untouched.

Sympathectomy, in contrast, would tend to destroy the small fibres, leaving a predominance of inhibitory large fibres which would decrease the tendency to summation and, consequently, the level of pain. Noordenbos' theory, like Livingston's, represents a major theoretical advance towards an understanding of the puzzle of pain.

Affect theory of pain

The theory that pain is a sensory modality is relatively recent. A much older theory, dating back to Aristotle, considers pain to be an emotion – the opposite of pleasure – rather than a sensation. Indeed, this idea of pain is part of an intriguing and usually neglected bit of history (Dallenbach, 1939). At the turn of the century, a bitter battle was fought on the question of pain specificity. Von Frey argued that there are specific pain receptors, while Goldscheider contended that pain is produced by excessive skin stimulation and central summation. But there was a third man in the battle – H. R. Marshall (1894), a philosopher and psychologist – who said, essentially, 'a plague on both your houses; pain is an emotional quality, or *quale*, that colours all sensory events'. He admitted the existence of a pricking-cutting sense, but thought that pain was distinctly different. All sensory inputs, as well as thoughts, could have a painful dimension to them, and he talked of the pain of bereavement, the pain of listening to badly played music. His extreme approach was, of course, open to criticism. Sherrington (1900), for example, noted that the pain of a scalded hand is different from the 'pain' evoked in a musicologist by even the most horrible discord. Marshall was soon pushed off the field. But if a less extreme view is taken of his concept, it suggests an important yet neglected dimension of pain. For pain does not have just a sensory quality; it also has a strong negative affective quality that drives us into activity (Figure 29). We are compelled to do something about it, to take the most effective course of action to stop it, and, of course, this behaviour is in the realm of emotion and motivation.

That pain is comprised of both sensory and affective dimensions was clear to Sherrington (1900) who proposed simply that

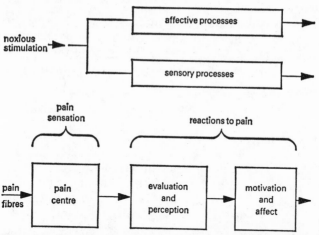

Figure 29. *Top:* diagram of Marshall's (1894) concept of pain as an affective quality or *quale*. Intense stimulation of the skin activates two parallel systems: one is the basis of the affective properties of the experience, the other underlies the sensory properties. *Bottom:* diagram of the concept, implicit in specificity theory, that motivation and affect are reactions to pain, but are not part of the primary pain sensation.
(from Melzack and Casey, 1968)

'mind rarely, probably never, preceives any object with absolute indifference, that is, without "feeling" . . . affective tone is an attribute of all sensation, and among the attribute tones of skin sensation is skin pain.' Introspectionist psychologists at the turn of the century also made a sharp distinction between the sensory and the affective qualities of pain. Titchener (1909–10) was convinced that there is a continuum of feeling in conscious experience, distinctly different from sensation, that ranges through all the degrees of pleasantness and unpleasantness. 'The pain of a toothache,' he wrote, 'is localized at a particular place, "in the tooth"; but the unpleasantness of it suffuses the whole of present experience, is as wide as consciousness. The word "pain" . . . often means the whole toothache experience.'

The remarkable development of sensory physiology and psychophysics during the twentieth century has given momentum to the concept of pain as a sensation and has overshadowed the role of affective and motivational processes. The sensory approach to pain, however, valuable as it has been, fails to provide a complete picture of pain processes. The neglect of the motivational features of pain underscores a serious schism in pain research. Characteristically, textbooks in psychology and physiology deal with 'pain sensation' in one section and 'aversive drives and punishment' in another, with no indication that both are facets of the same phenomenon. This separation reflects the widespread acceptance of von Frey's specificity theory of pain, with its implicit psychological assumption that 'pain impulses' are transmitted from specific pain receptors in the skin directly to a pain centre in the brain.

The assumption that pain is a primary sensation has relegated motivational (and cognitive) processes to the role of 'reactions to pain' (Figure 29), and has made them only 'secondary considerations' in the whole pain process (Sweet, 1959). It is apparent, however, that sensory, motivational, and cognitive processes occur in parallel, interacting systems at the same time. As we noted in Chapter 7, motivational-affective processes must be included in any satisfactory theory of pain.

Evaluation of the theories

When we consider all the theories examined so far, we see that the 'specific-modality' and 'pattern' concepts of pain, although they appear to be mutually exclusive, both contain valuable concepts that supplement one another. Recognition of receptor specialization for the transduction of particular kinds and ranges of cutaneous stimulation does not preclude acceptance of the concept that the information generated by skin receptors is coded in the form of patterns of nerve impulses. The law of the adequate stimulus can be retained without also accepting a narrow, fixed relationship between receptor specialization and perceptual experience.

It is clear that von Frey made an important contribution that must be retained in any theoretical formulation. He proposed that the receptors of the skin are not all alike but are differentiated with respect to lowest threshold to particular energy categories. This concept of receptor specialization continues to play a salient role in sensory physiology and psychology. Indeed, the recent evidence indicates a greater degree of receptor specialization than von Frey himself could ever have foreseen. The theory, however, encounters serious difficulties. It implies a narrow one-to-one relationship between psychological sensory dimensions and physical stimulus dimensions that is inadmissible in view of our current knowledge about pain.

Similarly, there can no longer be any doubt that temporal and spatial patterns of nerve impulses provide the basis of our sensory perceptions. The coding of information in the form of nerve impulse patterns is a fundamental concept in contemporary neurophysiology and psychology. Yet the peripheral pattern theory formulated by Weddell and Sinclair fails to provide an adequate account of pain mechanisms. It does not recognize the facts of physiological specialization. It does not specify the kinds of patterns that might be related to pain. It provides no hypothesis to account for the detection of patterns by central cells. Thus, because of its vagueness, the theory falls short of being a satisfactory formulation of pain phenomena.

In contrast, the concepts of central summation and input control have shown remarkable power in their ability to explain many of the clinical phenomena of pain. Goldscheider's emphasis on central summation mechanisms is supported by the clinical observations of extraordinary temporal and spatial summation in pathological pain syndromes. Livingston's theory of spinal reverberatory activity that persists in the absence of noxious input provides a satisfactory explanation of prolonged pain. Noordenbos' concept that large fibres inhibit activity in small fibres is supported by the evidence that pathological pain is often associated with a loss of large myelinated fibres. These theories, nevertheless, fail to comprise a satisfactory general theory of pain. They lack unity, and no single theory has yet been proposed that integrates the diverse theoretical mechanisms.

However, when all the theories – from specificity theory onward – are examined together (Figure 30), it is apparent that each successive theory makes an important contribution. Each

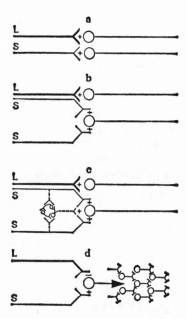

Figure 30. Schematic representation of conceptual models of pain mechanisms –
a, von Frey's specificity theory. Large (L) and small (S) fibres are assumed
to transmit touch and pain impulses respectively, in separate, specific, straight-
through pathways to touch and pain centres in the brain – b, Goldscheider's
summation theory, showing convergence of small fibres onto a dorsal horn
cell. Touch is assumed to be carried by large fibres – c, Livingston's (1943)
conceptual model of reverberatory circuits underlying pathological pain
states. Prolonged activity in the self-exciting chain of neurons bombards the
dorsal horn cell, which transmits abnormally patterned volleys of nerve
impulses to the brain – d, Noordenbos' (1959) sensory interaction theory, in
which large fibres inhibit (–) and small fibres excite (+) central transmission neurons. The output projects to spinal cord neurons which
are conceived by Noordenbos to comprise a Multi-synaptic Afferent
System. (from Melzack and Wall, 1970, p.3)

provides an additional mechanism to explain some of the complex
clinical syndromes or experimental data that were previously inexplicable. Despite the seemingly small differences, each change
contains a major conceptual idea that has had a powerful impact
on research and therapy.

On the concept of 'specificity'

The concept of 'specificity' lies at the heart of the controversy that surrounds the evolution of pain theories. It is essential, therefore, that we conclude by examining the concept in order to state unequivocally what we mean by it. Throughout this chapter, we have distinguished between *physiological specialization* and *psychological specificity*.The former is an indisputable fact; the latter is a theory for which there is no evidence. Neurons in the nervous system are *specialized* to conduct patterns of nerve impulses that can be recorded and displayed. But no neurons in the somatic projection system are indisputably linked to a single, specific psychological experience. Despite our attempts to establish this distinction (Melzack and Wall, 1962, 1965), many of our colleagues have failed to understand the distinction or continue to use the word 'specificity' in the sense of specialization but without saying so. If we can all agree that 'specificity' means physiological specialization, *without* implying that specialized neurons *must* give rise to the experience of pain and *only* to pain, or that pain can *never* occur unless they are activated, then we will have eliminated a major source of unnecessary controversy.

To help us move toward that goal, let us consider the term 'specificity' in the two ways in which it is used. The first is in the sense of 'diagnosis' and the second is in the sense of 'prognosis'. The first is correct; the second is wrong. Diagnosis means 'scientific determination' or 'a description which classifies precisely' (Random House Dictionary). When a scientist records the activity of a nerve fibre anywhere in the peripheral or central nervous system, and relates the activity to particular stimuli, he is carrying out a scientific diagnosis or classification. All neurons in the somatic sensory system can be classified in this scientific, objective way. However, when he makes a prognosis – that is, tries to *predict* the eventual psychological experience – he makes an untenable assumption. When he says that certain receptors or neurons inevitably give rise to the experience of pain, he attempts to predict the final outcome of the activity – and there are *no* experiments that demonstrate this relationship. For example, the stimulation of a single small-diameter nerve fibre *may* give rise to pain, but that demonstration does not show that the nerve fibre gives rise only to pain and is involved in no other experience. There is only one conclusion: 'specificity' in the diagnostic sense is scientifically correct; in the prognostic sense it is without scientific foundation.

10
The Gate-Control
Theory of Pain

The analysis of the strengths and weaknesses of the theories of pain described in Chapter 9 illuminates the requirements of a satisfactory new theory. Any new theory of pain, it is now apparent, must be able to account for:

1 The high degree of physiological specialization of receptor-fibre units and of pathways in the central nervous system.
2 The role of temporal and spatial patterning in the transmission of information in the nervous system.
3 The influence of psychological processes on pain perception and response.
4 The clinical phenomena of spatial and temporal summation, spread of pain, and persistence of pain after healing.

In 1965, we proposed the *gate-control theory* in the attempt to integrate these requirements into a comprehensive theory of pain. Basically, the theory proposes that a neural mechanism in the dorsal horns of the spinal cord acts like a gate which can increase or decrease the flow of nerve impulses from peripheral fibres to the central nervous system. Somatic input is therefore subjected to the modulating influence of the gate before it evokes pain perception and response. The degree to which the gate increases or decreases sensory transmission is determined by the relative activity in large-diameter (A-beta) and small-diameter (A-delta and C) fibres and by descending influences from the brain. When the amount of information that passes through the gate exceeds a critical level, it activates the neural areas responsible for pain experience and response. Like all theories, the gate-control theory has two facets: a *conceptual model* which is the basis of the theory, and particular *explanatory mechanisms* which are evoked to show how the model functions. The conceptual model will be described first, followed by a description of the impact of the theory and the status of recent explanatory mechanisms.

The conceptual model

The conceptual components of the gate-control theory can be described in a series of diagrams that reflect the increasing complexity of our knowledge of pain mechanisms. Each component represents a body of factual knowledge or, when there is a gap in our knowledge, a hypothetical construct. In these diagrams, the sign ⊢ on the end of a fibre system simply indicates the direction of flow of the effect from one system to the next. It is not meant to indicate a simple synapse or to imply that the effect is pre-synaptic or post-synaptic.

Any theory of pain must begin with the well-known fact that injury produces signals that are transmitted by the small-diameter (S) fibres – the A-delta and C fibres. These fibres penetrate the dorsal horns of the spinal cord and activate transmission (T) cells that project the signals to the brain. This component of the theory can be drawn as follows:

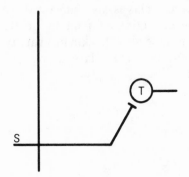

However, activity in small fibres also produces dorsal root potentials that reflect more complex, prolonged activity in the dorsal horn (Wall, 1964). Branches of the small fibres activate the cells of the substantia gelatinosa (SG) which are presumed to facilitate transmission from S fibres to T cells (Wall, 1964). The 'wind-up' effect (Mendell and Wall, 1965), in which successive stimuli produce increasingly larger and longer-lasting bursts of nerve impulses, suggests that complex arrangements of the SG cells may underlie these facilitatory effects. The activation of SG cells in addition to T cells is shown in the following diagram:

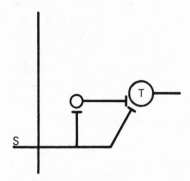

We also know that the large-diameter (L) fibres are able to fire one of the types of transmission cells that is activated by S fibres (Wall, 1978). In this case, the inputs from both the L and the S fibres will summate with each other. This is also suggested by clinical observations such as the elicitation of pain by gentle touches on hyperaesthetic (but otherwise normal) skin in a variety of neuralgic or referred-pain syndromes. These large fibres can be shown as impinging on T cells:

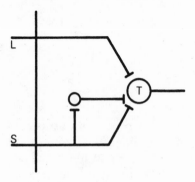

Large-fibre activity, we now know, also activates cells in the substantia gelatinosa (Wall, 1980 a, b) and, at the same time, inhibits transmission from afferent fibres to T cells (Wall, 1964; Hillman and Wall, 1969). It is assumed that this inhibition is mediated by SG cells. This inhibitory process can therefore be added to the conceptual model that has evolved as new evidence has accumulated:

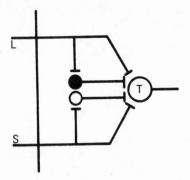

Finally, there is now indisputable evidence that cells in the brainstem, including those in the periaqueductal grey and nucleus raphe magnus, exert powerful inhibitory effects on transmission from afferent fibres to T cells, and that these act primarily on inputs evoked by injury or noxious levels of stimulation. It is assumed that these inhibitory effects are also mediated by inhibitory neurons in the substantia gelatinosa, and are therefore included in the last diagram of the series:

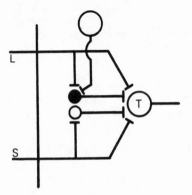

We now have all the ingredients of a conceptual model for pain. They are the basis of the gate-control theory of pain which was first proposed in 1965 and can now be revised on the basis of the recent physiological evidence described in Chapter 6.

Gate-control theory: mark 1

The first formulation of the gate-control theory in 1965 utilized the schematic model shown in Figure 31.

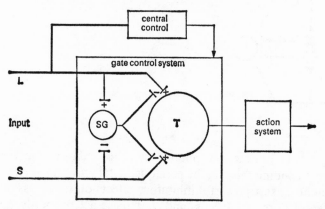

Figure 31. Schematic diagram of the gate-control theory of pain (Mark 1): L, the large-diameter fibres; S, the small-diameter fibres. The fibres project to the substantia gelatinosa (SG) and first central transmission (T) cells. The inhibitory effect exerted by SG on the afferent fibre terminals is increased by activity in L fibres and decreased by activity in S fibres. The central control trigger is represented by a line running from the large fibre system to the central control mechanisms; these mechanisms, in turn, project back to the gate-control system. The T cells project to the action system. +, excitation; −, inhibition. (from Melzack and Wall, 1965, p.971)

The model is based on the following propositions:
1 The transmission of nerve impulses from afferent fibres to spinal cord transmission (T) cells is modulated by a spinal gating mechanism in the dorsal horns.
2 The spinal gating mechanism is influenced by the relative amount of activity in large-diameter (L) and small-diameter (S)

fibres: activity in large fibres tends to inhibit transmission (close the gate) while small-fibre activity tends to facilitate transmission (open the gate).

3 The spinal gating mechanism is influenced by nerve impulses that descend from the brain.

4 A specialized system of large-diameter, rapidly conducting fibres (the Central Control Trigger) activates selective cognitive processes that then influence, by way of descending fibres, the modulating properties of the spinal gating mechanism.

5 When the output of the spinal cord transmission (T) cells exceeds a critical level, it activates the Action System – those neural areas that underlie the complex, sequential patterns of behaviour and experience characteristic of pain.

Spinal gating mechanism

The variable link between injury and pain described in earlier chapters indicates that a neural mechanism must exist which permits modulation of the input *before* pain is experienced. As we have seen, injury may occur without pain being felt, and pain is sometimes felt in parts of the body that have not been injured. Psychological factors can inhibit or enhance pain, and innocuous sensory inputs, such as gentle rubbing or heat, can similarly affect pain. For example, gentle massage of an injured area may decrease the pain, while even gentler touches of hyperalgesic skin of patients with post-herpetic neuralgia can produce excruciating pain. Obviously, the injury signals can be facilitated or inhibited by sensory inputs and by psychological factors so that pain is increased, decreased, or even abolished. In short, there appears to be a variable gate interposed between the sensory input and those areas in the brain that subserve the experience of pain.

The physiological evidence described in Chapter 6 suggests that the substantia gelatinosa is one of the likely sites of the spinal gating mechanism. It receives axons directly and indirectly from many of the large- and small-diameter fibres and the dendrites of cells in deeper laminae project into it (Figure 32). The substantia gelatinosa, moreover, forms a functional unit that extends the length of the spinal cord on each side. Its cells connect with one another by short fibres, and influence each other at

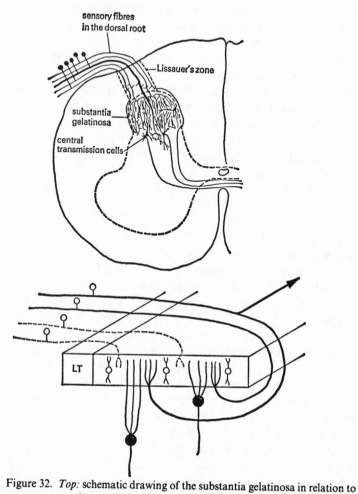

Figure 32. *Top:* schematic drawing of the substantia gelatinosa in relation to somatosensory fibres and dorsal horn cells that project their axons across the cord to the anterolateral pathway. (after Pearson, 1952, p.515)

Bottom: main components of the cutaneous afferent system in the upper dorsal horn. The large-diameter cutaneous peripheral fibres are represented by thick lines running from the dorsal root and terminating in the region of the substantia gelatinosa; one of these, as shown, sends a branch toward the brain in the dorsal column. The finer peripheral fibres are represented by dashed lines running directly into the substantia gelatinosa. The large cells, on which cutaneous afferent nerves terminate, are shown as large black spheres with their dendrites extending into the substantia gelatinosa and their axons projecting deeper into the dorsal horn. The open circles represent the cells of the substantia gelatinosa. The axons (not shown) of these cells connect them to one another and also run in the Lissauer tract (L T) to distant parts of the substantia gelatinosa. (adapted from Wall, 1964, p.92)

distant sites on the same side by means of Lissauer's tract and on the opposite side by means of commissural fibres that cross the cord (Szentagothai, 1964; Wall, 1964). The substantia gelatinosa, then, consists of a highly specialized, closed system of cells throughout the length of the spinal cord on both sides; it receives afferent input from large and small fibres, and is able to influence the activity of cells that project to the brain. Melzack and Wall (1965) have proposed, therefore, that it acts as a spinal gating mechanism by modulating the conduction of nerve impulses from peripheral fibres to spinal cord transmission cells.

The properties of the cells in lamina 5 suggest that they are the spinal transmission (T) cells that are most likely to play a critical role in pain perception and response (Hillman and Wall, 1969). They receive inputs from the small afferent fibres from skin, viscera and muscles, and their activity is influenced by fibres that descend from the brain. They respond to a wide range of stimulus intensities, and show increasing firing rates to increasing intensities of stimulation. Furthermore, their output is influenced by the relative activity in large and small fibres.

Effects of activity in large and small fibres
The theory proposes that sensory fibres transmit patterned information, depending on the specialized properties of each receptor-fibre unit, about pressure, temperature, and chemical changes at the skin. These temporal and spatial patterns of nerve impulses have two effects at the dorsal horns: they excite the spinal cord T cells that project the information to the brain, and they activate the substantia gelatinosa which modulates or 'gates' the *amount* of information projected to the brain by the T cells.

Hillman and Wall (1969) showed that activity in large fibres produces a burst of activity in lamina 5 cells followed by a period of inhibition. In contrast, activity in small fibres activates the cells and then produces prolonged activity and a facilitation of subsequent inputs (the 'wind-up' effect). The evidence, then, suggests that transmission in the dorsal horns is controlled by a spinal gating mechanism which is in turn controlled by the rival effects of large versus small afferent fibres.

There are two ways in which the cells of the substantia gelatinosa can act as a gating mechanism that influences the transmission of impulses from afferent fibre terminals to spinal cord cells (Melzack and Wall, 1970). They can act directly on the presynaptic axon terminals and thereby block the impulses in the terminals or decrease the amount of transmitter substance which they release; or they can act postsynaptically on the spinal transmission cells by increasing or decreasing their level of excitability to arriving nerve impulses. In 1965 we proposed that both effects occur, but emphasized presynaptic effects in the model because evidence for postsynaptic action was lacking. But it is now certain (Hongo, Jankowska and Lundberg, 1968) that modulating effects are also exerted postsynaptically on the spinal transmission cells. The evidence, in other words, indicates that the presynapatic control exists but that it is coupled with a simultaneous change in the postsynaptic transmission cells.

The small (A-delta and C) fibres, in this conceptual framework, play a highly specialized and important role in pain processes. They activate the T cells directly and contribute to their output. The activity of high-threshold small fibres, during intense stimulation, may be especially important in raising the T-cell output above the critical level necessary for pain. But the small fibres are believed to do much more than this. They facilitate transmission ('open the gate') and thereby provide the basis for summation, prolonged activity, and spread of pain to other body areas. This facilitatory influence provides the small fibres with greater power than any envisaged in the concept of 'pain fibres'. Yet at the same time the small-fibre impulses are susceptible to modulation by activities in the whole nervous system. This multifaceted role of the small fibres is consistent with the psychological, clinical, and physiological evidence.

Descending influences on the gate-control system

The evidence described in Chapter 2 shows that cognitive or 'higher central nervous system processes' such as attention, anxiety, anticipation, and past experience exert a powerful influence on pain processes. It is also firmly established (Chapter 7) that stimulation of the brain activates descending efferent fibres which can influence afferent conduction at the earliest synaptic levels of the somaesthetic system. Thus it is possible for brain activities subserving attention, emotion and memories of prior experience to exert control over the sensory input. This control of spinal cord transmission by the brain may be exerted through several systems.

Reticular projections. The brainstem reticular formation, particularly the midbrain reticular areas (Hagbarth and Kerr, 1954; Taub, 1964), exert a powerful inhibitory control over information projected by the spinal transmission cells. The inhibition of activity in lamina 5 cells by descending fibres from the brain (Hillman and Wall, 1969) is at least partly due to reticulo-spinal influences on the dorsal horn gating system. This descending inhibitory projection is itself controlled by multiple influences. Somatic projections comprise the largest input to the midbrain reticular formation. There are also projections from the visual and auditory systems (Rossi and Zanchetti, 1957). In this way, somatic inputs from all parts of the body, as well as visual and auditory inputs, are able to exert a modulating influence on transmission through the dorsal horns.

Cortical projections. Fibres from the whole cortex, particularly the frontal cortex, project to the reticular formation. Cognitive processes such as past experience and attention, which are subserved at least in part by cortical neural activity, are therefore able to influence spinal activities by way of the reticulo-spinal projection system. Cognitive processes can also influence spinal gating mechanisms by means of pyramidal (or cortico-spinal) fibres, which are known to project to the dorsal horns as well as to other spinal areas. These are large, fast-conducting fibres so that cognitive processes can rapidly and directly modulate neural transmission in the dorsal horns.

Concept of a central control trigger. It is apparent that the influence of cognitive or 'central control' processes on spinal transmission are mediated, in part at least, through the gate-control system. While some central activities, such as anxiety or excitement, may open or close the gate for all inputs from any part of the body, others obviously involve selective, localized gate activity. The observations by Pavlov (1927, 1928) and Beecher (1959) described in earlier chapters suggest that signals from the body must be identified, evaluated in terms of prior experience, localized, and inhibited *before* the action system responsible for pain perception and response is activated.

We have therefore proposed that there exists in the nervous system a mechanism, which we have called the *central control trigger*, that activates the particular, selective brain processes that exert control over the sensory input (Figure 31). We suggest that the dorsal-column–medial-lemniscal and dorso-lateral systems could fulfil the functions of the central control trigger. The dorsal column projection system in particular has grown apace with the cerebral cortex (Bishop, 1959), carries precise information about the nature and location of the stimulus, adapts quickly to give precedence to phasic stimulus changes rather than prolonged tonic activity, and conducts so rapidly that it may not only set the receptivity of cortical neurons for subsequent afferent volleys but may also act, by way of central-control efferent fibres, on the gate-control system. Part, at least, of their functions, then, could be to activate selective brain processes such as memories of prior experience and pre-set response strategies that influence information which is still arriving over slowly conducting fibres or is being transmitted up more slowly conducting pathways.

Action system

The gate-control theory proposes that the action system responsible for pain experience and response is triggered when the integrated firing level of the dorsal horn T cells reaches or exceeds a critical level. Pain, as we have seen, does not consist of a single ring of the appropriate central bell, but is an ongoing process comprising a sequence of responses by the action system, beginning with a series of reflex responses and continuing with complex strategies to terminate the pain.

We propose, then, that the triggering of the action system by the T cells marks the beginning of the sequence of activities that occur when the body sustains damage. The input has access to neural systems involved in affective as well as sensory activities. It is presumed that interactions occur among all these systems as the organism interacts with the environment.

We believe that the interactions between the gate-control system and the action system described above may occur at successive synapses at any level of the central nervous system in the course of filtering of the sensory input. Similarly, the influence of central activities on the sensory input may take place at a series of levels. The gate-control system may be set and reset a number of times as the temporal and spatial patterning of the input is analysed and acted on by the brain.

The impact of the gate-control theory

The immediate effect of the theory was to evoke controversy among scientists and clinicians in the field of pain. One group accepted the theory as a major breakthrough while a second group considered it a dangerous threat to the established specificity theory. The gate theory received accolades and vituperation. The eminent anaesthesiologist John J. Bonica called the theory 'undoubtedly one of the major revolutions in our concept of pain in the last 100 years' (Cherry, 1977, p.13). Liebeskind and Paul (1977, p.41), in the attempt to find reasons for the recent explosion of interest in pain research, wrote that, 'Probably the most important was the appearance in 1965 of the gate-control theory of pain by Melzack and Wall. This theory . . . has . . . like none before it, proved enormously heuristic. It continues to inspire basic research and clinical applications.' The interest generated by the theory is reflected by the fact that, of more than 2 million articles in all basic (non-applied) medical fields published in the 1960s, the paper that described the gate-control theory is among the 100 most cited papers. It is eighth of the 11 most cited papers in the neurosciences (Garfield, 1980).

However, while the theory had its proponents, it also provoked outrage in believers of the old specificity theory. A welcome nine-teenth-century virulence appeared in the literature. 'The gate-control theory of pain: an unlikely hypothesis' was the title of one paper (Schmidt, 1972). In another we find the sentence, 'I think therefore that one ought at this stage to strongly support Schmidt in his attempt to prevent the Gate Hypothesis from taking root in the field of neurology' (Iggo, 1972, p.127). These responses were modified when this group of careful experimenters observed modulation of spinal signals evoked by injury-detecting afferents (Cervero *et al.*, 1976; Handwerker *et al.*, 1975).

Spirited defences by the 'Old Believers' still appear in textbooks (Mountcastle, 1980), but the facts are available in the literature for those who prefer them to propaganda. It is perhaps a little tedious that one must refer to the original papers or to the phenomena themselves. In a lyrical review, Dykes (1975) attacked the gate-control theory: 'In addition to its dubious veracity, the theory is incomplete.' To prove his point, he quoted Denny-Brown *et al.* (1973) twice as arguing that 'the input of both large and small fibres to the dorsal horn regulate relays through the region without requiring a gate mechanism'. A glance at the papers in the series (Kirk and Denny-Brown, 1970; Denny-Brown *et al.*, 1973) shows that the authors in fact are quite specific in using the exact gating mechanism we adopted. One may hope that this period of vituperation will pass into a more mundane but constructive time.

We formulated a hypothesis that seemed to us to bring together all the facts available in 1965. Since that time much has changed. Some of the 'facts' were wrong. Much more is now known.

Gate-control theory: mark II

A simple diagram of pain mechanisms is the barest reflection of the beautiful and purposeful complexity of the real nervous system. It involves simplification of the detailed facts revealed by our work and by the many outstanding teams of researchers whose work was briefly reviewed in Chapters 6 and 7. Since we are the authors of an old, frequently reproduced diagram, we will now attempt to modify it to incorporate new facts and ideas. We need to make three changes (Figure 33), and later we must add a completely new dimension. First, we need to emphasize the multiple functions of the SG by showing that it contains both excitatory and inhibitory links. Therefore, we show (Figure 33) two types of SG cells: an excitatory one (white circle) and an inhibitory one (black circle). Second, since we still do not know the mechanism of this inhibition and since the original diagram was read incorrectly as implying a purely presynaptic mechanism, we place a bar on the end of the inhibitory link to emphasize that its action could be presynaptic, postsynaptic or both. Lastly, the growing evidence of a powerful brainstem inhibitory system which is influenced by the sensory input after transmission through the gate and which projects back to the dorsal horn is emphasized by including it as a separate input to the gate.

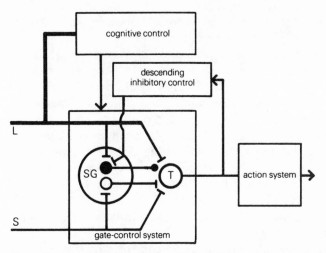

Figure 33. The gate-control theory: Mark II. The new model includes excitatory (white circle) and inhibitory (black circle) links from the substantia gelatinosa (SG) to the transmission (T) cells as well as descending inhibitory control from brainstem systems. The round knob at the end of the inhibitory link implies that its action may be presynaptic, postsynaptic, or both. All connections are excitatory, except the inhibitory link from SG to T cell.

Figure 33, therefore, presents the revised conceptual model of the gate theory (Mark II) that incorporates some of the recent evidence. The new dimension will be discussed at the end of this chapter. However, it must be kept in mind that the field is still in a state of flux and further revisions of the explanatory mechanisms may be necessary. Despite the revisions, the conceptual model of gating and the propositions that underlie it remain valid. Clearly, we do not imply that the gate theory is the final 'truth' about pain. However, a satisfactory alternative to the theory has not yet been proposed. Those who wish to abolish the gate theory have not come up with a reasonable alternative that advances the field but, rather, have sought to return to the comfort of the orthodox specificity model.

We wish to emphasize that the assumption that the substantia gelatinosa is the primary vehicle for gating remains an assumption and is not yet fact. The anatomical evidence accumulated since 1965 (and described in Chapter 6) confirms and extends the possible role of SG cells as modulators in the transfer of impulses from peripheral nerves to the large dorsal horn cells whose axons transmit the information to the ventral horn, to distant segments and to the brain. In addition, physiological recording in the substantia gelatinosa of the cells' responses to peripheral stimuli shows that the cells have many interesting characteristics which do not themselves seem to be transmitted along the long-range pathways. Stimulation of the Lissauer tract produces changes of the membrane potential of afferents, changes of reflex excitability, and inhibition of transmitting cells. Lesions of the Lissauer tract influence the excitability and size of dermatomes in monkeys. This combination of effects would seem to add up to strong supportive evidence that the substantia gelatinosa constitutes a gate control. However the most fascinating questions remain.

If the substantia gelatinosa is a gate control, why is it so complex? If the only function of the substantia gelatinosa is to modulate the transmission of nociceptive impulses, this could surely be carried out by a small number of cells. A simple gain control mechanism would need very little circuitry. It is important to speculate on the complexity in the region because only in this way will hypotheses and their testing experiments be generated. We must not make the mistake of isolating nociceptive impulses and the sensation of pain from all other aspects of somatosensory mechanisms. To do so would be as silly and illogical as to study the perception of the colour red as though the underlying mechanism could be discovered in isolation from mechanisms involved with other colours, shapes and intensities which combine to make the richness of the visual world. We should therefore expect a gate control to be operating on all aspects of the arriving information. Furthermore, it is highly unlikely to be a simple gain control but more likely to control and emphasize different aspects of the arriving messages with the emphasis changing from moment to moment.

In our initial paper we spoke for simplicity of the antagonism between large and small fibres. This physiological observation has been extended to all the examples so far discovered of cells which receive nociceptive afferents. However this is an arbitrary fact and what is needed is some biologically useful function. Hillman and Wall (1969) showed for lamina 5 cells that the meaning of the antagonism was to generate an inhibitory surround. It is reasonable to assume that such a mechanism increases the spatial resolution of the transmission system just as it does in the eye. Furthermore, they showed that the intensity of the action of the inhibitory surround was under descending control. Evidently the control mechanism is likely to be involved not only in modality and intensity control but also in spatial resolution.

One apparent complexity of the substantia gelatinosa (SG) rapidly leads to a considerable simplification. There is now good anatomical and physiological evidence that far from being a loosely organized neuropil, the SG and the underlying large cells are highly spatially organized in a somatotopic map. Entering afferent fibres give rise to ascending and descending branches that run in rostrocaudal directions. These run in remarkably straight lines emitting clusters of terminals as they proceed. Matching this organization of afferents, the cells of lamina 4 send dendrites into laminae 2 and 3, and these dendrites form a flat fan which is also rostrocaudally oriented. If the receptive fields of the SG cells or lamina 4 or 5 cells are plotted, it is found that the most lateral cells are concerned with the most proximal part of the dermatome and the most medial cells have their receptive fields in the most distal part of the dermatome. Thus an electrode moving from lateral to medial encounters first cells with proximal receptive fields and then cells with more and more distal receptive fields. If an electrode penetrates vertically through lamina 2, clusters of small cells are found with small receptive fields grouped on the same region of skin. Then a large cell is encountered immediately ventral to the small cells and its receptive field encompasses all those of the small cells. A picture is emerging of the SG with a series of mediolateral compartments each one handling a small area of skin.

Systems known to descend in the dorsolateral pathway which might send terminals into the SG originate from a wide variety of brain structures: raphe nuclei, reticular formation, trigeminal nuclei, vestibular nuclei, cerebral cortex and hypothalamus. Many of these are, of course, highly differentially organized systems and it would be quite wrong to assign to each a single, simple task. Therefore descending orders could be quite specific in terms of how they modulate particular modalities of afferent input and in terms of their spatial effect. The area is potentially structured to establish a detailed filter or template which selectively transmits particular types of information from particular locations.

The new dimension

We would like to raise what seems to us to be a paradox. Why is it that vertebrates retain unmyelinated afferent fibres when they are clearly capable of growing myelinated fibres. All of the information collected by the unmyelinated fibres is also present in myelinated fibres. Yet the two types exist and apparently terminate in different areas of the cord. The paradox is particularly peculiar when one considers large animals such as the horse or giraffe, whose unmyelinated fibres take several seconds to deliver information from foot to spinal cord. A possible solution to this paradox is that our sensory experience derives from fast and slow systems which have quite different functions. Just as every motor movement starts from a platform – the posture – so, too, the rapid signalling of events must also occur on a background setting of the sensory systems. The rules and mechanisms of this sensory background setting would be very different from those of the fast signalling system. One of the possible rules might be that it could change relatively slowly and hold its setting for long periods. Under these circumstances where speed is not at a premium, C fibres might be quite adequate. Furthermore, we might expect long lasting changes and should design our experiments to detect them. Could it be that the substantia gelatinosa is the first stage of just such a sensory background setting system rather than being itself a fast transmission system?

Models of the adult brain classically depict streams of nerve impulses which flow and interact over stable anatomical structures. We now suspect that there is a further dimension which could explain slow changes and plasticity of connections. Nerve fibres carry not only nerve impulses but also chemical substances which are transported and released relatively slowly. The unmyelinated afferent fibres are particularly rich in peptides and the concentrations of these substances change slowly for several days following a peripheral nerve injury. The substantia gelatinosa also contains a galaxy of peptides including the enkephalins and at least eight others. When peripheral nerves are damaged or poisoned, there is a slow change in the terminals of the fine fibres in the spinal cord and a coincident disappearance of inhibition; at the same time, there is an enormous expansion of the receptive fields of the transmitting cells. It seems highly likely that nerves are able to control the routing of nerve impulses into the central nervous system by a mechanism which depends on the slow transport and release of chemicals, in addition to the very rapid transport and action of nerve impulses. This may mean that much of the stable anatomical substrate over which nerve impulses could flow is kept inactive by these slowly shifting processes. The concept of ineffective synapses (Wall, 1977) which can be made effective and released by the slowly shifting action of cells of the substantia gelatinosa adds a new dimension to the gate-control theory.

11
Implications of the Gate-Control Theory

The major impact of the gate-control theory, initially, was to free the field of pain from the straitjacket of specificity theory. Physicians who knew perfectly well that pain in the clinic often failed to conform to the rigid textbook model felt freer to describe unusual cases or inexplicable phenomena. Psychologists suddenly found a model which placed psychological observations and techniques in the mainstream of pain research. Physiologists began to explore regions of the spinal cord and brain that were previously held to play no role in pain and discovered complex mechanisms and relationships that were hitherto unsuspected. The transmission of pain signals to the brain was no longer restricted to a single pathway and it became possible to speculate on the functional relations among different ascending and descending systems. The main beneficiary of all this activity has been the suffering person, and the impact of recent discoveries on the treatment of pain will be discussed in later chapters. This chapter will deal with the basic implications of the gate theory.

Parallel processing systems: the dimensions of pain

One of the first effects of the gate theory was to destroy the idea that pain is a simple sensation subserved by a direct transmission line to a pain centre. The concept of pain as purely a sensory experience long overshadowed the affective and cognitive dimensions of the total pain experience. Typically, physiological and psychological textbooks dealt with 'pain' in one chapter and 'aversive drives' in another, as though both were entirely different processes. The gate theory, however, with its emphasis on parallel processing systems, provided the conceptual framework for integration of the sensory, affective and cognitive dimensions of pain.

The gate-control theory proposes that the action system responsible for pain experience and response is triggered when the integrated firing level of the dorsal horn T cells reaches or exceeds a critical level. Melzack and Casey (1968) have noted that the output of the T cells is transmitted towards the brain primarily by fibres in the ventrolateral spinal cord and is projected into two major brain systems: via neospinothalamic fibres into the ventrobasal thalamus and somatosensory cortex, and via medially coursing fibres into the reticular formation, the medial and intralaminar thalamus and the limbic system. Stimulation at noxious intensities evokes activity in both projection systems, and discrete lesions in each may strikingly alter pain perception and response (Chapter 7).

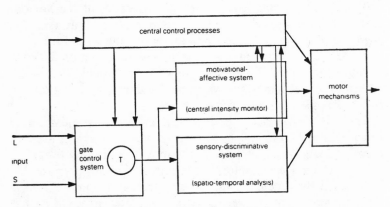

Figure 34. Conceptual model of the sensory, motivational and central control determinants of pain. The output of the T cells of the gate-control system projects to the sensory-discriminative system (via neospinothalamic fibres) and the motivational-affective system (via the paramedial ascending system). The central control trigger is represented by a line running from the large fibre system to central control processes; these, in turn, project back to the gate-control system, and to the sensory-discriminative and motivational-affective systems. All three systems interact with one another, and project to the motor system.
(from Melzack and Casey, 1968)

Behavioural and physiological studies led Melzack and Casey (1968) to propose (Figure 34) that:

1 The selection and modulation of the sensory input through the neospinothalamic projection system provides, in part at least, the neurological basis of the sensory-discriminative dimension of pain.

2 Activation of reticular and limbic structures underlies the powerful motivational drive and unpleasant affect that trigger the organism into action.

3 Neocortical or higher central nervous system processes, such as evaluation of the input in terms of past experience, exert control over activity in both the discriminative and motivational systems.

It is assumed that these three categories of activity interact with one another to provide *perceptual information* regarding the location, magnitude, and spatiotemporal properties of the noxious stimulus, *motivational tendency* toward escape or attack, and *cognitive information* based on analysis of multimodal information, past experience, and probability of outcome of different response strategies. All three forms of activity could then influence motor mechanisms responsible for the complex pattern of overt responses that characterize pain.

There is a convincing body of evidence that stimulation of reticular and limbic system structures produces strong aversive drive and behaviour typical of responses to naturally occurring painful stimuli (see Chapter 7). Melzack and Casey propose that portions of the reticular and limbic systems function as a *central intensity monitor*: that their activities are determined, in part at least, by the intensity of the T-cell output (the total number of active fibres and their rate of firing) after it has undergone modulation by the gate-control system in the dorsal horns. The cells in the midbrain reticular formation are capable of summation of input from spatially separate body sites (Bell *et al.*, 1964); furthermore, the post-stimulus discharge activity of some of these cells lasts for many seconds (Casey, 1966), so that their activity may provide a measure of the intensity of the total T-cell output over relatively long periods of time. Essentially, both kinds of summation transform discrete spatial and temporal information into intensity information. Melzack and Casey propose that the output of these cells, up to a critical intensity level, activates those brain areas subserving positive affect and approach tendency. Beyond that level, the output activates areas underlying negative affect and aversive drive.

The complex sequences of behaviour that characterize pain are determined by sensory, motivational, and cognitive processes that act on motor mechanisms. By 'motor mechanisms' (Figure 34), Melzack and Casey mean all of the brain areas that contribute to overt behavioural response patterns. These areas extend throughout the whole of the central nervous system, and their organization must be at least as complex as that of the input systems we have primarily dealt with so far. Even 'simple' reflexes, which are generally thought to be entirely spinal in their organization, are now known to be influenced by cognitive processes: if we pick up a hot cup of tea in an expensive cup we are not likely to simply drop the cup, but jerkily put it back on the table, and *then* nurse our hand.

Ascending-descending interactions

By eliminating the concept of a single, straight-through pain pathway, the gate theory opened the way to speculation about the interactions among ascending and descending systems. Dennis and Melzack (1977) propose that the laterally projecting pathways (described in Chapter 7) – the spinocervical, neospinothalamic, and dorsal column postsynaptic tracts – are eminently suited for rapid transmission of *phasic* information, such as the onset of injury or sudden changes in a damaged area. This information can be precisely localized and quickly bring about responses to prevent any further damage. In contrast, the medially projecting pathways – the spinoreticular, paleospinothalamic and propriospinal systems – seem best adapted to carry *tonic* information about the state of the organism. They signal the actual presence of peripheral damage and continue to send that message as long as the wound is susceptible to re-injury.

An intriguing question is why there are three rapidly conducting systems which are all capable of carrying information about pain, touch and proprioception. Dennis and Melzack (1977) sug-

gest that these pathways may be individually inhibited or facilitated depending on the ongoing behavioural state or particular
behavioural activity. Injury or attack may occur under many
circumstances – while the person or animal is asleep or awake,
eating, working, exploring, or grooming. In all of these activities,
the brain must continue to receive proprioceptive and tactile information in addition to nociceptive inputs. Since neurons in a
given pathway cannot carry information about all three at the
same time, it is possible that a pattern of differential inhibition
and facilitation may be imposed on the pathways. Thus, the
same noxious stimulus, occurring during different behaviour patterns, might evoke impulses in different pathways. A nociceptive
message ascending in one pathway may trigger different responses
than the same message ascending in another pathway. In this
way, depending on the behavioural state and activity at the
moment of injury, the brain can always extract the proprioceptive
and tactile information necessary for adaptive responses and still
continue to receive information about the nature and extent of
the injury. The particular pathways which are activated would
depend on descending controls from the brain as well as interactions among the pathways.

Hypotheses on the functions of the various ascending pathways
are not mutually exclusive. The possibility that the fast and slow
pathways have a differential role in phasic and tonic types of
pain does not exclude them from playing a role in sensory-
discriminative and motivational-affective processes. In fact,
people who receive a sudden injury use few affective words on the
McGill Pain Questionnaire while prolonged pain is usually characterized by a high proportion of such words (Melzack, Wall and
Ty, 1982). It is best to consider the fast and slow systems the same
way we consider the large and small fibres in the gate theory: in
terms of their *relative* activity. Both are always active in pain-
related events, but the nature of the experience and the behaviour
may be determined by the relative activity in each system.

Convergence and summation

The gate-control theory proposes that fibres from the skin, the viscera and other structures converge onto central transmission (T) cells. The net result of all the facilitatory and inhibitory effects determines the output of the T cells. Pain associated with peripheral nerve lesions is characterized by hyperalgesia and hyperaesthesia, which are presumably due to excessive summation. Originally, in 1965, we proposed that this summation is the result of a selective loss of large fibres, which should diminish inhibition at the gate. But it is now evident that there is no simple relationship between the type of fibre loss and the presence or absence of pathological pain (or even pain insensitivity).

Wall (1978) has reviewed the recent evidence that a selective loss of large fibres is not necessarily accompanied by pain. There are even two reports (Schoene *et al.*, 1970; Comings and Amromin, 1974) of hereditary insensitivity to pain associated with a loss of large- and medium-sized myelinated fibres and with normal, preserved C fibres. It is possible that pain following a peripheral nerve lesion is due to ongoing degeneration of nerve fibres (Dyck, Lambert and O'Brien, 1976), but this cannot be the case for pain that persists several years after nerve damage. The simplest explanation is that the loss of any type of fibre sets the stage for pathological pain. As we have seen, deafferentation is typically accompanied by abnormally high firing frequencies and bursting activity. However, descending inhibition could be expected to act as a 'governor' or regulator to offset the central effects of deafferentation. That is, if there is excessive T-cell firing, the output would activate descending inhibitory fibres which would decrease firing below the critical level for pain. These compensatory inhibitory mechanisms would explain why most people, after peripheral nerve injury, have little or no pain. Happily, the majority of people do *not* develop causalgia, phantom limb pain, or post-herpetic neuralgia. But, then, why do some people develop these syndromes?

There are several possible explanations. First, the amount of fibre loss may be critical. A very large loss of fibres could produce such massive levels of central firing that they cannot be kept under control even by maximal descending inhibition. Second, the amount of sparing is important. Abnormal bursting does not occur after total section of all roots from a limb; some fibres must be spared for the abnormal firing to occur (Loeser and

Ward, 1967). This observation fits well with the fact that many of the neuralgias occur after partial nerve injury, and causalgia occurs more frequently after partial than after total peripheral nerve lesions (Sunderland, 1978). Third, the level of descending inhibition may not be sufficient to control the pathological firing activity. This may be due to individual differences in the amount of available neurotransmitters, in which factors such as aging, with its concomitant loss of peripheral and central neurons, may play a role. Fourth, some people may be more susceptible than others to developing pain after a peripheral nerve lesion. Injured fibres, as we have seen, are easily fired by noradrenalin. However, Inbal *et al.* (1980) observed that one strain of rats readily developed pain-related behaviour after a nerve lesion while another strain did not. It is possible, therefore, that genetic factors determine some aspect of the noradrenergic influence on injured fibres.

Whatever the reason why central neurons generate pain signals in some people and not in others (or at one time and not another time), it is a fact that deafferented cells have abnormal physiological properties, and – in some patients – it is reasonable to infer that inhibitory influences are insufficient to prevent summation of inputs from a variety of sources. In terms of the gate theory, the 'gate is open' (or at least unchecked), thereby providing the conditions for summation, delays, referred pain, and other characteristics of pathological pain syndromes.

The gate theory provides a conceptual basis for spontaneous pain in the absence of injury and for the convergence of inputs to allow spatial and temporal summation. The convergence of nerve impulses from the skin, viscera or muscles onto the T cells would contribute to their total output. In the absence of adequate inhibitory control after the initial T-cell discharge, successive stimuli would produce a more intense and prolonged barrage of nerve impulses after each presentation (Mendell and Wall, 1965). These mechanisms may account for the fact that non-noxious stimuli, such as a series of gentle touches or applications of a warm test-tube, can trigger severe pain in patients suffering phantom limb pain, causalgia and the neuralgias.

Spontaneous pain, which occurs in the absence of any obvious stimulation, can also be explained. The spontaneous activity generated by deafferented central cells would be transmitted unchecked and would produce spontaneous pain. These mechanisms can also account for the long delays between stimulation and pain experience that are frequently observed after peripheral-nerve or dorsal-root lesions. Because the total number of peripheral fibres is reduced, it may take considerable time for the T cells to reach the firing level necessary to trigger pain, so that pain perception and response are delayed.

In addition to the sensory influences on the gate-control system, there is a tonic inhibitory influence from the brain. Thus, any lesion that impairs the normal downflow of impulses to the gate-control system would open the gate. Central nervous system lesions associated with hyperalgesia and spontaneous pain (Head, 1920; Cassinari and Pagni, 1969) could have this effect.

The gate-control theory also suggests that psychological processes such as past experience, attention, and emotion may influence pain perception and response by acting on the spinal gating mechanism. Some of these psychological activities may open the gate while others may close it. A woman who one day discovers a lump in her breast, and is worried that it may be cancerous, may suddenly feel pain in the breast. If anxiety is prolonged, the pain may increase in severity and even spread to the shoulder and arm. Later, the mere verbal assurance from her doctor that the lump is of no consequence usually produces sudden, total relief of pain.

In some cases, the presence of pain may be determined to a large extent by personal psychological needs. They may produce facilitiation of all inputs from an area so that nerve impulses generated by pressure or thermal stimuli, or by circulatory activities within the tissue, will be summated to evoke pain (Szasz, 1968). In contrast, they may close the gate to all inputs from a selected body area. Thus, a person may develop 'glove anaesthesia' – total loss of sensation, including pain, from the whole hand. The pattern of sensory loss makes it apparent that there is no neuropathology to account for the symptoms (Walters, 1961; Merskey and Spear, 1967). Psychotherapy may relieve the glove anaesthesia, only for it to return months later, perhaps even at the other hand.

Inadequate inhibitory control may also help explain some intriguing laboratory observations. Stimulation of the skin with a small warm stimulator (with a tip diameter of one to two millimetres) often produces reports of stinging pain, even though stimulation of a larger area of skin with a probe of the same temperature produces only reports of warmth sensation (Melzack, Rose and McGinty, 1962). These observations appear to be related to 'after-sensations' or 'afterglows', which have a long, fascinating history in research on pain (Hayes, 1912; Boring, 1942). Touching the skin, especially the lip, with a hair or thread frequently sets off a tingling or 'afterglow' sensation that may persist for several minutes (Melzack and Eisenberg, 1968). The afterglow sometimes spreads beyond the site of stimulation, and may continue as a prolonged, heightened awareness of the area that can be evoked at will by intense concentration.

Two possible mechanisms may underlie the stinging pain that is sometimes evoked by stimulation with a small-tipped warm probe. First, the small stimulating surface may occasionally activate the excitatory centres of receptive fields with minimal activation of their inhibitory surrounds. The decreased inhibition would permit maximal transmission of impulses, without the inhibitory 'turn-off'. The ensuing prolonged summation could bring about stinging pain of long duration. Second, it is possible that when insufficient or ambiguous cutaneous information is applied to the skin, the tonic inhibitory control exerted by the brain is decreased so that the input undergoes maximal summation and is perceived as pain.

Phenomena of convergence, summation and inhibition are demonstrated in other laboratory experiments. Melzack, Wall and Weisz (1963) found that a slap on the skin decreases the level of perceived pain when it either precedes or follows an electric shock by as long as fifty milliseconds. Halliday and Mingay (1961), furthermore, have found that the threshold for shock on one arm is raised by a shock delivered as long as a hundred milliseconds later to the other arm. This phenomenon, which is known as 'metacontrast', is powerful evidence that pain results after prolonged monitoring of the input pattern by central cells. It is assumed that this monitoring may take even longer in pathological pain syndromes, since pain often occurs after delays as long as thirty seconds or more after stimulation. Such long delays simply cannot be explained in terms of slowly conducting fibres.

These data also indicate that the pain-signalling pattern can be influenced by stimulation at distant body sites. Shock applied to one arm influences pain felt in the other (Halliday and Mingay, 1961). Vibration of one wrist influences the level of itch perceived at the opposite wrist (Melzack and Schecter, 1965). Care was taken in both of these studies to rule out distraction of attention as the cause of the effect; rather the changes in pain or itch appear to reflect temporal and spatial interactions of somatic inputs in the central nervous system.

Referred pain

We have already discussed the neural mechanisms that underlie many forms of referred pain (p.124). Cells in lamina 5 of the dorsal horns receive a convergence of fibres from skin and viscera (Pomeranz, Wall and Weber, 1968), and the projection of the outputs of these cells to the brain would produce pain felt in both areas. Thus, cardiac patients, during an anginal attack, often feel pains in the upper chest and left shoulder and arm as well as a diffuse pain in the mid-chest region. However, the story is more complex. Within or near (or occasionally at a considerable distance from) the area of referred pain, it is often possible to find small 'trigger points' which are exquisitely sensitive and trigger severe pain when pressed on by a finger or punctured by a needle.

Examination of cardiac patients by Kennard and Haugen (1955) revealed that most of them show a common pattern of trigger spots (Figure 35) in the shoulder and chest. Pressure on the trigger spots often produces intense pain that may last for hours. Astonishingly, similar examination of a group of subjects who did not have heart disease revealed an almost identical distribution of trigger spots. The application of pressure produced marked discomfort which sometimes lasted for several minutes and even increased in intensity for a few seconds *after* removal of the stimulus.

The patterns of referred pain are so consistent from person to person that physicians often diagnose the diseased structure on the basis of the pain pattern. It is not surprising, therefore, that

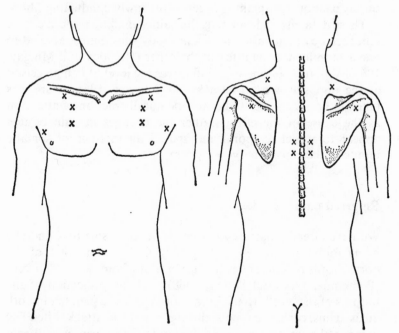

Figure 35. Kennard and Haugen's (1955, p.297) chart of trigger spots (marked by Xs) in cardiac patients, showing the areas that are most frequently sensitive. Firm pressure on the trigger spots produces discrete, stabbing, 'hot' pain that sometimes persists for as long as several hours. Pressure at the same spots in non-cardiac patients often produces mild pain for several minutes.

many trigger points are located in approximately the same place in most people (Travell and Rinzler, 1946, 1952). Pressure on these trigger points evokes pain in the referred area and, usually, pain in the related diseased visceral structure. Even more remarkable is the fact that injection of an anaesthetic drug in the trigger points removes the referred pain and, very often, the pain of the diseased visceral structure. The frequency of painful attacks may decrease significantly after a single such injection. Sometimes, the pain may disappear permanently (Travell and Rinzler, 1946). There is a characteristic sequence to many of these referred pains. For example, in some cases of chronic coronary insufficiency which produces anginal pain, the pain referred to the arm and shoulder becomes the outstanding symptom. The person protects the arm and tends to keep it in a rigid, fixed position. After anaesthetic injection of the trigger points, the pain relief allows the patient to use the arm and shoulder normally.

These observations are part of a large body of data on painful trigger points associated with muscles and the fibrous membrane (fascia) that covers them (Figure 36). The nature of these myofascial trigger points is poorly understood. Some points, particularly those found in the lower regions of the back, are associated with definite nodules of fibrous tissue. Simons (1975, 1976) has reviewed evidence that these nodules may develop after several kinds of trauma, including virus infections and other fever-producing diseases. Korr, Thomas and Wright (1955) propose an additional cause. They suggest that trigger points develop during the course of growth as a result of musculoskeletal stresses and strains, particularly associated with the muscles of the back. It is also possible, as Kennard and Haugen have suggested, that the areas at which blood vessels and nerves lie close to the surface, rather than hidden under muscles and other tissues, are particularly susceptible sites for the formation of trigger points.

Trigger points appear to be involved in a variety of pain phenomena (Glyn, 1971; Simons, 1975, 1976). They have been implicated in conditions such as muscle pain (myalgia), muscular (non-joint) rheumatism, muscle inflammation (myositis or myofascitis), and inflammation of the white fibrous tissue that comprises muscle sheaths and fascial layers of the whole muscle-joint-tendon-ligament system (fibrositis or myofibrositis). Valuable evidence has been obtained by studies of 'fibrositic' areas of the low back (Brendstrup *et al.*, 1957) and of tender nodular areas in the shoulder and arm (Awad, 1973). In both cases, the excised tissue (compared to normal control tissue) showed marked oedema, characteristic chemical changes, and an accumulation of mast cells (see p.115). Awad (1973) inferred from his observations that trauma of some kind triggers a chemical process in which localized oedema occurs and produces the breakdown of mast cells, thereby releasing free histamine. Histamine has a number of local effects on circulation in the area and is a potential pain-producing agent. The oedema could be the basis of a nodule (in some cases), and the chemical sequence just described could be the basis of localized circulatory, thermal,

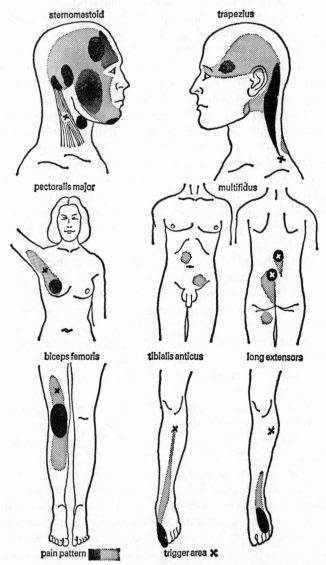

sternomastoid

trapezius

pectoralis major

multifidus

biceps femoris

tibialis anticus

long extensors

pain pattern ▨▨▨   trigger area ✖

Figure 36. Typical myofascial pain patterns and their related trigger areas reported by Travell and Rinzler (1952, p.425). When the referred pain pattern of a muscle is known, it can be used to locate the muscle that is the source of pain. The name of the muscle associated with each pain pattern is shown.

sudomotor (sweating) and other changes. One effect could well be to produce local muscle spasm. Indeed, a recording electrode inserted into a trigger point elicits a sharp, severe, persistent pain and abnormal, high-frequency discharges in the muscle that persist for thirty minutes or more. No such activity is seen in normal muscle.

The kinds of trauma that initiate these activities are not fully documented, but it is clear that there is a variety of them (Simons, 1975, 1976). Loss of local blood flow (ischemia) due to a sudden sprain, unusual mechanical pressure, toxins, extreme cold or heat, and fever-producing diseases appear to be some of the causes. Persistent pressure on nerves at exit points, including nerve entrapment (Kopell and Thompson, 1976), is another. Scar tissue remaining from an earlier injury or even surgery may be yet another trauma that initiates the sequence of events that produces trigger points or larger trigger zones. Some of these causes, such as muscular stresses and strains, would produce patterns of trigger points common to most people, while others, such as scars, would vary from person to person. As Glyn (1971) notes, such 'insults' cause painful lesions which tend to heal spontaneously; but in the elderly, and in others in whom there may be a constitutional chemical abnormality in muscle or connective tissue, these trivial lesions perpetuate themselves until they become chronic.

Yet it is astonishing how easily many of these trigger point diseases are relieved (Travell and Rinzler, 1952; Simons, 1975, 1976). Injection of an anaesthetic or saline into the trigger point, or simply needling the area with a dry needle may produce total relief of pain. It is essential (Bonica, 1957) to find *the* trigger point; that is, it is often highly localized, and stimulation must occur precisely at the point to produce the sharp pain and the sudden or gradual cessation of the vicious cycle of changes that produced it. Simons (1976) observes that the precise point is often found by the characteristic sharp pain and by a localized muscle spasm (not seen in normal muscle) which grips the tip of the needle as it penetrates. Why these simple procedures work is not clear. Possibly, the sharp, severe pain may activate descending inhibitory mechanisms which temporarily decrease or abolish the pain signals. This, in turn, may decrease the sympathetic outflow that appears to be an essential component of the whole cycle

(Glyn, 1971). The simplicity of these procedures is especially startling when we consider the severity and crippling nature of many of these myofascial pains, such as muscular rheumatism and low back pain (Glyn, 1971), torticollis ('stiff neck'), and a variety of other disabling myofascial syndromes.

Trigger points may involve only myofascial structures (Travell and Rinzler, 1952) or may become associated with pathological visceral activity (Simons, 1975, 1976). It is reasonable to assume that trigger points produce a continuous input into the central nervous system. Diseased viscera, then, may evoke an input which summates with the input from the trigger points to produce pain referred to the larger skin areas which surround the trigger points. Conversely, stimulation of the trigger points may evoke volleys of impulses that summate with low-level inputs from the diseased visceral structure, which would produce pain that is felt in both areas. These phenomena of referred pain, then, point to summation mechanisms which can be understood in terms of the gate-control theory.

Two types of mechanisms may play a role. The first involves the spread of pain to adjacent body areas. The T cell has a restricted receptive field which dominates its 'normal activities'; in addition, however, it is also affected by electrical stimulation of afferent nerves that cover a much larger body surface (Mendell and Wall, 1965; Devor, Merrill and Wall, 1977). This diffuse input is normally inhibited by gate mechanisms, but may trigger firing in the T cell if input is sufficiently intense or if the gate is opened. Anaesthesia of the area to which the pain has spread, which blocks the spontaneous impulses from the area, is sufficient to reduce the bombardment of the cell below the threshold level for pain. The discovery that the small visceral afferents project directly or indirectly onto lamina 5 cells (Pomeranz, Wall and Weber, 1968) provides the gate-control theory with still further power in explaining referred pain.

The second mechanism to explain referred pain involves the spread of pain and trigger zones to regions at a considerable distance, including visceral structures as well as cutaneous and myofascial areas. These referred pains suggest that the gate can be opened by activities in distant body areas. This possibility is consistent with the gate model, since the substantia gelatinosa at any level receives inputs from both sides of the body and (by way of Lissauer's tract) from the substantia gelatinosa in neighbouring body segments. Mechanisms such as these may explain the observations that anginal pain, or pressure on other body areas such as the back of the head may trigger pain in the phantom limb.

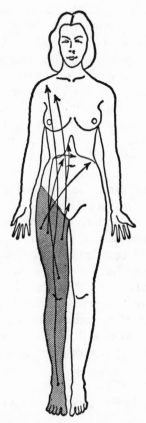

Figure 37. Patterns of referred sensation after cordotomy. The stippled area shows the region of analgesia produced by cordotomy in this woman. Heavy pressure applied to the analgesic skin produced 'an unpleasant form of tingling' that was felt at a non-analgesic part of the body. The sites of stimulation are indicated by dots, and the arrow from each dot indicates the point to which sensation was referred.
(from Nathan, 1956, p.88)

Referred pains may also occur after lesions of the central nervous system. Nathan (1956) studied patients who had undergone unilateral or bilateral cordotomy, mostly for the relief of cancer pain, and found that pinpricks applied to analgesic parts of the body such as the leg evoked pain that was felt at distant sites on the same or opposite side of the body (Figure 37). He also observed that, in some patients, the pain was referred to the site of an earlier injury. It is possible that the decreased input to the reticular formation after cordotomy brings about a release from inhibition at all levels of the spinal cord. Consequently, the impulses produced by noxious stimulation at analgesic areas would tend, via the substantia gelatinosa, to open the gates at other levels. It is conceivable that the low-level inputs from trigger zones or sites of earlier injury at distant areas of the body would then summate to produce the level of T-cell firing necessary for the perception of pain.

Phenomena of mis-referral of sensation are also familiar to a small number of people who, for reasons unknown but presumably because of aberrant connections in the nervous system, find that when they scratch a body area (such as the knee) they feel a curious itchy or tickling sensation in a distant body area, such as the upper shoulder. Observations such as these (Sterling, 1973) underscore the complexity of central neural connections and take us far away from simplistic concepts of the nervous system as little more than an old-fashioned telephone switchboard that has one plug-in connection for each telephone. Like our more complicated telecommunications networks, errors in connection occur, sometimes with trivial consequences and sometimes with painful, crippling, disastrous ones.

Prolonged activity in the nervous system

The gate-control theory, by eschewing a straight-through pain pathway and a rigid relationship between injury and pain, is able to give serious consideration to prolonged neural activities related to pain. There is little doubt that such mechanisms are necessary to explain several fascinating clinical and experimental observations. Nathan (1962) reviewed several cases which indicate that somatosensory input may produce long-lasting effects similar to memories produced by visual and auditory stimulation. In one case, stimulation of the stump of an amputee who, five years before amputation, had sustained a severe laceration of the leg by an ice skate, later produced vivid imagery of the pain of the skating accident: 'It was not that he remembered having had this injury; he felt all the sensations again that he had felt at the time.' Similarly, phantom limb pain is sometimes felt in areas that had been painful prior to amputation. The pain of a sliver of wood under a fingernail or a tight cast on a foot have been reported as persisting in the phantom after amputation of the limb (Bailey and Moersch, 1941; White and Sweet, 1969).

The concept of a memory-like mechanism in pain is also supported by convincing experimental evidence. The most fascinating study (Hutchins and Reynolds, 1947; Reynolds and Hutchins, 1948) originated when dentists in the United States Air Force, during World War II, observed that aircrew often complained of toothache in a recently filled tooth when they flew in semi-pressurized airplanes. The first hypothesis – that air-pockets were trapped under the filling and exerted pressure on the tooth-pulp – was eliminated by carefully drilling and refilling the offending tooth, and finding that the painful episodes still persisted. It was then observed that the aircrew complained when they also had a sinus infection, so that changes in air pressure may have been exerting their effects by stimulation of receptors in the sinuses. In an ingenious set of experiments, volunteer aircrew underwent drilling and filling of diseased teeth, without local anaesthetics, on both sides of the mouth. It was then observed that pinpricks of the nasal mucosa, as long as seventy days later, produced pain in the treated teeth on the stimulated side. The effect was permanently abolished on one side by a single novocaine block of the trigeminal nerve, but persisted in the opposite, non-blocked side (Hutchins and Reynolds, 1947; Reynolds and Hutchins, 1948). These referred pains necessitate the assumption of a long-term central neural change. The data suggest that the treatment of the teeth evoked inputs that produced changes in firing patterns in the central nervous system. These changes, once initiated, were somehow capable of summating the continuous, low-level input from the treated teeth with inputs from more distant sources. The single block of a peripheral nerve, which could not have affected the teeth, permitted resumption of normal neural activity and the end of pain. That the *input* as such, rather than conscious awareness, was essential in initiating the abnormal central activity is evident in the observation that a' subject who had four teeth extracted under nitrous oxide anaesthesia felt pain referred to the jaw when the nasal mucosa was pricked thirty-three days after treatment.

Similar observations were made by Cohen (1944) who studied patients who had anginal-effort syndrome, with pain referred only to the left side. He injected a small amount of hypertonic saline under the skin of the right side of the back which gave rise to a diffuse, deep-seated pain that soon disappeared. Two hours later, long after the pain had passed, exertion and anginal pain again caused its appearance.

Cohen (1944) also observed events involving a much longer timespan. Two of his patients were men who had each lost a leg and reported that they had never felt pain in the phantom leg. More than twenty years after amputation, both men developed anginal pain and each suffered severe pain in the phantom leg during the anginal attacks.

The gate-control theory is able to explain some kinds of prolonged pain after a peripheral nerve lesion or other nerve pathology. The loss of fibres would tend to promote abnormal, prolonged activity and therefore provide the basis for persistent pain. Furthermore, the pain would tend to limit movement of the affected area, which in turn would decrease the normal firing patterns produced by motor activities. A single anaesthetic block could bring about prolonged relief of pain. By decreasing or abolishing input to the hyperactive neuron pools, the total firing level of the T cells would fall below the critical level that produces pain. As a consequence, the person would move normally and produce normal patterns of input from muscles and other tissues. These patterns, which would include a higher proportion of impulses from the remaining large fibres, would tend to maintain the gate in a more closed position and prevent pain from returning.

This explanation, however, is not always satisfactory. For example, it does not explain why teeth that have been drilled and filled without local anaesthetic may be the site of referred pain when the nasal sinuses are stimulated as long as seventy days later, or why a single anaesthetic block of the appropriate nerve from the jaw abolishes the phenomenon permanently. This effect cannot be attributed to a loss of fibres. Nor can it be due to a chronic local irritation after the dental manipulation: the anaesthetic block could not have affected the teeth themselves. The effect, instead, points to prolonged changes in central neural activity which may be initiated by a brief, painful input and stopped permanently by a single anaesthetic block.

There are many clinical observations which lead to the same conclusion. Momentary pressure on trigger areas in cardiac patients produces severe pain for several hours, and a single anaesthetic block of the areas may abolish recurrent cardiac pain for days, weeks, or longer. How can a single, brief input produce such long effects, and how can a temporary block of input stop it? Similarly, injections of anaesthetic drugs into trigger areas or sympathetic ganglia in people suffering phantom limb pain may produce pain relief that long outlasts the duration of anaesthesia, even though the stump is used little more than it had been prior to treatment.

The explanation of these prolonged effects, which are among the most puzzling features of pain, requires the assumption that prolonged, intense, or otherwise abnormal somatic input may produce long-term changes in activity in the central nervous system. These neural substrates of prolonged activity may activate the T cells to produce persistent pain.

The neural mechanisms that underlie prolonged, memory-like activity related to pain remain a mystery. There is striking behavioural and physiological evidence (see Melzack, 1973) that brief sensory input may produce prolonged neural changes. For example, intense, high-frequency stimulation of sensory fibres for twenty minutes produces a dramatic change in a simple spinal cord reflex that persists for more than two hours (Spencer and April, 1970). Pain produced by dilute formalin injected under the skin of a rat's paw for an hour prior to total deafferentation of the paw affects the animal's tendency to bite the paw as long as weeks later (Dennis and Melzack, 1979). Still more striking is the observation that mild electric shocks applied to a hindleg ankle during a conditioned-learning experiment in cats produce a three-to fourfold increase in the size of the cortical area to which the ankle afferents project (Metzler, 1980). These studies leave no doubt that brief periods of intense stimulation may produce dramatic, persistent changes in central neural activity. The speculation that they are subserved by reverberatory activity in closed, self-sustaining neuron loops (Livingston, 1943) has failed to receive any confirmation. However, it is possible that changes occur within neurons or in the synaptic connections among neurons as a result of prior sensory inputs. Despite considerable research, the nature of the neural changes that subserve memory-like processes in pain remains unknown.

The gate-control theory in retrospect

In 1965 we made a general proposal about the way in which nerve impulses that arrive at the spinal cord interact with each other and are controlled by impulses that descend from the brain. The substantial advances in knowledge since 1965 have led to modifications and a reformulation of the gate-control theory. We now know far more about the small cells of the substantia gelatinosa and believe that they include a variety of different excitatory as well as inhibitory interneurons. Our expectation that the chemistry and pharmacology of the area would turn out to be unusual has been more than vindicated by the discovery of the huge array of peptides including enkephalins. A major problem of detailed mechanisms remains. The original scheme stressed presynaptic control but we now know with certainty that postsynaptic inhibition also occurs. We still do not know the relative role of presynaptic and postsynaptic mechanisms or even if they should be separated. There are severe technical problems because of the small size of the components and their admixture in tiny areas. The predicted control endings on the incoming sensory afferents have rarely been found and instead there is evidence of more complicated mechanisms which could intrude both pre- and postsynaptically. We now know that the receptive fields of the transmitting cells have a complex excitatory-inhibitory organization, which can explain the tendency of large fibres to inhibit the excitation of small fibres (Hillman and Wall, 1969). While tremendous advances have been made on the morphology of the area (Gobel, 1979; Wall, 1980 a, b), the correlation of anatomy and physiology represents a huge technical challenge. For example, the terminals containing enkephalin have been located, as have the axons containing opiate receptors, but unfortunately the presumed emitting and the presumed receiving structures do not make contact (Hunt *et al.*, 1980). The descending controls which are an inherent part of the scheme have been found to originate from a number of structures and to be dependent on different chemicals for their action, but here again the details remain to be unravelled. However, the original concept of a gate control stands as a powerful summary of the phenomena observed in the spinal cord and brain, and has the capacity to explain many of the most mysterious and puzzling problems encountered in the clinic.

Part Four
The Control of Pain

'Perhaps few persons who are not physicians can realize the influence which long-continued and unendurable pain may have upon both body and mind . . . Under such torments the temper changes, the most amiable grow irritable, the soldier becomes a coward, and the strongest man is scarcely less nervous than the most hysterical girl.'

S. Weir Mitchell, 1872

12
The Challenges of Pain
and the Search for Drugs

Anyone who suffers pain tries to stop it as soon as possible by his own actions or with the help of others. As the pain's severity and duration increase, the person's behaviour is increasingly dominated by his condition and this gives rise to a series of challenges. We need first to analyse these challenges before we proceed to examine the methods of control.

Challenges to the person who suffers

As pain appears, so does a very natural anxiety (Wall, 1979). What is the cause of the pain? What will be the consequences? What is the best treatment? If the pain persists, the initial anxiety is likely to be replaced by a state of quiet withdrawal. The person's life becomes increasingly dominated by the pain, which refuses to go away and which resists the best treatments available. This state of misery brings with it three pressing needs, each with its problems. First, there is the need to communicate with others, and those others may have difficulty in understanding the nature of the suffering. Second, injury, sickness and pain trigger in the victim a need for the behaviour best suited to recovery. This includes rest, sleep, and a general decrease in activity. These needs often conflict with the need to communicate and with the activity forced on the patient by well-meaning helpers. Sleep is a particular problem. The pain itself, and sometimes the therapeutic drugs, interfere with the natural sleep patterns so that the patient becomes exhausted just at a time when sleep is most needed. Third, and most urgent, is the search for treatment and relief. Each new treatment is approached with great expectations and consequent despondency if it fails. As time goes by, the alternation of hope and despair leads to a change in the character of the patient and his way of thinking. Drastic measures are accepted without complaint. Bizarre proposals which would quickly be rejected by critical thought in calmer times become immensely attractive. The stage is set for the appearance of the quack.

Challenges to friends and relatives

The sound of a baby's cry and the quiet moan of an old person produce an imperative reaction in those who hear them. We are impelled to move toward the one who suffers, to offer help, sympathy and treatment. But what if the pain persists in spite of our best efforts? We quite correctly feel inadequate and therefore, in some sense, also feel guilty. We have developed many tactics for dealing with feelings of guilt and inadequacy. Irritation, denial and withdrawal are the most common. Everyone close to a patient in prolonged pain battles with the conflicting tendencies to approach and withdraw.

Challenges to the medical profession

The physicians, surgeons and associated health professionals who take part in the treatment of pain are first of all human beings and therefore subject to the same pressures of guilt and inadequacy as other people. In addition, they have received special training, but we must analyse the direction of that training. The development of medicine over the past two centuries has been directed above all at the cure of disease. This would seem reasonable, but this attitude has brought with it less concentration on – even a lack of respect for – the control of symptoms. The medical phrase 'mere symptomatic treatment' is used to condemn a superficial approach to medicine which fails to come to grips with the fundamental problem of the underlying disease which caused the symptom. There is obviously good reasoning and sense in this approach but it has in general diverted attention, thought, research and training away from the problems, such as severe pain or nausea, of those patients with diseases which have yet to be curable.

Similarly, even in the case of diseases that are curable either by time or by the doctor there has not been the same massive effort applied to the relief of symptoms during the recovery process as is applied to a search for diagnosis and cure. Social pressure to cure is as much responsible for this state of affairs as the attitude of the medical profession. Patients and relatives often expect a doctor eventually to say, 'I am sorry, there is nothing more to be done.' What is meant is that no known therapy will cure or arrest the disease but the statement makes no mention of the symptoms. The point at which this statement is made depends on the personality and training of the specialist and on the finances of the society and of the patients. Kings and presidents are in considerable danger of rigorous curative therapies terminated only by the closure of the coffin lid.

There are interesting exceptions to this generalization about the fixation of medical attention on cure. Anaesthetists have developed a strong speciality over the past century without ever attempting to cure anything. Their attention was directed to signs and symptoms, especially pain, and they have made, as we shall see, some of the most important advances. Similarly, the field of physical medicine, frequently held in low repute by academic medicine just because it concentrates on symptom relief, has made significant advances. The same may be said for psychiatrists and clinical psychologists who teach methods of coping, of self-control and of self-understanding. These developments have considerable relevance for patients in prolonged pain.

A further tendency in medical practice which affects pain patients has been the development of specialization which was necessitated by the increased complexity of knowledge. In some countries, particularly the United States, this has been accompanied by the virtual disappearance of the generalist – the family doctor. This means that the patient must make his own initial diagnosis and choose the speciality which most obviously fits his condition. Let us consider a common type of case.

A middle-aged woman develops low back pain followed a few days later by vaginal bleeding. She reasonably decides that she has a uterine problem and goes to her gynaecologist. He, finding fibroids (firm masses) in the uterine wall, carries out a dilation and curettage of the uterus, thinning down its inner wall. We must understand that (1) uterine problems may occasionally cause low back pain; (2) the patient had presented herself for relief to an expert on the uterus; (3) the doctor accepts the patient's challenge to his special knowledge and obliges her with the practice of his skill. Let us follow this case further. The pain disappears as is often the case with low back pains (with or without dilation and curettage) and, as is also often the case, the pain later recurs. The patient and the doctor have been through a learning experience in which the back pain is apparently related to the uterus. The gynaecologist advises a more radical approach, the removal of the uterus, since he finds that the fibroids have grown since his last examination. The total removal of the uterus – a hysterectomy – is carried out, but the pain does not disappear.

The disappointed patient now believes, reasonably, that the target was wrong and feels that the trouble is in her bones and muscles. She knows that chiropractors and osteopaths believe that readjustment of the relations of vertebrae cures a number of conditions and she decides to visit one. There is again a period of relief but then a recurrence which is made worse by further manipulation. After visiting an orthopaedic surgeon she is told that a slightly displaced disc might be the cause. The patient, now growing desperate, begs the orthopaedic surgeon to remove the intervertebral disc. This operation is followed by a further increase in the pain which is clearly related to movement and seems to involve the articulation of the vertebral bones. The orthopaedic surgeon, of course, specializes in bones and joints and operates on the patient to fuse several vertebrae together to prevent movement of one vertebra against the other. The patient now has a stiff back which is more painful than ever. At this point the patient is referred to a neurosurgeon for an operation on the sensory roots. Although we will not describe her case any further, it is evident that she may decide to embark on an entirely new cycle of treatments.

This common story can clearly occur only in a very affluent society which has sufficient money to support specialists who are capable of performing difficult operations and who have sufficient time to consider them. Poorer societies may escape the phenomenon of multiple surgery by isolated specialists; instead the patient may pass less dramatically and more economically from one doctor to another, whose practices may consist of herbal remedies, acupuncture or other common procedures of folk medicine.

Each of the operations described above was based on a theory of the cause of a disease, each had been 'shown' to work in certain cases, and each was directed at a cure of the condition. After each failure, the patient was naturally sad and disappointed, and more determined than ever to find a solution. But how did the specialists feel? They too felt sad and disappointed – and threatened. For each specialist, the threat is to his working hypothesis and to his professional standing and self-respect as well as to his common humanity. As the patient moves from one hospital clinic to another, the thickness of the medical file builds up. The doctors become more cautious as this patient shows a history of failure by his colleagues. Depending on several factors – including his confidence in his special area of diagnosis and treatment, his respect for his colleagues, and his financial need to take on another patient – the doctor may approach or withdraw from the patient. If he withdraws, the patient's anger is certain to rise and the insistence and vigour of the search for treatment may also rise, increasing the pressure on the specialists.

In this part of the book (Part Four), we will describe and evaluate the current methods of pain control. There are presently four major approaches to relieving pain and suffering: pharmacological, surgical, sensory-modulation, and psychological. Prior to the formulation of the gate-control theory, sensory-modulation and psychological approaches were simply sideshows outside the mainstream of pain therapy. Only two medical procedures had the stamp of approval of conventional medical wisdom for the control of severe, intractable pain: the use of drugs, and, if they failed, the destruction of the pathways in the spinal cord or brain that were believed to carry pain signals. We will discuss the pharmacological approaches to pain control in this chapter and the surgical methods of control in the next one.

Pharmacological control of pain

It may come as a surprise to readers that ninety-nine per cent of drug prescriptions for pain come from only two families of compounds, the aspirin type and the opium type. This fact tends to be hidden by enthusiastic advertising for some new variant of one or the other family. The confusion is increased by the labelling of simple chemicals with trade-names and by selling mixtures of compounds with yet another trade-name. While these two families have survived, they are historically not the only anti-pain drugs. Plants were long the fávourite source of medicine and these gave us the mandrake – a relative of the potato – which contains atropine and scopolamine which cloud consciousness. Henbane contains hyoscamine, another of these compounds. Hemp produces cannabis or hashish which has certain analgesic effects. Hemlock was used as a general soporific but was also thought to have a local action and was applied as a local poultice. Many plant oils such as clove oil have a strong local anaesthetic action. Of all plant derivatives, alcohol has surely been used and abused more than any substance for numbness and oblivion. But extracts of willow and of poppy have led to the most specific and useful drugs.

The salicylates, including aspirin

In 1763 a country clergyman from Chipping Norton in England, Edward Stone, wrote to the Royal Society in London to tell them that the extract of willow was good for rheumatism and bouts of fever. In 1827, Leroux isolated the active compound from the willow, Salix Alba, and named it salicin. Throughout the nineteenth century, many variations of this molecule were produced and used, and by 1899, Dreser produced acetylsalicylic acid. This was marketed by Bayer under the trade name of Aspirin. Many more variants have been produced in this century and the names of those commonly used include, in addition to the salicylates, the following: phenylbutazone, indomethacin, mefanamic acid, ibuprofen, acetaminophen (paracetamol) and phenacetin. This remarkable group has three therapeutic actions: (1) against pain; (2) against inflammation; and (3) against fever. They vary in their relative power to produce these three desirable effects and also in the unfortunately large number of side effects.

Rationale. The site of action of these drugs appears to be entirely on the injured tissue itself and there is no convincing evidence that therapeutic doses have any effect directly on peripheral nerves or in the central nervous system. The most likely proposal to explain the action of aspirin-like compounds comes from the work of Vane, first reported in 1971. In the 1930s, an active compound was discovered in semen and, since the fluid comes from the prostate gland, it was called prostaglandin. It was later discovered that there is a large family of these compounds and that they are synthesized from a fatty acid, arachidonic acid. When tissue is damaged, prostaglandins are synthesized and released into tissues where they play a part in triggering the three classic signs of inflammation: (1) the blood vessels dilate, producing redness; (2) they leak fluid, producing swelling; and (3) nerve endings are sensitized so that they produce nerve impulses more easily and therefore increase pain. Aspirin blocks the synthesis of prostaglandins and therefore prevents the appearance of this crucial substance which announces that tissue is damaged. The aspirin family intrudes at various different stages of the chain of synthesis. This proposal that aspirin acts within damaged tissue itself and not on the nervous system explains two important puzzles. Locally administered aspirin is rapidly effective for both pain and swelling; it is not necessary for the brain to receive aspirin. Secondly, aspirin given to a normal person without injury is not an analgesic for the usual test stimuli, such as electric shocks, which do not immediately harm tissue and therefore do not produce the tissue breakdown products on which aspirin acts. It is evident that these drugs are ideal – in that they specifically select only the areas from which pain originates while leaving other systems unaffected. Unfortunately, the prostaglandins are involved in normal body regulations and interference with them produces unwanted side effects.

Uses. The site of action in damaged tissue defines the uses of these drugs. Sudden injury sets off a chain of reactions related to pain. First, small molecules such as histamine and serotonin are released. Then, larger peptides such as bradykinen appear. Finally the prostaglandins are synthesized and released. Therefore, these drugs are effective against slow, prolonged tissue damage and its pain wherever it occurs. A broken leg, the socket of an extracted tooth, and an arthritic joint all have in common the same tissue reactions and, therefore, the same sensitivity to these drugs. Pain triggered by events which do not produce inflammatory reactions does not respond to the drugs.

Side effects. Some people develop an extreme sensitivity to aspirin and show severe side effects to normal therapeutic doses. The commonest of these is gastric irritation and bleeding. Unfortunately, the development of sensitivity to one is accompanied by sensitivity to all. Aspirin also affects the blood clotting mechanism and is used intentionally for this purpose. Two aspirin tablets (650mg) approximately doubles the mean bleeding time in normal adults. An all too common example of adding insult to injury is to drink enough alcohol to produce a mild gastritis after which aspirin is taken for the hangover. Every hospital emergency room is familiar with this combination as the trigger for massive gastric haemorrhage. There is only a narrow range in normal people between the effective dose and the onset of side effects. Since every household contains an array of aspirin-like compounds, accidental or intentional overdoses are common. These affect brain, liver, kidney and blood chemistry. Fortunately, intensive care units have become skilled at the reversal of these toxic effects if treatment is started rapidly.

The opiates, also known as narcotics

Opium, the extract of poppy, was known to the Sumerians in 4000 BC, but we know little about the uses to which it was put. The first medical document, the Ebers Papyrus of 1550 BC, recommends it for crying children. The Greeks dedicated it to the gods of night, death, sleep (Hypnos) and dreams (Morpheus) – hence the name 'morphine'. Hippocrates prescribed it as a hypnotic. However, in Roman times, it was used specifically against pain by Galen in the second century AD. The use of opium spread from Rome and so did its abuse. Avicenna, the greatest of the Arab physicians, died in 1037 from an overdose of opium and so did Clive of India in the eighteenth century. The export of opium partly for medicine but largely for pleasure became big business, particularly for the British East India Company. Their right to import opium into China was the cause of the Opium Wars in 1820. China was by no means the only customer: 90,000 lbs of opium were officially imported into Britain in 1870 and all rich nations were on a similar binge.

As was apparent in the description of aspirin and local anaesthetics, the nineteenth century was rich in analysis and synthesis of simple organic molecules. In 1803, morphine itself was isolated by Sertürner from opium. Opium contains about ten per cent morphine and also smaller amounts of many other alkaloids, two of which are related to morphine. These are codeine and thebaine. From these three molecules, a very large number of synthetic compounds have been generated. At least twenty-five different compounds are listed in the pharmacopoeia and their most famous trade names include heroin, dilaudid, percodan, palfium, and demerol (pethidine). The individual members of this group differ widely in their potency, duration, penetration and side effects but they are fundamentally similar in their mode of analgesic action. All produce analgesia and, as the dose rises, varying degrees of drowsiness, change of mood and mental clouding.

Rationale. The site of the analgesic action of the opiates is undoubtedly in the central nervous system and has been discussed in Chapters 6 and 7. These compounds act by imitating the natural opiates, the endorphins and the enkephalins, which are produced in areas of the brain and spinal cord. There are two clearly different sites of action with respect to pain. One of these is in the midbrain, where a system in the periaqueductal grey matter triggers a nearby system of descending controls which, in turn, inhibits the ability of the spinal cord to transmit messages about injury. The second area of action is in the spinal cord itself where high concentrations of enkephalins and opiate receptors exist in the substantia gelatinosa. The opiates are capable of producing local control of the transfer of messages about tissue damage from afferent fibres to the transmitting cells which send messages to the brain. There are undoubtedly many other brain areas which are directly or indirectly affected by opiates.

Uses. Narcotics may be given by mouth, by intramuscular injection or, for very rapid action, by intravenous injection. Oral administration is obviously the most convenient, even though absorption may be slow and erratic. Since narcotics are all very bitter tasting, they are taken with honey or a syrup to mask their awful taste.

Narcotics are most commonly used in emergencies with rapid onset of severe pain. They are injected for severe injuries, heart attacks and abdominal crises. They are also widely used to control post-operative pain and labour pain. Finally, they play a crucial role in the management of pain in terminal disease (which we will discuss in Chapter 16).

The discovery that narcotics have a direct action on the spinal cord has led to a new method now under extensive trial. One tenth of the normal dose is injected into the fluid around the lumbar cord. This produces a profound and long-lasting analgesia of the legs and pelvis without any of the psychedelic effects. It has also been found that morphine placed outside the cord in the epidural space produces analgesia in the nearest segments. While these methods still have their problems, they open the way to the possibility of local analgesia without the anaesthesia and paralysis produced by local anaesthetics. Narcotics never produce a complete analgesia, so that it is not possible to operate using them alone unless the dose is raised to levels that produce unconsciousness. However, not all pains respond to epidural morphine, and the failures may tell us something of the mode of action. When pains originate from denervation, as in brachial plexus avulsion, the terrible pain is not in any way ameliorated, presumably because the narcotic receptors on the spinal terminals of the incoming sensory fibres are destroyed.

Addiction. More nonsense on narcotic addiction is written by both doctors and the press than on any other medical matter. The undoubted occurrence of addiction has led to a mass hysteria about its danger which has been very harmful for patients as well as for addicts. The reaction to intravenous narcotics by the great majority of normal experimental subjects who are not in pain is one of discomfort. One of the present authors has experienced this a number of times during pain tests and found the sudden onset of a flying drunken feeling with nausea and headache to be distinctly unpleasant and not at all fitting the popular expectation of a pleasant dream state. Patients in acute emergency pain frequently receive one or more injections and they experience a powerful relief of both their pain and anxiety and often drift off to sleep. A survey was made of the consequences of such injections given to the many thousands of Israeli casualties in the Yom Kippur War. Not a single case of narcotic addiction was found among these men in spite of the fact that most were in the age range most commonly at risk for social addiction.

But what of the patients who get narcotics over long periods of time? The usual hospital routine is to give a dose every four hours and this may continue for weeks or months in terminal cancer patients with multiple metastases. However, this intermittent medication may have disadvantages because the drug is gradually metabolized and the pain level varies over the four hours. To overcome this, a number of techniques of self-paced administration have been developed in which the patient is free to give himself regulated small doses at short intervals (Keeri-Szanto, 1979). When these methods were introduced, there was of course considerable fear that the patient would rapidly overdose himself since he could administer the very drug which is supposed to induce addiction with all its associated irresponsible behaviour. Therefore, narrow limits were built into the system, with continuous monitoring in order to follow patients' behaviour when given free access to injected narcotics. The result is very clear. Patients do not push their drug intake to the highest permitted dose. On the contrary, they bring their pain down to a bearable level at which they do not have mental clouding. Then they continue to give themselves the narcotic at the doses required to maintain this desired state. The overall result is that the patient gives himself less than the medical staff would administer.

Who then are the self-destructive and socially undesirable addicts? Let us look at the less emotional subject of alcoholism. Most of us are not alcoholics and do not have an internal struggle not to become addicted. Most of us have been drunk, usually on social occasions, while seeking release and euphoria. A few people feel miserable and inadequate all the time and have only felt pleased with themselves on certain rare occasions when drunk. Even fewer seek continuous escape, oblivion or dependency. Turning back to narcotics, one can see that their illegal use and abuse has marked similarities with alcohol. The Singapore Chinese merchant, just as clever and successful as his American counterpart, smokes opium before dinner or as a nightcap while the American drinks a martini or a brandy. Biographies reveal many distinguished Westerners as having been regular secret users of narcotics with no apparent effect on their health or effectiveness. A few people, who always show serious personality problems before using narcotics, feel a sense of fulfilment for a few seconds or minutes only after a sudden surge of narcotics. Some seek escape and oblivion. These people are generally sick, and are unhappy with or without narcotics or alcohol. Their existence is no reason for the doctor to withhold medicine from normal people in the fear that he will create monsters.

Tolerance. The most common rational reason given by physicians for withholding opiates from those in pain due to terminal illness is that patients develop such rapid tolerance to the drugs that narcotics should be saved until some extreme and final crisis. However, Twycross (1978) found that cancer patients require a gradually increasing dose only during the first few days of stabilization. After this initial period, the required dose levels out at a safe and acceptable level and from then on remains as stable as the patient's condition. If the patient's disease spreads, it may be necessary to increase the dose to some higher level which again stabilizes. If the patient's condition improves, spontaneously or due to therapy, the dose of morphine can be decreased without any objection from the patient. There is no evidence of tolerance in these patients who take steady doses of narcotics for months, even for years.

Most drugs have multiple effects and the onset of tolerance differs for each of the different effects. This is also a common problem with alcohol, in which the amount taken to produce a particular effect rises rapidly day by day. Unfortunately, the amount needed to produce euphoria rises much more rapidly than the amount needed to produce oblivion. This partly explains the number of pathetic alcoholics who can no longer achieve the desired happiness before they fall off their bar-stools. Similarly, the dose needed by the social narcotic addict to produce the sudden psychedelic effect is extremely large and approaches the lethal dose. This tolerance of the psychedelic effect actually works to the advantage of the cancer patient. During the first few days of regular narcotic administration, the patient may feel drowsy and have muddled thoughts. These unwanted effects pass but the desired analgesia continues.

This type of differential tolerance has been shown in studies with animals by Abbott (1980). In rats, a test is used in which the tail is dipped in hot water and the time is measured until the animal flicks its tail out of the water. With rather high doses of morphine, the time which the animal leaves its tail in the water is prolonged. On repeated testing it is found that higher and higher doses of morphine are needed to produce this prolongation. However, in another test discussed in Chapter 7, a small amount of the irritant formalin is injected under the skin of a rat's paw and its prolonged behavioural reactions are recorded. Morphine in quite small doses decreases the animal's reaction to the irritant. In this test, unlike the tail-flick test, repeated testing and treatment with narcotics does not lead to tolerance. It therefore seems that the formalin test better imitates the chronic pain patient's failure to develop tolerance, whereas the tail-flick test better imitates those aspects of human response to narcotics which develop tolerance.

Tolerance is a widespread phenomenon which goes far beyond drugs. We have already noted (and will see again in later chapters) that chronic pain may recur even though the initial treatment is successful. This is particularly true after neurosurgical procedures. The body possesses a host of homeostatic mechanisms which maintain a stable level of many body functions. If some event occurs which disturbs the level of function, these mechanisms react to push the function back to the 'normal' level. For example, if the air temperature drops, skin vessels constrict to decrease heat loss and metabolism increases to raise heat production. If these measures fail to return the body temperature to normal, more vigorous and sophisticated reactions occur; shivering starts, a fire is lit, migration to Florida begins. Each of these reactions has a limited power which may be overwhelmed. If a man falls into the Arctic Sea, the heat loss exceeds the ability of the homeostatic mechanisms to protect the body, and temperature falls to a level where even the restorative mechanisms themselves fail.

We have continually stressed that pain, too, is under control by factors other than the input from injury. Some pains are best understood as a failure of control. When pain exists and a drug, a surgical lesion, physiotherapy or psychotherapy are initiated, the remaining control mechanisms will react in an attempt to re-establish the pain. This reaction may provide an explanation common to all eventual failures of therapy. A placebo which initially produces an excellent response fails on repeated administration. Many physiotherapies may do the same. An initially satisfactory dose of morphine may not be effective on the third application; but if the dose is raised, the effect may be strong enough to overwhelm the counter-reaction of the control mechanisms. The failure of surgery such as a cordotomy to control pain after some months of success may also be seen as due to a slow readjustment of control, in which there is enhanced use of previously minor pathways so that they can produce major effects.

Withdrawal. It is a common belief that the failure by those who take narcotics to maintain regular narcotic medication leads immediately to an intense and intolerable yearning, anxiety and terror. As with the fear of tolerance, this fear also turns out to be a gross exaggeration. We have already mentioned that a survey of several thousand military casualties given narcotics failed to identify a single case of addiction attributable to brief therapeutic exposure. Patients in severe chronic pain treated with narcotics may on occasion be successfully treated by a cordotomy, a nerve block or by physiotherapy. The common picture seen in such patients is that as soon as they obtain relief of their pain they request no further narcotics. Since they are indeed quite restless and jumpy, they are tapered off to normal within one or two days with rapidly decreasing doses of sedatives.

Side effects. All drugs have multiple actions. This is especially true of the narcotics which will affect any of the narcotic receptors found throughout the body. Normally, nerve impulses release endogenous opiates at selected sites in the nervous system and in this way achieve a specificity of action. When a narcotic is injected or ingested to act on the whole body, all receptors come into action simultaneously producing not only the desired analgesia but also other results. Some of these are desirable, such as the decrease of anxiety. Outside the central nervous system there are mixed effects, good and bad. The narcotics tend to paralyse smooth muscle. The coronary arteries dilate so that morphine has two beneficial actions in a heart attack, in which the pain drops and blood flow to the heart increases., Similarly the pain of renal colic is relieved by a direct action on smooth muscle as well as on pain. Constipation always occurs and nausea may be serious so that these side effects have to be treated with other drugs.

Other pharmacological treatments

By mentioning other treatments briefly, we can bring together the general principles we have been proposing. Let us consider, as an example of acute pain treatment, the highly contentious issue of drugs in childbirth. First, there is the right of the mother to experience her life without the enforced intrusion of drugs which will muddle her thinking. Second, if the mother decides that the suffering is or will be intolerable, the procedures must not interfere with the ease of delivery. Third, the baby is a passive bystander in these decisions at a time when passage through the birth canal and the switch-over to air breathing is hazardous and makes the child particularly susceptible to the side effects of drugs intended for the mother.

Early in labour, the mother is almost always given an atropine-like drug to control vomiting in case narcotics or general anaesthesia are to be given later. These sedate the mother and may slightly alter her memory of the experience. Low, safe doses of a general inhalant anaesthetic, which the mother administers to herself, are sometimes available for use at the height of contractions. Short-acting narcotics are frequently given, but the dosage has to be limited because they are likely to depress the child's respiration. Local anaesthetics can be infiltrated epidurally around the lumbar and sacral spinal cord, which provides spectacular comfort for the mother while leaving her mind clear. However, since this also produces a partial paralysis and therefore a weakening of contractions, labour is slightly prolonged. Furthermore, the local anaesthetic reaches the baby by way of the placenta, but safe doses are recognized and the baby's condition is continually monitored (by recording its heart rate) so that any signs of foetal distress can be promptly recognized and, if need be, the birth is hurried by a number of emergency procedures. Here, then, we see that each well-meaning action has its potentially harmful reactions and each needs social and technical debate to achieve an acceptable balance between the two. This balance can be achieved, and the mother must not feel that she is a traitor to herself and her baby if she cannot tolerate the pain.

Turning to more chronic pains, we have discussed (Chapter 5, p.113) the role of inflammation as a reaction to injury associated with pain. There are very powerful anti-inflammatory agents such as the steroid hormones. However, the attack on inflammation also diminishes a crucial body defence mechanism. Infections normally held in check can suddenly emerge. Reparative scar formation may be impeded. In spite of these dangers, the steroids play an important role in limiting inflammation and pain in certain carefully supervised states. A number of cancers, particularly some from the prostate and breast, are dependent for their growth on the presence of hormones. This led to a number of therapies to slow cancer growth by starving them of the required hormones. The most radical approach was to destroy the entire pituitary gland since this indirectly controls the other hormones. Its destruction can be achieved surprisingly easily since the pituitary is in the base of the skull and is covered by thin bone which can be penetrated by a stout hypodermic needle directed through the nostril (Moricca, 1974). It was noticed that, in some cases, there is a rapid and profound relief of pain (Moricca, 1974; Katz and Levin, 1977; Corssen *et al.*, 1977; Lipton *et al.*, 1979). The mechanism of pain relief remains obscure because the pain may decrease without any apparent change in the tumour. It is suspected that the treatment may affect the hypothalamus which, apart from its control of the pituitary, has powerful interconnections with the limbic system and with descending control systems.

We have often mentioned depression as a concomitant of chronic pain and it is therefore natural that the many types of anti-depressant drugs now available should be prescribed. They help the patient's natural depression but they also sometimes have a surprisingly powerful effect on pain which appears to be independent of their action on the depression. These drugs act by increasing the concentration in the brain and spinal cord of the amine transmitters such as serotonin. These amines are thought to play a role in the inhibitory mechanisms, especially the descending controls. It may therefore be that the anti-depressant drugs have a double action, one to help depression and one to increase the effectiveness of existing inhibitory mechanisms. Here, then, we see a final example of drugs having widespread actions which may limit the drugs' usefulness or, as in this case, may fortuitously complement each other.

Drugs and the market place

Pharmaceutical companies are under general humane pressures to help people in pain but they are also under commercial financial pressures to capture the largest possible fraction of the market. This means that the money available to them must be divided among research, production and advertising. While a few large companies make substantial basic-research efforts to discover new compounds or to develop old ones, the majority of companies carry out little or no research and are, therefore, dependent on the research efforts of the universities and larger companies. Many companies sell identical compounds which are required by law to be identical since all governments maintain a strict control over the composition and purity of drugs. If identical compounds have to be sold by many different companies, they can only succeed by giving them different names and by mounting massive promotional and advertising campaigns. Let us see how this works out in practice by examining the medicines against pain available in two countries. Countries A and B are large and small respectively, both with a high standard of medical care, but we will not identify them because they do not differ substantially from other developed countries. The data in Table 5 are taken from the list of drugs which are available to all doctors for prescription to their patients.

If we look at the 56 general anti-pain drugs (analgesics) in country B, we find that the contents of the drugs fall into two classes: 39 of them are aspirin-like compounds alone or in various mixtures, and 17 of them are narcotics alone or in various

Country A: Large developed country with extensive medical services

Total number of companies making anti-pain drugs	87
Total number of names for anti-pain drugs	270
for abdominal pain	77
for inflammation (non-steroid)	58
for angina	35
for migraine	16
for skin	12
for pain in general	72

Country B: Small developed country with extensive medical services

Total number of companies making anti-pain drugs	33
Total number of names for anti-pain drugs	187
for abdominal pain	69
for inflammation (non-steroid)	27
for migraine	17
for pain in general	56

Table 5.

mixtures. Aspirin-like compounds include aspirin, paracetamol (acetaminophen) and phenacetin. Aspirin by itself is sold under six different names by six companies and paracetamol is also sold by itself with five different brand names. Paracetamol and phenacetin have analgesic effects similar to those of aspirin. Therefore, it is apparent that not only is the same drug being sold under different names but, in addition, mixtures of drugs with similar properties are being sold under other different names. One may reasonably ask if this proliferation of similarly effective compounds in many combinations has any proven medical reason or if these were introduced without proper research and maintained on the market for purely commercial reasons. In country B, which we examined in 1980, we find that 10 of the analgesics contain either dipyrone or amidopyrine. These are highly active aspirin-like compounds but they were banned in the United States in 1938 because they tended to produce a blood disease called agranulocytosis. How can it be that 42 years after one country has prohibited a drug, it is still available and very widely used in another modern, responsible country? Is it ignorance or commercial pressures, or was the United States wrong in its assessment of the drug? Interestingly, phenacetin may no longer be prescribed in country A.

If we turn to the 17 medicines containing the other class of analgesic, the narcotics, we find a similar proliferation of identical drugs with different brand names and of mixtures of drugs with similar analgesic properties. The conclusion of the world's most respected book on pharmacology (Goodman and Gilman, 1980) on the difference between the narcotics is as follows: 'The differences between morphine and its semisynthetic and synthetic surrogates have been considerably overestimated. In equianalgesic doses, most of these drugs produce approximately the same incidence and degree of unwanted side effects.' If this is the case, how is it that there are seven different narcotics listed? The strength of the narcotics and anti-pain compounds varies enormously and the weakest, codeine, is 12 times less effective than morphine, milligram for milligram, even if given by injection. Codeine is the most common narcotic used in analgesic tablets and the dose varies from 8 to 15mg per tablet. Considering that 120mg of injected codeine is needed to produce an apparent analgesia, it is highly doubtful that 15mg of swallowed codeine will have any effect at all on pain – and we can find no clear evidence in the literature that it does. Therefore, with the 9 mixtures containing codeine, we are faced with the question of whether the dose is sufficient to be effective or whether it is included for show. Of the remaining 8 powerful narcotic medicines, we find that 4 are identical with different brand names and that the remaining 4 are different but all have approximately the same effect.

An example of the tendency to sell the same compound under different names is provided by an examination of the pharmacopoeia of country A:

Number of names for drugs containing:

aluminium hydroxide (for stomach pains)	44
aspirin	26
codeine (including cough mixtures)	33
ergotamine (for migraine)	8
paracetamol	46

It is reasonable, then, to question whether this multiplication of compounds, mixtures and brand names has anything to do with therapeutic effectiveness and how much of it is the chicanery of the market place, where doctors and patients are subject to the same show from pharmaceutical companies as was put on by the old-fashioned salesmen of snake oil and other popular nostrums.

13
Neurosurgical Approaches to Pain Control

While drugs are able to keep most kinds of pain under control, there are nevertheless several pain states which are not helped or which require such large doses that the person becomes confused or drowsy and finds it impossible to function normally. Until recently, the most common medical procedure for the control of severe, chronic pain which could not be helped by drugs was to destroy selected peripheral nerves or pathways in the central nervous system. Before we evaluate the general effectiveness of these procedures, we will first describe a few of the most common ones.

Permanent block or destruction of peripheral nerves

Pain may sometimes be so severe that both patient and doctor are forced to accept the option of a permanent destruction of nerves supplying a region despite the fact that, even if successful, this will result in a complete numbing of the region, and, in certain cases, in paralysis. It is evident in Figure 26 (p.204) that there is a choice of site of the procedure from the periphery to the roots entering the spinal cord. Each site has its advantages and disadvantages. If the painful area is small and is supplied by a single nerve, a peripheral procedure is chosen and the operation is simple. If the area is large or is close to the spine, then it is necessary to move towards central structures. One possible operation is to section only the sensory roots (rhizotomy), leaving the ventral roots intact. This has the advantage of leaving movement intact, but involves major surgery. In rhizotomy, the ganglion which contains the cell bodies of the sensory nerve is separated from the spinal cord, so that the nerves degenerate and are permanently lost.

Much ingenuity has gone into the destruction of nerves. Nerves can, of course, be exposed in open surgery but with the advent of techniques to bring needles close to nerves, less drastic operations become possible. After a temporary test of the effectiveness of the proposed destruction by injection of local anaesthetic, it is possible to inject a toxic substance which will destroy nerve fibres. Alcohol and phenol have been the most commonly used compounds. Another method is to burn a nerve by passing a high-frequency current through the tip of a needle, which produces intense heat. A prolonged block of nerves can also be achieved by cooling the nerve sufficiently to freeze it.

A common site of nerve destruction has been in the face, which is supplied by its own special cranial nerve, the trigeminal nerve. The sensory part of this nerve has three divisions which supply the forehead, the nose and maxilla (upper jaw), and the lower jaw. The cell bodies of this nerve lie in a shallow depression on the floor of the skull. This ganglion is the facial equivalent of the dorsal root ganglia which supply sensory nerves to each of the body's segments. A peculiarly unpleasant disorder of this nerve is trigeminal neuralgia, which we have discussed earlier. It occurs in older people and consists of attacks of stabbing pain of devastating intensity originating from a relatively small area of the face or inside of the mouth. The gentlest movement over this area triggers an attack of pain. Fortunately, most of these cases respond to a drug, carbamazepine ('tegretol'), which specifically suppresses this type of pain. However, some patients do not respond or have serious side effects of the drug and remain candidates for surgery. In some cases it is possible to cut a single branch of the main nerve which supplies the trigger area, but even here there is a tendency for regeneration. Usually the area is too wide for this procedure and therefore it is necessary to move centrally.

The next target for attack is the sensory ganglion. This can be approached by needle through one of the foramina (openings) in the base of the skull through which branches of the nerve exit in order to innervate the tissues. Alcohol injections of the ganglion were common and relatively easy to perform but left the entire face numb and were frequently followed by regeneration and recurrence of the pain. The numbing of the entire face is an unpleasant feeling at best, as one can guess from the temporary numbing of a small area of the face after dental anaesthesia. However, it has particularly serious consequences to the cornea of the eye which is no longer protected by the blink reflex and tears, and therefore tends to ulcerate from minor injury. In order to avoid this, attempts are made to destroy only a fraction of the nerve by positioning a needle in the ganglion, testing with low-level stimulation to see if the needle lies among the sensory fibres coming from the area of pain and then passing a high-frequency current through the needle until a portion of the fibres is destroyed.

The most general operation, however, continues to be an open exposure of the ganglion by turning down a flap of skull under the temporal muscle. Then the temporal lobe and its dura are elevated to reveal the ganglion on the floor of the skull. Usually the nerve roots flowing toward the brain from the ganglion are cut. This exposure has allowed a number of new techniques and ideas to be tested.

The origin and nature of trigeminal neuralgia is uncertain but there are many guesses. It occurs in older people, on the right side of the face (61%) more commonly than on the left, and in women (58%) more often than in men. The cause of trigeminal neuralgia must be subtle since no consistent anatomical changes have been found and the syndrome may mysteriously appear and disappear. It appears to depend on properties that are unique to the trigeminal nerve. In about 2% of the cases it is part of multiple sclerosis – a demyelinating disease of the central nervous system. All this points to some minor disorder of the nerve or perhaps some of its terminals in the medulla which produces this explosion of sensation following a gentle stimulus. Recently, several neurosurgeons have developed unusual surgical therapies, all of which work at least temporarily (Loeser, 1977). Some firmly massage the ganglion, while others decompress the ganglion by removing the dura which covers it. Most recently, the trigeminal nerve has been cushioned from the pulsation of the carotid artery which runs close by and is thought to be producing mechanical damage. The temporary success of all these operations indicate the complex role of the sensory input. It is possible that simply the stimulation of tissues during these procedures activates inhibitory mechanisms that may abolish the pain permanently or for at least long periods of time.

A more selective approach to the abolition of pain in the face without affecting other senses derives from the clinical observation of patients who had blockage of a small artery at the lower end of the medulla, the inferior cerebellar artery. It was noticed that, although these patients were completely analgesic on one side of the face while they could still appreciate light touch applied to the area. As the fifth nerve enters the brainstem, it sends sensory nerve fibres downwards to connect with cells in the medulla. There were reasons to think that these descending fibres on the surface of the medulla were the ones responsible for triggering pain. Sjöqvist therefore exposed the medulla by an approach from the back of the head below the cerebellum and cut the descending tract. The operation is itself dangerous, but if the patient survives there is a long-lasting selective facial analgesia reminiscent of the results of a spinal cord tractotomy which produces analgesia of a part of the body.

All surgical lesions of nerve roots and ganglia bring with them the disadvantage of total anaesthesia rather than selective removal of the pain. In addition, particularly with root sections, some of the patients develop unbearable new types of sensation of a peculiar nature which may be worse than the original pain and which are very resistant to treatment and to spontaneous cure. The mechanisms of these pains induced by nerve section have been discussed in Chapter 8. They lie partly in the region of the injured nerve which begins to generate abnormal nerve impulses and to produce unusual sensitivities. Furthermore, the cutting of peripheral nerves induces changes in the central nervous system, and the cutting of roots produces a major loss of nerve fibres which degenerate in the spinal cord following the lesion. The spinal cord cells which have lost their input begin to fire spontaneously and the nearest intact nerves increase their central influence. This means that an ongoing sensation is felt from the region which is totally anaesthetic while gentle stimulation of the edge of the anaesthetic area produces sharp pain. In seven cases of severe, chronic pain originating from peripheral nerve injury, Noordenbos and Wall (1981) have shown that meticulous surgery which excises the injured area in the peripheral nerve, including careful grafting of a section of new nerve, failed to remove the pain and in some cases made it worse. Here it is apparent that the peripheral nerve surgery was aimed at the wrong target because the seat of the trouble had already been transferred to the spinal cord.

Surgical or chemical destruction of spinal roots

We have seen that the site of neurosurgical attack moves toward the spinal cord as the site of origin of the pain becomes more diffuse. Unfortunately, this is a fairly common occurrence when cancer spreads to the thorax, abdomen or pelvis, or to the vertebral column and the adjacent roots and nerves. The large nerves peripheral to the ganglia contain a mixture of sensory and motor nerve fibres, so that cutting them results not only in an area of complete numbness but also in paralysis and wasting of muscles. The paralysis can be avoided by taking advantage of the divergence of the sensory nerves into dorsal roots as they approach the spinal cord, leaving the motor fibres to run in the ventral roots. Open surgery, which involves removal of the bony vertebral arches and opening of the dura mater, allows the surgeon to see the dorsal roots and to cut them. Because the body area served by one root overlaps with its neighbours, it is always necessary to cut at least three roots in order to achieve a complete anaesthesia of any part of the body. It can be seen that this involves major surgery which is clearly to be avoided, particularly in patients who may be desperately ill from the disease which is causing their pain. An alternative, much simpler method is to inject into the cerebrospinal fluid a solution of phenol and thick glycerine which can be made to soak the desired nerve roots by positioning the patient so that the viscous globule runs over one group of dorsal roots on one side. The most common roots to be approached in this way are the sacral roots supplying the pelvis, a frequent source of pain in cancer patients which can be treated by a simple lumbar puncture. This method is less accurate and less long-lasting than direct surgical section but is obviously far less disturbing to the patient.

There are unfortunate side effects of these procedures in a high percentage of patients who survive for long periods of time. When a dorsal root is destroyed either by a knife or by chemicals, the nerve fibres central to the cut are isolated from their cell bodies which lie in the dorsal root ganglia in the bony canal between the vertebrae. These isolated central parts of the nerve root degenerate and there is never any regeneration, unlike the regenerative process which can take place in peripheral nerves. This means that nerve cells in the spinal cord permanently lose the nerve fibres which normally activate them. Nerve cells which lose their normal drive demonstrate one of the many types of homeostatic mechanism, in this case called *denervation hypersensitivity*. It is as though the cell recognizes that it no longer receives its normal excitatory signals and therefore raises its own excitability to a stage where the cell begins to generate nerve impulses when no input signal is received. The consequence to the patient is that he first experiences the desired total anaesthesia in the region supplied by the cut roots, then develops a pins-and-needles feeling which may gradually grow in intensity until he is in continuous pain. The surgeon has created on a small scale the same disorder which occurs with the common motorbike accident of brachial plexus avulsion in which, as we have described earlier (p.21), the majority of patients with extensive root damage suffer severe pains.

Surgical or chemical destruction of the sympathetic system

All parts of the body are supplied by a special set of efferent nerves which originate in the chain of sympathetic ganglia which run on each side of the vertebral column from the top of the chest to the upper abdomen (Figure 6, p.77). These nerves supply the blood vessels, glands and viscera and control their activity. In 1889, François-Franck first suggested that sensory afferent nerves probably run along with this efferent system and that it might be possible to stop some pains by cutting the ganglia. This idea was taken up particularly by the French surgeon, René Leriche (1879 – 1956), who wrote one of the first surgical textbooks on pain. He believed that there are certain types of pain which are particularly influenced by the sympathetic system and proceeded to prove this by taking out the sympathetic ganglia related to the painful part, and often producing dramatic pain relief. The success of this operation, particularly in causalgia, does not definitively demonstrate why it works. François-Franck (1899) proposed that it was simply due to cutting a special type of sensory fibre. Leriche proposed that the sympathetic efferents were responsible for stimulating damaged nerve fibres and further suggested that there was an abnormal reflex pathway mediated through the sympathetic ganglia rather than through the spinal cord.

The direct surgical approach to the sympathetic ganglia is always difficult and sometimes dangerous. As a result, anaesthesiologists have learned to insert long needles that reach the sympathetic ganglia. They then inject a test dose of local anaesthetic and, if the effect is satisfactory, the ganglia are injected with a destructive fluid such as alcohol or phenol. However, it was the anaesthesiologist, Hannington-Kiff (1974), who solved the problem of how a sympathectomy works by taking a new approach. Pharmacologists have developed a large number of chemicals which block the action of noradrenalin, which is emitted from the sympathetic efferent fibres. One of these, guanethidine, has a particularly long-lasting action and effectively blocks the ability of the sympathetic fibres to release noradrenalin. After a guanethidine block of the painful limb by means of Hannington-Kiff's technique (Chapter 8, p.184), the pain is often relieved even though sensory fibres are not blocked by this drug. The success of this treatment supports the observation by Wall and Gutnick (1974) that damaged sensory fibres become highly sensitive to noradrenalin. It therefore appears that certain types of nerve damage allow the sympathetic system to trigger impulses in sensory nerve fibres.

The sympathetic system is involved in pain in a second way. It controls the diameter of blood vessels and therefore affects blood flow and blood pressure. If blood flow becomes inadequate for the needs of a muscle, pain occurs as in a cramp or in angina pectoris. In most of these conditions, the blood flow regulation mechanisms have done the best they can to deliver the maximum available blood flow to the region. However, on occasion, the sympathetic system is still active or over-active and it is possible to obtain an improved blood flow by removing the vasoconstricting effect of the sympathetic fibres either surgically or chemically.

Cordotomy: the cutting of tracts in the spinal cord

In the terrible days when tuberculosis was a universal scourge, patients would sometimes have widespread infections extending far beyond the lungs – which are the commonest site of infection. Around a nest of bacteria, the tissue reacts to produce a nodule called a tuberculoma. One location of these slowly expanding small spheres is on the surface of the spinal cord. The tuberculoma presses against the spinal cord and may cut the white matter by pressure, thereby producing a quite localized lesion. In 1905, Spiller saw a tubercular patient who had lost the ability to feel pain and temperature in the lower half of his body. At autopsy it was found that tuberculomas had cut across the ventral lateral white matter of his spinal cord at the thoracic level. At Spiller's instigation, in 1911, Martin exposed a patient's spinal cord and intentionally cut across these ventrolateral fibres. This was followed by a rapid development of technique and application, particularly for patients with cancer pain. If the operation is carried out on one side, the patient is strikingly analgesic to pinprick on the opposite side of the body below the level of the lesion. In this area he cannot identify a touch by the tip or the head of a pin. He is also unable to differentiate between warm and cold objects. The patient's sense of touch is much less disturbed, with only minor changes of threshold and ability to recognize if he was touched by two points or by one. However, it must be stressed that the operation does not entirely abolish the ability to feel pain from the affected area. If a blood pressure cuff is put on an affected leg and the blood supply is blocked, exercise still evokes a severe cramping pain.

It has been known since the last century (Edinger, 1889) that the white matter cut in this operation contains axons which run directly from the spinal cord to the thalamus – the spinothalamic tract. This finding seemed so compelling that the operation is often called a spinothalamic tractotomy, with the implication that it cuts the spinal 'pain pathway'. It was the simplest rationale for the operation and, in spite of later facts which make the idea highly unlikely, the concept has persisted. The main end-station of these fibres is the ventral posterior lateral nucleus (part of the ventrobasal complex) of the thalamus, and destruction of this nucleus is singularly unsuccessful in producing a long-lasting analgesia. Furthermore, of the hundreds of thousands of nerve fibres cut in this very extensive section, Mehler (1962) estimates that only about 1,500 are destined for the thalamus. In fact, this quadrant of cord carries many ascending fibre systems and the most massive of these which might be concerned with pain terminates in the reticular formation in the pons and medulla. Moreover, the area contains descending control systems which could affect sensibility as well as motor control.

The major problem with the operation is that the effect fades as months go by. While fully justified in patients who are in the terminal stages of cancer from which they will die in weeks or months, the operation should not be done in patients who are likely to survive for longer times – partly because the pain returns, frequently accompanied by a variety of unpleasant sensations. These are presumably generated by nerve cells whose normal input has degenerated as a consequence of the operation. When pains are often felt on both sides of the body, it is necessary to cut the tracts on both sides of the spinal cord. If that is done, the sectioning of descending pathways can produce distressing consequences. The control pathways to bladder and rectum run in the ventral quadrants so that patients may have incontinence added to their miseries. In the cervical cord, respiratory control pathways are likely to be cut or damaged in bilateral operations leading to periods of paralysis of the diaphragm.

Many of the patients who are candidates for a cordotomy are desperately ill from the disease which is the cause of their pain and are therefore extremely poor risks in their ability to withstand the anaesthesia and major surgery which are necessarily involved in exposing the spinal cord. To solve this problem, Mullan (1966) introduced the much less intrusive technique of percutaneous cordotomy. Here, under X-ray control, a needle is inserted between the cervical vertebrae until it lies in the cerebrospinal fluid on the ventral side of the cord. Its tip is located with respect to the cord by injecting a fluid which can be seen by X-rays. When the position is considered satisfactory, a thin wire is pushed into the cord and it is again tested as being in a proper location by using gentle electrical stimulation and asking the patient what he feels. Once verified as being in ventral white matter, a heat lesion is produced around the tip of the wire by means of an electric current. While the immediate complications of this simple operation are less than those of open surgery, the neurological complications are slightly more frequent because of difficulty of control of the location and extent of the lesion.

Cerebral operations for relief of pain

There are three major reasons why surgeons have operated on the brain in an attempt to produce analgesia. The first and simplest is that pains may originate from the upper chest, head and neck so that even bilateral cordotomies would fail to produce temporary analgesia in these areas. Second, in the face of actual or expected failure of cordotomies to produce prolonged relief, it was thought possible that more radical sections of presumed pain pathways in the brain would produce a more profound and prolonged analgesia. Third, there has been a general belief that somewhere there must exist a specialized pain centre whose destruction would specifically abolish pain. This 'centre' would be expected, on the basis of the simplistic nineteenth-century thinking of classical neurosurgery, to be in the thalamus or cortex.

Mesencephalic tractotomy

A very tempting target for operation for those convinced that the spinothalamic tract is the 'pain pathway' is the confluence of spinothalamic fibres, just before arriving in the thalamus, on the lateral surface of the midbrain just below the inferior colliculus. White and Sweet (1969) report on thirty cases in whom this tract was cut at seven of the most distinguished centres of neurosurgery in the world. The appalling death rate of forty-one per cent shows the difficulty and danger of lesions in this region. While there was temporary pain relief reported in the survivors, forty-six per cent developed dysaesthesias described as more severe than the original pain. These abysmal results led to the operation being abandoned but do not appear to have influenced in any way the thinking of those who moved on to the next target, the thalamus.

Thalamotomy

One of the founders of neurosurgery was Sir Victor Horsley, an extraordinary and eccentric man who also made major discoveries in anatomy and physiology at the turn of the century. He realized that the brain has a very constant relationship to the skull in which it rests. He measured the distance of various deep-brain structures from several fixed and obvious skull points – the midline, the ear canal, and the lower edge of the eye socket – and found the measures to be highly repeatable. He and Clarke then developed a coordinate system and maps of the brain which allow wires to be lowered into the brain to end in the desired structure. This stereotactic method has become a major technique for placing electrodes in deep-brain nuclei and tracts for recording or for lesion-making. Stereotactic surgery allows an approach to any part of the midbrain and forebrain in man with the needles inserted through a small hole drilled in the skull. The technique has become widely used by neurosurgeons to make lesions in the basal ganglia for movement disorders (such as Parkinson's disease) and obviously allowed lesions to be made in the thalamus for sensory disorders. Since 1948, when Spiegel and Wycis began to carry out thalamotomy for pain, a large number of patients have had many different thalamic areas destroyed, often with multiple lesions. These have included destruction of the pulvinar, a nucleus not known to be related to somatosensory inputs. The results are disappointing and educational.

Many of the lesions produced analgesia and pain relief but the usual picture is of a fading of the effect at a faster rate than after cordotomy (Spiegel and Wycis, 1966). As might be expected, these lesions produce a wide range of other effects on mood and motivation, but no case has been reported of a prolonged inability to feel pain while other sensations were left intact. Clearly, there is no evidence that the thalamus contains *the* pain centre. On the contrary, any of a series of widespread lesions temporarily disturbs the patients' ability to feel pain, but pain rapidly returns if the patients recover their general intellectual abilities. These operations have not in the least deterred those who are convinced that all human sensations are located in the cerebral cortex, whose major input and output is the thalamus. Therefore, surgeons have turned to the cortex.

Cortical lesions

Valuable information about cortical function has been revealed by the study of epileptic fits. They begin as local, massive, synchronized over-activity of discrete areas of cerebral cortex. During this early stage of a fit, the patient may report any of a large variety of sensations, mood changes or motor movements, but never frank somatic pain. Stimulation of the cortex has frequently been carried out by neurosurgeons in conscious man, but has rarely evoked pain. Destruction limited to the cortex has not been reported as producing analgesia but it may produce a radical change in thought processes. In spite of this negative evidence, which suggests that the cortex is not the site of a pain centre, operations on the cortex are still performed. Various types of frontal lobectomy and lobotomy (or leucotomy) have been carried out on pain patients. These operations isolate all or part of the frontal lobes from the rest of the brain. The patients are not analgesic in any ordinary sense. That is to say, they respond or sometimes over-respond to a normally painful stimulus and on direct questioning they say that their original pain is still present. However, in the successful patients, the pain appears to worry them less and they can shift their attention on to other matters. It seems that the patients' assessment of the significance of the pain has changed. The successes, as measured by less complaint, are achieved at the cost of a general change of ways of thinking. With small lesions, the overall shifts of personality may be quite small but, as with all forms of psychosurgery, there are subtle changes so that the patients' friends and relatives recognize that they are no longer the same as they were.

Summary of surgical approaches

It may seem to the reader that we have adopted a negative approach to these therapies. It is certainly true that acceptable long-term control of pain is rarely achieved by surgery. Not only does the pain eventually recur but additional unpleasant sensations appear as a result of denervation. Nevertheless, short-term control can on occasion be achieved, particularly with cordotomy, and is fully justified in patients with a short time to live, such as people in the terminal stages of cancer. However, neurosurgical attempts to abolish other forms of chronic pain are often a disaster. One tragic case will suffice to show what can happen. A man developed phantom limb pain as a result of a brachial plexus avulsion. The arm was amputated – an unnecessary operation which was done in the incorrect belief that the paralysed arm was abnormally affecting healthy, sensitive tissue. He then had a high cervical cordotomy. When this failed, it was repeated a second time in the belief that the first operation was not sufficiently extensive. He then had two operations on his frontal lobes which produced a definite, though temporary, psychological change but with no reduction of his pain. After destruction of the ventrobasal nucleus (Fig. 21, p. 156) of the thalamus also failed, this unfortunate man committed suicide.

Our increasing knowledge of pain mechanisms now makes it clear that cutting the peripheral or central nervous system does not simply stop an input from reaching the brain. Surgical section of a peripheral nerve has multiple effects: it permanently disrupts normal input patterning; it may result in abnormal inputs from irritating scars and neuromas; and it destroys channels that may be potentially useful to control pain by input modulation methods. Similar consequences occur after cordotomy, which is perhaps the most common operation to relieve pain. Cordotomy does much more than just destroy pain-signalling fibres. It also has multiple effects (Melzack and Wall, 1965): it reduces the total number of responding neurons; it changes the temporal and spatial relationships among all ascending systems; and it affects the descending fibre systems that control transmission from peripheral fibres to dorsal horn cells. The reduction of input to the central nervous system, we now know, produces highly abnormal, bursting activity in the deafferented central cells – a condition that may persist long after the surgical section and which is conducive to prolonged pathological pain (Melzack and Loeser, 1978).

The complexity of brain activity also defies simple surgical solutions to pain problems. Pain signals project to widespread parts of the brain. If one area is surgically eliminated, there are others that still continue to receive the input. The nervous system, moreover, is able to form new connections and thereby provide new pathways for the sensory input. This plasticity is evident in physiological studies which show that after destruction of fibres to a central neural structure, the branches of neurons from adjacent areas now dominate the activity of the structure. These branches are normally kept under control but are unmasked by denervation (Wall and Egger, 1971). Plasticity is also demonstrated in studies on the effects of lesions of the central grey matter (Melzack *et al.*, 1958). The animals failed to respond to noxious heat a month after the lesions were made; nevertheless they began to respond within a few days after onset of testing with noxious stimuli until they became indistinguishable from normal animals. The nervous system appears to have undergone some kind of reorganization so that the input, blocked from ascending through one pathway, is now projected through another.

Happily, the role of the neurosurgeon in the treatment of pain has been changing rapidly in recent years. Fewer rhizotomies and cordotomies are now being carried out, and neurosurgeons are turning increasingly to non-destructive approaches such as the use of devices to electrically stimulate nerves, spinal cord and discrete areas of the brain. A small number of neurosurgeons are carrying out pioneering work in these fields, and the results so far – which will be described in the next chapter – are highly exciting. They hold great promise for the patient in severe, intractable pain who is not helped by the traditional drug therapies.

14
Sensory Control of Pain

The gate-control theory, after its publication in 1965, had a powerful impact on the treatment of pain. Its emphasis on a dynamic balance between excitatory and inhibitory influences, including feedback interactions between spinal and brain levels, has been the basis of new conceptual approaches to pain therapy and has suggested new forms of treatment. The gate theory, in recent years, has opened the way for a search for techniques to modulate the sensory input. It suggests that pain control may be achieved by the enhancement of normal physiological activities rather than their disruption by destructive, irreversible lesions. In particular, it has led to attempts to control pain by activation of inhibitory mechanisms.

The gate theory suggests four general methods to control pain by modulation of the input:

1 The use of anaesthetic blocking agents to decrease the number of nerve impulses that impinge on the T cells.

2 Low-level stimulation which selectively activates the large fibres that inhibit transmission from peripheral fibres to T cells.

3 Intense stimulation which activates brainstem mechanisms that exert an inhibitory influence on the spinal gate-control system and at higher synaptic transmission levels.

4 The direct activation of descending control systems by electrical stimulation or by pharmaceutical agents.

While the first three methods have a fascinating history that pre-dates the gate-control theory, the theory provided a scientific rationale for them that led to their widespread use and acceptance. It is clearly far preferable to attempt to decrease excitation by anaesthetic blocks or to increase inhibition by stimulation of nerves than to destroy nerve tissue with the possible consequence of unpleasant sensations and motor loss.

Temporary local anaesthesia

For millennia, the leaves of *Erythroxylon coca* have been chewed by those who live in the Andes for its psychedelic effect. These leaves, which contain cocaine, were well known to produce a numbing of the mouth but this was generally ignored as an unwanted side effect. The pure alkaloid was isolated by the middle of the nineteenth century and in 1884 Sigmund Freud and Karl Köller in Vienna made a general study of the physiological effects of cocaine, including the fact that it produced a local anaesthetic effect if it penetrated into tissue. Freud, as might be expected, was most interested in its mental effects and went on to wean a colleague from morphine by giving him cocaine, thereby producing the first iatrogenic (physician-induced) cocaine addict. Köller, however, immediately saw the practical possibilities of the use of cocaine as a local anaesthetic and instilled it into the eye. General anaesthesia with ether or chloroform were well established by this time but the serious toxic side effects of these compounds were becoming apparent, so that an alternative form of anaesthesia was immediately exploited. Thus, in 1884, Hall introduced local anaesthesia to dentistry, and in 1885 Halsted produced nerve blocks by injecting cocaine around nerves.

Halsted was chief of surgery at Johns Hopkins Medical School, at that time the most important centre of surgery in the world since it was developing the technique of aseptic surgery from which all modern surgery evolved. Members of the department gained experience on themselves by injecting the area around various nerves and invented the idea of regional anaesthesia. In the process, many of these men, who had distinguished careers as professors of surgery, became steady cocaine addicts. By 1905 the first synthetic local anaesthetic, procaine, was produced, which does not have the psychedelic effects of cocaine. Since 1948, procaine has largely been replaced by lidocaine which is more powerful and less toxic, and by a family of related compounds with slightly varying properties but all having '-caine' at the end of their names.

This may not be the end of the story. Just as cocaine is a naturally occurring plant compound which blocks nerve conduction, other nerve-blocking compounds are found in different species. For example, some fish and salamanders have developed a nerve blocker of extraordinary potency – tetrodotoxin. Similarly, a family of dinoflagellates, found in sea water and eaten by shellfish such as clams, produces one of the most potent poisons known – saxitoxin. These compounds block nerve impulses by some mechanism which differs from the -caines and, while they are presently used (with considerable caution) only by scientists, they might generate another family of local anaesthetics.

Procedure and uses. Local anaesthetics do not penetrate unbroken skin. While they are often a component of sunburn sprays and lotions, there is considerable doubt that they have any effect on the surface and it is generally believed that the relief they produce comes from cooling of the skin. Cooling is an effective way to control pain after minor superficial injury and is the basis for the various sprays used, especially in athletics, as a first-aid treatment for kicks and bruises.

Local anaesthetics are able to penetrate mucous membrane tissue and are therefore incorporated in the innumerable nostrums for sore throats and haemorrhoids, and are even swallowed for hiccups. However, by far the commonest use of local anaesthetics is by needle injection. Here the aim is to squirt the anaesthetic onto a nerve, or sometimes just to infiltrate a general area which one wishes to make numb. Most of us have experienced this technique in the hands of dentists who inject close to one of the nerves supplying the teeth on which they are to work. The injection is usually given in combination with adrenalin, which constricts the local blood vessels and slows down the absorption of the anaesthetic into the blood stream, thereby prolonging its local action.

Anaesthesiologists have become highly skilled in approaching most of the peripheral nerves in the body. They are now often aided in this procedure by using image-intensified X-rays so that they can follow the course of the needle tip with respect to bony structures. It is possible in this way to give a regional anaesthetic to a whole limb, but this involves extensive infiltration with quantities of local anaesthetic which approach the toxic limits. For the legs, chest, abdomen and pelvis a more economical approach can be used in which advantage is taken of the confluence of the sensory nerves as they pass into the spinal cord. As we have already mentioned, there is a space – the epidural space – between the inner side of the bony vertebral canal and the dura mater which covers the spinal cord. The nerve roots have to pass through this space and it is possible to place a fine catheter in it and to flood the region with local anaesthetic. Since these catheters can be manoeuvred to any segment of the spinal column, large areas of the body can be anaesthetized on both sides by this skilled but simple procedure of epidural block.

A more direct approach to achieve spinal anaesthesia for pain in the abdomen, pelvis or legs involves injection of the anaesthetic by way of a lumbar puncture needle. The needle is pushed through the skin in the midline of the lower back so that it slips between the vertebrae, passes through the epidural space, punctures the dura and enters the cerebrospinal fluid. In the adult, the spinal cord does not fill the entire spinal canal and the lowest part is filled with a bundle of nerve roots which supply the lower lumbar and sacral segments. This bundle, the cauda equina ('horse tail'), can be safely penetrated by a needle since the roots move out of the way and it is possible to soak the entire region in local anaesthetic. As the amount of anaesthetic is increased, the level of anaesthesia on the body surface rises upwards. The limit is determined by the danger of paralysing the respiratory muscles in the chest. Here, then, we see that by taking advantage of the specialized anatomical flow of sensory fibres, it is possible to anaesthetize small or large areas of the body without interfering with other systems or with the patient's thinking processes.

The rationale. Local anaesthetics act by stabilizing the membranes of nerve and muscle cells which produce action potentials. After an injection, a high concentration of the anaesthetic is built up around the target nerve. The nerve membrane at rest maintains the separation of specific ions so that potassium ions accumulate on the inside and sodium ions on the outside. If the normal membrane is slightly disturbed by changing the voltage across it, this mechanism to separate ions is briefly altered, and sodium ions rush in while potassium ions flow out. This explosive flow of ions produces the nerve impulse and the impulse runs along the nerve membrane followed in a few milliseconds by the restoration of the resting state. Local anaesthetics block the triggering mechanism by which these impulses are generated so that the nerve remains fixed in its resting state for as long as the local anaesthetic is present in a high enough concentration.

Side effects. Great as this advance has been, there are certain limits to its usefulness. Local anaesthesia usually involves a complete block of all nerve fibres in the region. This results in a complete numbness of the area supplied by a nerve, but also in paralysis since the motor fibres are also blocked.

If the amount of anaesthetic rises generally in the body, other impulse-generating structures, such as the heart, begin to be affected by showing a decrease in excitability. In fact, local anaesthetics are so effective in stabilizing heart muscle that they are used intentionally as a general intravenous drug to decrease the heightened excitability of heart muscle when abnormal contractions occur. Similarly, the brain is exposed to rising levels of the drug and its first reaction is to increase its excitability, presumably because inhibitory mechanisms are most easily affected.

Since local anaesthetics produce such a satisfactory abolition of pain for an hour or more even if they cause local paralysis, there has been a search for methods of prolonging their action. Such drugs have been discovered but, unfortunately, they have toxic effects, including damage to the nerve which is blocked. The alternative approach has been to devise methods for continuous application of the short-acting drugs. This procedure succeeds over periods of days by using an indwelling catheter, and is utilized in some hospitals to suppress the worst of the pains after an operation or a wound. However, complications eventually set in and the treatment must end. One of the most interesting side effects of these drugs is that in addition to blocking nerve impulses they also block the transport of substances along nerve fibres. This transport is necessary for the integrity of the nerve and for its target organs, and this secondary effect may therefore forbid the dream of a long-term local anaesthetic derived from this family of -caines.

Recently, morphine has been used in an unorthodox fashion for the relief of chronic pain. Normally, of course, it is injected into muscles such as the buttock or it is ingested orally. There is now evidence that morphine may bring about dramatic relief of some kinds of pain if a small amount is injected epidurally. Extremely severe pain due to spreading cancer in the pelvic region can sometimes be relieved to a significant extent by injection of a few milligrams of morphine in the lumbar epidural space. The results of this procedure, like all new techniques, seem extremely exciting. However, the method is new and requires more carefully controlled research before it can be recommended without reservation.

Despite the short-acting effect of an anaesthetic agent, anaesthetic blocks of the sensory input often produce pain relief that outlasts the duration of the blocks (Livingston, 1943; Kibler and Nathan, 1960). Successive blocks may relieve pain for increasingly long periods of time. Anaesthetic blocks of tender skin areas, peripheral nerves, or sympathetic ganglia would have the effect of diminishing the total sensory input that bombards the spinal transmission cells. They would, therefore, reduce the spinal cell output below the critical level necessary to evoke pain. These blocks, moreover, could bring about a cessation of self-sustaining, memory-like activity, so that temporary blocks would produce long periods of relief. Furthermore, the relief of pain would permit increased use of the body, allowing the patient to carry out normal motor activities. These, in turn, would produce patterned inputs (particularly from muscles) that would contain a high proportion of active large fibres that would further close the gate and delay the recurrence of pain. In addition, the motor 'commands' that descend from the brain to the spinal cord are accompanied by inhibitory descending control impulses which would also reduce the sensory input during movement.

The varieties of physical therapy

A multitude of techniques are practised by physiatrists (doctors of physical medicine and rehabilitation) and physiotherapists. The following (Zohn and Mennell, 1976) is a partial list:

1 Manual therapy: exercise; massage; manipulation; relaxation.
2 Mechanical therapy: traction; compression.
3 Heat: superficial heat: dry; wet.
4 Heat: deep heat: shortwave diathermy; microwave diathermy; ultrasound.
5 Cold: vapocoolant spray; ice packs; ice massage; hypothermia.
6 Electrotherapy: alternating current (Faradism); sinusoidal current; transcutaneous nerve stimulation.
7 Electrotherapy: direct current (galvanism); interrupted galvanism.

These are the more commonly used among many physical procedures, most of them requiring elegant and complicated-looking equipment. There is no doubt that they are effective for a wide variety of pains. However, their mechanism of action is poorly understood. The common feature of most of them is that they produce a sensory input – they generate nerve impulses that enter the spinal cord and brain and produce their pain-relieving effects for reasons that we will later try to understand. We will first consider several of the procedures briefly, and then examine some of them in detail.

Massage and manipulation

Almost all societies practise mixtures and variations of these two techniques in which mechanical pressure is used against pain. While they are generally practised by highly skilled, carefully trained professionals, there is not one of us who does not scratch an itch, stretch an aching back, or rub an area that hurts. These are our own, almost instinctive, manoeuvres which have developed into the various anti-pain procedures we are now discussing. Some people take them seriously, with an almost religious awe, while others treat them in a more matter-of-fact way.

Massage

Clearly, there are many massage techniques, each with its enthusiastic following. Some therapists move only skin with light repeated movements while others massage deep structures so vigorously that they produce pain. Massage may be given at the site of pain or at a considerable distance. Light mechanical vibrators driven by electricity and oscillating at the frequency of the mainline voltage are being used more frequently. Deep massage involves heavy pressure and the stretching and pinching of ligaments, tendons and muscles. One of the main problems for an analysis of this and the following procedures is to know exactly what it is the therapist is doing and which of all the various pressures and movements are most effective.

Manipulation

Here the patient is subjected to a variety of stretchings, twistings and pullings. Some are gentle, some are quite violent. There are many practitioners, including osteopaths and chiropractors. However, physiotherapists, physiatrists and orthopaedists (bone specialists) also practise forms of manipulation. There are, in addition, faddist groups that practise special manipulations and massages. Each school operates on its own theoretical target. Some claim to be placing bones, especially the vertebrae, in their correct alignment but there is no X-ray evidence that the bones are out of place before the manipulation or that they are changed afterwards. Others claim to be releasing trapped pockets in joint cavities but there is no evidence that there are such pockets trapped or released. Some say they are breaking up scar tissue which is trapping nerves while others state that they are putting muscles in their correct tensions. It is a pity that there is such a plethora of untested hypotheses since these manipulations on occasion produce quite dramatic relief. Yet the manipulators, the patients and the rest of us remain ignorant of exactly what was done to produce the disappearance of the pain or, for that matter, how to explain the many failures.

Heat therapy

General heating

Since neolithic times, people in all parts of the world have found ways of raising the body temperature and have used them for treatment of their pains. The North American Indians' hodown, the Finnish sauna, the innumerable spas of Europe around hot springs (especially the thermae of Italy), the Roman baths with their hot and tepid rooms, the Russian and Turkish versions of the steam room, and the Japanese hot soaking tub all produce intense heat. The body temperature is allowed to rise in spite of the body's attempts to lose heat by sweating and by opening the superficial blood vessels. The surrounding air or the water is so hot that the body takes in more heat than it can get rid of and so the body temperature rises.

Local superficial heat

Great ingenuity has been used through the ages to apply and sustain local superficial heating. The poultice is an ancient art in which some substance is heated to the highest safe temperature and is then allowed to transfer its heat slowly to the skin. T. S. Eliot in 'Prufrock' has the nice couplet:

'Here comes the nurse with the red hot poultice,
Slaps it on and takes no notice.'

Since ancient times, heated clay, stones, bread, dough, and towels have been shaped and placed on painful areas to heat them. In our modern age, we use electrically heated pads. We also produce vasodilation by rubbing herbs or drugs into the skin or by applying plasters made of mustard or cantharides (which is an extract of Spanish flies). Friar's Balsam and many liniments similarly produce a vasodilation of the blood vessels in the skin and, consequently, a feeling of warmth. Since the skin turns red as the blood vessels open up, these compounds are called rubifacients, or 'red makers'.

Local deep heat

Ultrasound. One of the uses of this modern technique is to raise the temperature in deep structures. The sounds that we hear consist of pressure waves in the air, and the highest tones we can hear are produced by wave frequencies of about fifteen to twenty thousand cycles per second. Pressure waves produced at high frequencies beyond our hearing range are called ultrasound just as ultraviolet is a type of light with a frequency beyond our ability to see. An ultrasound frequency of over one million cycles per second takes on a number of characteristics like light. It can be focused and beamed. It travels through water and soft tissues and, like an intense beam of light, it heats whatever absorbs it. The sound is produced by a rapidly vibrating crystal, like a crystal loudspeaker, which is placed on the skin. The sound enters the body and passes through the soft tissue with very little loss of energy. However, when the sound hits something solid like bone, it is absorbed and turned into heat. In this way, it is possible to warm gently the surface of bones and especially joints. (A more modern use of ultrasound is to record echoes reflected back from deep structures so that pictures can be made of hard and soft tissues. It is particularly useful to examine a baby in the mother's uterus since ultrasound is harmless, unlike X-rays which may produce genetic damage. In an entirely different application, ultrasound echoes are also used to locate submarines.)

Diathermy. This is a method of heating a part of the body or a limb from the middle outward and it uses electromagnetic radiation rather than the pressure waves used in ultrasound. Visible light is electromagnetic radiation at frequencies which do not pass through the body, so that a person who stands in front of a light casts a shadow. Radio waves are electromagnetic radiation at frequencies that pass through the body and most other structures, including walls in homes. The frequencies used in diathermy pass into the body but are absorbed in the deep tissues where the electromagnetic energy is transformed into heat. This property is used to the patient's advantage in diathermy where the middle of a limb can be gently warmed while leaving the skin virtually unaffected. (Another use of this principle is in the microwave oven, which also cooks food from the middle outward.)

Mechanisms of action

Heat appears to be most effective for low-to-moderate levels of pain due to deep-tissue injuries such as bruises, torn muscles and ligaments, and arthritis. Whether it speeds up repair is not known, but it is doubtful. Despite the widespread use of heat to relieve pain, we do not know why it works. There are two hypotheses which both need to be tested. The first relates to the obvious vasodilation and the consequent increase of blood flow. It seems reasonable that, if there is damaged tissue or infection, the blood must bring cells and chemicals needed for the repair of injured or inflamed tissues and must sweep away the breakdown products of injury – such as histamine, bradykinin and prostaglandins – which we know contribute to pain. Even in the use of superficial heat for the relief of pain in deep structures, it is possible that deep blood vessels are dilated by 'somato-visceral' reflexes evoked by skin stimulation. This vascular hypothesis merits investigation because anti-inflammatory agents such as prostaglandin inhibitors are often effective analgesics, which suggests that the substances produced by inflammation and injury are built up at faster rates than they can be carried away by the blood flow.

The second hypothesis proposes that the heating of tissues generates nerve impulses which play a role in the afferent barrage and have an inhibitory effect by closing the gate in the spinal cord. This would explain how the application of heat at a distance from the source of the damage and pain can be effective. The nerve impulses stimulated by heating the skin travel into the spinal cord and, at convergent synapses, inhibit impulses that originate in damaged tissue much deeper than the heated skin. Therefore, it is possible that heat counteracts pain by stimulating nerve impulses which decrease the effectiveness in the spinal cord of the pain-producing nerve impulses.

The mechanisms that underlie the pain-relieving effects of most of the procedures of physical therapy remain a mystery. The most plausible hypothesis for all of them is that they produce sensory inputs that ultimately inhibit pain signals ('close the gate'). As we have seen, the gate theory proposes that this may occur (1) by activation of large fibres by gentle stimulation which has inhibitory effects at segmental levels; or (2) by activation of small fibres which project signals to brainstem areas which, in turn, send messages to the spinal cord that close the gate. Different procedures in physical medicine may be explained by either or both mechanisms. There is now considerable evidence about these mechanisms which has been revealed as a result of the dramatic growth of interest in transcutaneous electrical stimulation.

Electrical stimulation of nerves, spinal cord and brain

The most obvious prediction of the experiments that led to the gate-control theory was that a rise of pain threshold should occur after stimulation of large, low-threshold fibres since their central action is accompanied by an inhibition of cells which transmit injury signals. The large fibres in a peripheral nerve can be preferentially stimulated by passing electric currents through the nerve. The reason for this selective stimulation is that large-diameter fibres have a lower longitudinal electrical resistance than small fibres, so that current can flow through them more easily. The sensation produced by gentle electrical stimulation of normal peripheral nerves is a buzzing, tingling feeling which becomes painful only if the strength of stimulation is greatly increased to stimulate small fibres.

Wall and Sweet (1967) therefore set about stimulating the large fibres in peripheral nerves first in themselves and then in patients. They used three different methods: (1) stimulation of nerves through electrodes on the skin; (2) stimulation by electrodes surgically implanted around nerves and activated by subcutaneous radio-stimulators; and (3) stimulation of sensory roots entering the spinal cord. Each of these methods has developed into widely used therapies and they will be described separately.

Transcutaneous electrical nerve stimulation

All nerves within about four centimetres below the surface of the skin can be stimulated by placing electrodes on the skin surface. These include the large nerves in the upper and lower arm, the nerves in the lower leg, and any superficial skin nerves. The electrodes, these days, are usually made of flexible conducting silicone and they make contact with the skin through a conducting paste. The electrodes are connected to a pocket-sized, battery-operated stimulator which puts out a continuous series of electrical pulses. The frequency and duration of the pulses vary among different stimulators, but in all of them the strength (amplitude) of the pulses can be varied by the patient himself. The patient raises the strength of stimulation until a comfortable tingling is felt in the area supplied by the nerve which is being stimulated.

This technique has now been used by hundreds of thousands of patients with machines made by more than forty companies. There is usually a decrease of pain during the stimulation and this is satisfactory for the continuous control of the pain in a substantial percentage of the cases. The most clearcut responses have been obtained when there is skin tenderness associated with nerve damage or disease, or when there are tender muscle points. In patients with causalgia – the most dramatic example of pain associated with localized nerve damage – stimulation central to the area of damage produces a striking decrease in the skin's sensitivity while stimulation peripheral to the damage increases the pain. In post-herpetic neuralgia, patients whose main complaint is an unbearable sensitivity of the skin report a satisfactory return of normal sensitivity when the main affected nerves are stimulated (Nathan and Wall, 1974). Since the procedure is so simple and free of side effects, it has come to be used as an initial treatment for many chronic pain syndromes. It is also used in many centres for acute pains by applying the electrodes around the incision scar at the time of surgical operations; it often increases the patient's comfort and decreases the amount of narcotic needed to control post-operative pain. Similarly, the technique is used widely in Sweden during the first stages of childbirth when the mother frequently feels surges of low back pain during uterine contractions.

The mild increase of pain threshold, particularly in cases of skin tenderness, is sufficient to control pain in many patients during the stimulation. Of even more interest to some patients, particularly those with damage to nerves, the relief outlasts a brief period (15–30 minutes) of stimulation by many hours. This is a remarkable phenomenon in which a brief action produces a very prolonged relief.

There is no longer any doubt that transcutaneous electrical stimulation (TES) is an effective way to treat chronic pain. It is significantly more effective than a placebo machine when stimulation is administered within the painful area, over a related nerve, and even at a distance from the nerve (Thorsteinsson *et al.*, 1977). In a study of joint pain in patients with rheumatoid arthritis, stimulation near the painful joint at low intensity produced significant pain relief in 75% of patients. When the stimulation intensity was increased, pain relief was obtained by 95% (Mannheimer *et al.*, 1978). Intensity is clearly an important factor, and so is the frequency of the stimulation, although it may depend on the kind of pain. In a study of rheumatoid arthritis (Mannheimer and Carlsson, 1979), high-frequency (70Hz) stimulation was more effective than low-frequency (3Hz). Of 20 patients, 18 reported pain relief with 70Hz, but only 5 with 3Hz. Furthermore, the average duration of pain relief with 70Hz was 18 hours, while for 3Hz it was only 4 hours. In contrast, in a study of 123 patients who had pain due primarily to lesions of the nervous system, low-frequency stimulation was better (Eriksson *et al.*, 1979). High-frequency (10–100Hz) stimulation produced significant pain relief in about 35% of patients, and an additional 20% were helped by low-frequency (1–4Hz) stimulation. The intensity was below painful levels in all cases, but was sufficiently intense to activate deep structures and produce muscle contractions. The good effects persisted in most patients: after 3 months, 55% of patients continued to use the treatment. After 1 and 2 years, 41% and 31% continued to obtain satisfactory relief from the stimulation. An intriguing finding in this study is that the pain relief by low-frequency stimulation was abolished by naloxone (an opiate inhibitor), while relief by high-frequency stimulation was not. This, of course, suggests that each type of relief is mediated by different neural mechanisms.

Perhaps the most exciting feature of TES is that it produces relief in patients who received little or no relief by other methods, including neurosurgical procedures, anaesthetic blocks and so forth. In a group of 30 patients with post-herpetic neuralgia, Nathan and Wall (1974) observed that 11 were helped more by TES than by any other treatment. In 9 patients, pain relief outlasted stimulation by 1 to 2 hours, and 2 patients were cured. It is not yet possible to state the optimal frequencies or intensities of stimulation for each kind of pain problem, or the percentages of people helped. But it is clear that a high proportion is helped by appropriate stimulation, that TES is more effective than any other form of treatment for many patients, and that the proportion may become higher when the correct form of stimulation is found for each pain syndrome, probably for each patient.

The original reason for introducing the technique still appears valid as a partial explanation of its success. Sensory nerve impulses have mixed effects in the central nervous system, producing both excitation and inhibition. A predominant effect (discussed in Chapter 6) is for the large-diameter afferents to raise the threshold of cells which respond to injury signals. As the continuous stimulation is applied, there is a gradual rise of the threshold of spinal cord cells in their ability to respond. Some writers, at the early stages of this work, suggested that the electrical stimulation was having a direct effect on the peripheral nerve fibres by blocking them; but, although this effect is possible when stimulation is at intense levels, there is no evidence that it explains the effects produced by gentle stimulation, which appears to leave normal nerves unaffected in their ability to carry nerve impulses. However, Wall and Gutnick (1974) discovered a new factor which may play a role in the stimulation of damaged nerves. Direct stimulation of a normal sensory nerve fibre at a distance from its receptive field generates nerve impulses which run in the normal direction towards the central nervous system, as well as nerve impulses which travel antidromically towards the periphery. As we noted in Chapter 8, the new sprouts which grow from the ends of damaged nerves take on several new properties. One of these is that nerve impulses that invade a sprout from the parent fibre tend to silence the sprout and raise its threshold to stimuli for a long time. Therefore, it may be that electrical stimulation of peripheral nerves, in addition to producing a central inhibition, also may decrease the abnormal excitability of the damaged parts of the peripheral nerve.

Dorsal column stimulation

Wall and Sweet, (1967) realizing that it was essential to stimulate central to an area of nerve damage, implanted electrodes around major nerves in order to test the usefulness of the technique. While this is possible in the case of nerves to the limb, it is not possible where the location of disease is extensive or is so close to the spinal cord that no anatomical possibility exists either of reaching nerves by skin stimulation or even of reaching all the relevant nerves by surgical exposure. Therefore, as a trial, they stimulated large numbers of sensory roots as they enter the spinal cord. An anaesthesia needle was placed in the cerebrospinal fluid at the site where the roots run from the pelvis into spinal cord. An electrode was then run in through the needle to lie among the roots. For brief periods, these patients were given mild stimulation and they reported that their pain decreased while the stimulation was applied. These test results were sufficiently encouraging for Shealy *et al.* (1967) to develop a more radical procedure which would allow prolonged, permanent stimulation of the dorsal columns of the spinal cord. The dorsal columns receive branches of many of the large nerve fibres which enter the spinal cord through each sensory root and carry them towards the brain. To stimulate the dorsal columns in man, Shealy and his colleagues took the same equipment previously used to implant stimulators around peripheral nerves and inserted the electrodes directly onto the dorsal columns. The wires to the electrodes were led out through the dura and were attached to a radio stimulator apparatus.

This procedure obviously involves major surgery and was plagued by equipment breakdowns and by leakage of the cerebrospinal fluid through the hole in the dura through which the electrodes ran. Furthermore, a number of patients who initially responded very well for periods of weeks or months began to experience a return of their pain. For these reasons, this radical form of dorsal column stimulation has become less common and has been replaced by a much less intrusive technique – percutaneous dorsal column stimulation. In this method, electrodes are inserted through special epidural needles until they lie on top of the dura just above the dorsal columns. This is a highly skilled yet simple technique which requires no anaesthesia or major operation. Furthermore, the electrodes and the wires that lead to the surface of the body can be left in place for some weeks so that prolonged testing can be carried out. If the results are disappointing, the electrodes are simply pulled out. But, if the patient shows marked pain relief, the wires can be buried and attached to a radio stimulator during a relatively minor operation. A recent study (Urban and Nashold, 1978) has shown that of twenty patients who tried percutaneous epidural stimulation of the dorsal columns, seven reported excellent relief over a two-week trial period and were then given a permanently implanted receiver system. All but one of these patients experienced continuing pain relief throughout a long follow-up time of up to two years. What is impressive here is that the procedure is relatively simple, allows rapid identification of patients who will be helped, and produces excellent results in those for whom it is effective.

While this development was proceeding, surgeons tried dorsal column stimulation for the pain which may accompany multiple sclerosis of the spinal cord. To their surprise, and the patients' gratification, not only was the patients' pain improved but there was also an improvement of movement and bladder control. This procedure is now being explored actively in many centres in large numbers of patients with various types of spinal cord and peripheral nerve lesions.

It is presumed that the major effect of this treatment is explained by the same factors we have described for peripheral nerve stimulation. The afferent sensory fibres in the dorsal columns all send branches into the spinal cord dorsal horn where they enter the cord. Each electrical pulse applied to dorsal columns sends impulses toward the brain, and other impulses which descend and enter the dorsal horn. It is assumed that the impulses entering the dorsal horn trigger an inhibition. It is known from clinical observation that the dorsal columns are the crucial structures which must be stimulated to get the effect. In cases of brachial plexus avulsion, where sensory roots are torn from the cord, there are no sensory fibres entering the cord and therefore none in the dorsal columns originating from the arms. These unfortunate cases have extremely severe phantom pain which does not respond to dorsal column stimulation presumably because there are no relevant sensory fibres to stimulate, although in other respects the spinal cord is intact. However, successful effects of dorsal column stimulation have been reported by Lindblom and his colleagues (1975) in patients with chest pain following the damage to nerves which may occur during chest surgery. In a beautiful series of careful tests, they showed that the effect is to readjust sensitivity to gentle stimuli which produce intolerable pain, while the normal actions of unaffected nerves are very little disturbed. As with successful gentle nerve stimulation, it seems that the successful effects of dorsal column stimulation are more to re-establish a normal balance of excitation and inhibition rather than to enforce a powerful blockade.

Brain stimulation

The discovery that electrical stimulation of the periaqueductal grey matter in animals produces a profound analgesia, which we described earlier, led to attempts to relieve chronic pain in human patients by similar stimulation. Some patients suffering chronic pain have now had electrodes implanted stereotaxically in the periaqueductal grey matter in the upper (rostral) portions of the brainstem and generally the results have been mixed. In one study of six patients (Hosobuchi *et al.*, 1977), five with cancer received complete relief of pain until they died three to eighteen months after implantation. The sixth patient, with facial anaesthesia dolorosa (severe pain in the face even though the skin is insensitive to stimulation), had only partial relief. Interestingly, although the chronic pain was relieved to some degree in all cases, pain due to pinprick or intense radiant heat was relatively unaffected except when the brain stimulation was at very high levels. There are limitations to the procedure, however. First, continuous periaqueductal stimulation soon shows adaptation effects (tolerance), so that the stimulation becomes ineffective. Occasionally, effectiveness is restored and the stimulation is given for a few hours at a time, with rest intervals of at least three or four hours. Second, the electrical stimulation produces tolerance to narcotic drugs such as morphine, so that much higher doses are needed to be effective. The underlying mechanisms are presumed to be the same as those involved in stimulation-produced analgesia in animals; that is, descending inhibitory fibres are activated to 'close the gate'. This assumption is supported by the observations that endorphins in the cerebrospinal fluid are increased by stimulation, and that naloxone (the morphine antagonist described earlier) abolishes the analgesia produced by the stimulation. This neural system, then, clearly contains the naloxone-sensitive type of opiate receptors.

Stimulation of another area of the brain can also provide excellent relief of chronic pain. In a recent study, eighteen patients with severe pain received electrodes implanted in the thalamic somatosensory relay nucleus (Turnbull *et al.*, 1980). Complete or partial pain relief occurred in twelve patients as a result of repeated periods of stimulation. Remarkably, the pain disappeared completely in a thirteenth patient. As in peripheral nerve stimulation, stimulation of the thalamus produces a tingling feeling in the affected body areas when it effectively relieves pain. This procedure is promising because pain is often suppressed for long periods of time after stimulation is stopped – as long as twenty-four hours in some patients. Interestingly, patients who receive partial relief report that intermittent attacks of sharp pain may disappear altogether, while the underlying constant ache tends to recur when stimulation is stopped. Resumption of stimulation again produces partial or complete relief. The mechanism of action of stimulation in the sensory thalamus is not clear. It is possible that descending inhibitory systems are activated indirectly by thalamic and cortical fibres that are known to project to the reticular formation. Another possible mechanism is that, because most of these patients have pain due to lesions of the nervous system, impulses evoked by stimulation disrupt abnormal firing in neuron pools in the brain that have been deprived of input and are therefore firing at excessive rates.

These procedures, so far, appear to be hopeful, and many of the problems have been overcome. The rapid development of tolerance to stimulation seems to be prevented or slowed down by reducing the duration of the periods of stimulation. Whether this strategy will work indefinitely, and for all patients, is not known. All surgeons have had failures and some have had no success at all. This may be due to the small and ill-defined nature of the target. In some cases, analgesia was achieved but was unacceptable because it was accompanied by abnormal eye movements or sleep disturbances, presumably due to spread of the stimulus. It is clear that this technique is very hopeful and we must await developments. Since no destruction of brain tissue occurs, even those who fail to respond are not harmed – whereas surgical lesions may leave the patient in worse condition than before.

The role of the market place

It is important to examine the role of the market place in the development of transcutaneous stimulation just as we did in the case of drugs. In 1967, Wall and Sweet showed that gentle, electrical stimulation of nerves in some patients would relieve their pain. The equipment needed to do this was of the simplest type imaginable and involved standard electronic circuitry. Many new electronic components which have become available since then have made it possible to make several equivalent variations of the same theme. The components in the most elaborate circuits can be bought for about $25 from any electronics shop. A great deal of effort and ingenuity by medical electronics companies went into the packaging of the bits to make a convenient box which the patient could carry and operate. The equipment sells for about $500 in the United States and by 1979 there were over 40 companies selling $28,000,000 worth of these transcutaneous stimulators in the United States alone.

One may ask what the contribution of the companies was to this bonanza. The original research was carried out in universities and was financed by public funds. The electronics was common knowledge. The companies packaged and promoted. In some companies, promotion included education of doctors and nurses. Some of this promotion could genuinely be called a help to the doctors and patients. With forty companies making essentially the same product, it became necessary for them to fall back on the advertising techniques used to sell toothpaste. The advertisements tend to be bombastic and each stimulator is described as though it is novel and unique. The advertisements exaggerate the stimulator's effectiveness in the same way that aspirin advertisements are suitably vague but imply that all types of pain respond. One company at least has been involved in setting up a chain of so-called 'pain clinics' in which the major mode of treatment is, of course, its particular model of transcutaneous stimulator. Here, as with the pharmaceutical companies, we find that industry has made valuable and essential contributions but financial competitive pressures have tended to produce an escalation in cost and confusion to doctor and patient.

Acupuncture and other forms of folk medicine

The study of folk medicine by anthropologists and medical historians has revealed an astonishing array of ingenious methods to relieve pain (Brockbank, 1954; Wand-Tetley, 1956). Every culture, it appears, has learned to fight pain with pain: in general, brief, moderate pain tends to abolish severe, prolonged pain. One of the oldest methods is cupping, in which a glass cup is heated up (by coals or flaming alcohol) and then inverted over the painful area and held against it. As the air in the cup cools and contracts, it creates a partial vacuum so that the skin is sucked up into the cup (Figure 38). The procedure produces bruising of the skin with concomitant pain and tenderness. Cupping was practised in ancient Greece and Rome as early as the 4th century BC, and was also practised in ancient India and China. Over the centuries, the

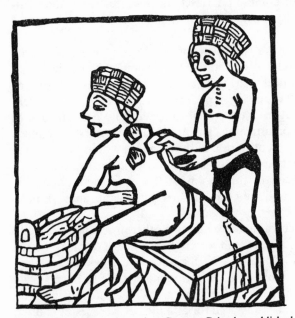

Figure 38. Cupping, shown in a German Calendar published in 1483. Note that the attendant holds a lighted lamp in his left hand. (reprinted in W. Brockbank (1954) from the Wellcome Historical Medical Library)

method spread to virtually all parts of the world, and cups of various sizes, shapes and materials have evolved. Cupping has been used – and is still widely practised – for a large variety of ailments, including headaches, backaches and arthritic pains.

Scarification is another ancient practice in which the skin is cut by a sharp knife or by awesome devices such as lever-driven multiple blades. Scarification has a widespread practice in its own right. Sometimes, it became part of 'wet cupping', in which a hot cup was placed over the cut skin and sucks out blood. Wet cupping and scarification, like leech-induced bleeding, were often used to reduce the amount of fluid in the body, especially in cases of congestive heart failure. In addition, they were used to produce pain as well as local irritation and inflammation to combat disease and severe, chronic pain. Old medical texts describe the methods in great detail, and it is evident that they were used not only for common diseases but specifically for the treatment of headache, backache and sciatica, and other forms of chronic pain.

Cauterization is yet another ancient method. Generally, the end of an iron rod was heated until it was red-hot, and was then placed on the painful area, such as the foot in the case of gout, or on the buttock, back or leg in patients with low back pain. Often, however, the cautery was applied to specifically prescribed sites distant from the painful area. The procedure, of course, produced pain and subsequent blistering of the area that was touched by the cautery. The great Arabic physician, Avicenna, warned that when the cautery is used in the region of the head, care should be exercised 'not to boil the brain or shrivel its membranes' (Elliott, 1962).

The same effect was achieved by two other procedures: rubbing blistering fluids into the skin, or applying a cone of moxa (made from the leaves of the mugwort plant) to a site on the body, setting the tip of the cone aflame, and allowing it to burn slowly until it approached or reached the skin. Again, the procedure produced pain and, while used for all kinds of diseases, was often prescribed specifically for painful conditions.

There are countless other methods that resemble the ones just described. It is evident that the one factor common to all of them is that they produce pain to abolish pain. The pain was usually brief and moderate but its effect was to relieve or abolish a much more severe, chronic pain. These methods, of course, did not always work, but they obviously worked well enough to have survived as procedures of folk medicine throughout the world for thousands of years. Do these procedures work better than a placebo? There are no experimental studies, but the evidence from studies of acupuncture – a related procedure – suggests that they do.

The methods we have just described are generally known as 'counter-irritation', and some are still frequently used although there has not been (until recently) any theoretical or physiological explanation for their effectiveness. Suggestion and distraction of attention are the usual mechanisms invoked, but neither seems capable of explaining the power of the methods or the long duration of the relief they may afford. Because they involve painful or near-painful levels of stimulation to relieve pain, these methods have also been labelled as 'hyperstimulation analgesia' (Melzack, 1973).

This interest in folk medicine gained enormous impetus in recent years by the rediscovery of the ancient Chinese practice of acupuncture, which has been in continuous practice for at least 2,000 years. Basically, the procedure involves the insertion of fine needles (made of steel, gold or other metals) through specific points at the skin and then twirling them for some time at a slow rate. The needles may also be left in place for varying periods of time. The practice of acupuncture is part of a complex, fascinating theory of medicine in which all diseases and pains are believed to be due to disharmony between Yin (spirit) and Yang (blood) which flow in channels called 'meridians'. Acupuncture charts are extremely complex and consist, traditionally, of 361 points which lie on 14 meridians, most of which are named after internal organs, such as the large intestine, the heart, or the bladder (Kao, 1973). A great deal of mystery surrounds the practice of acupuncture in China, and the points chosen for treatment of a given malady are held to be influenced by the time of day, the weather and a multitude of other variables. The mystery, however, may hide one or more basic physiological principles.

Acupuncture was first described in the western world by the Dutch physician Willem ten Rhyne in 1683. After great initial enthusiasm, interest in acupuncture soon diminished. Since that time, acupuncture has been 'rediscovered' in the west about two or three times a century. In recent years, the major cause of the renewed interest in acupuncture was the description of its use in modern China to produce analgesia in order to carry out surgery. This was a new application of the method, and often involved electrical stimulation of body tissues through needles hooked up to battery-driven stimulators (electroacupuncture). Films of such operations are extremely dramatic, and the feeling arose that if acupuncture could produce sufficient analgesia for surgery, it must surely be effective for chronic pains of all kinds.

Two major findings soon put the picture in perspective. First, it became evident that the use of acupuncture to produce analgesia for surgery is relatively rare and undependable. In China, it is used for no more than five to ten per cent of surgical operations, and it is carried out on selected patients who have been thoroughly exposed to acupuncture methods (Bonica, 1974). In western countries acupuncture is rarely effective for surgery. As a result, the initial enthusiasm for the use of acupuncture for surgery dropped rapidly. However, visitors to China became more aware of its traditional use for various aches and pains, and often observed impressive results in cases of low back pain, myofascial pain, and some of the neuralgias. Second, the discovery by outstanding physiologists in China that the nerves (rather than meridians) are essential for effective pain relief by acupuncture placed the practice on a firm scientific basis.

Several kinds of evidence, obtained in western countries as well as in China, reveal the nature of acupuncture's action on pain. The first is the demonstration, in carefully controlled studies, that acupuncture has significantly greater effects on pain than placebo stimulation (Chapman *et al.*, 1976; Anderson *et al.*, 1974; Stewart *et al.*, 1977). However, an impressive number of studies show that acupuncture stimulation need not be applied at the precise points indicated on acupuncture charts. It is possible, for example, to achieve as much control over dental pain by stimulating an area between the fourth and fifth fingers, which is not designated on acupuncture charts as related to facial pain, as by stimulating the Hoku point between the thumb and index finger which *is* so designated (Taub *et al.*, 1977). The decreases in pain obtained by stimulation at either site are so large and occur in so many patients that it is unlikely that the pain relief is due to placebo effects. Rather, the results suggest that the site that can be effectively stimulated is not a discrete point but a large area, possibly the whole hand.

The same conclusion can be drawn from another study – a double-blind experiment on the efficacy of acupuncture on osteoarthritic pain – in which the control patients received 'placebo' acupuncture stimulation at sites just adjacent to the 'real' acupuncture points (Gaw *et al.*, 1975). Patients in both groups showed significant improvement in tenderness and subjective report of pain as evaluated by two independent observers, as well as in activity of the joint. Because there was no difference between the two groups, the improvement was attributed to a placebo effect. It is more likely, however, that it is stimulation within a large area and not merely at a point that has an effect. Similar conclusions can be drawn from an excellent study of acupuncture control over pain in patients with sickle-cell anaemia (Co *et al.*, 1979). In fact, intense stimulation at many sites of the body may be effective. It is the intense stimulation rather than the precise site that appears to be the crucial factor. This is exactly the conclusion drawn by several writers (Ghia *et al.*, 1976; Lewit, 1979) who showed that acupuncture stimulation of the painful area is as effective as stimulation at designated distant points. From all this it may be concluded that intense stimulation is the necessary factor, and the precise site of stimulation is less important than the intensity of the input.

That the pain relief produced by acupuncture cannot be attributed simply to a placebo effect is also indicated by the fact that partial analgesia can be produced in animals such as monkeys and mice (Vierck *et al.*, 1974; Pomeranz *et al.*, 1977; Sandrew *et al.*, 1978), and that acupuncture stimulation inhibits or otherwise changes the transmission of pain-evoked nerve impulses at several levels of the central nervous system (Kerr *et al.*, 1978). However, acupuncture needles are not essential to produce these effects. They are also produced by intense electrical stimulation, heat, and a variety of intense sensory inputs (Le Bars, Dickenson and Besson, 1979a, b). The effectiveness of all of these forms of stimulation indicates that acupuncture is not a magical procedure, but only one of many ways to produce analgesia by an intense sensory input which may be labelled generally as 'hyperstimulation analgesia'.

Hyperstimulation analgesia

Intense transcutaneous electrical stimulation

The concept that acupuncture is only one of many ways to deliver intense stimulation led Melzack and his colleagues to administer transcutaneous electrical stimulation the same way as acupuncture – for brief periods of time at moderate-to-high stimulation intensities. Consequently, they carried out a series of studies to determine whether acupuncture and transcutaneous electrical stimulation are comparable procedures.

The first study (Melzack, 1975b) examined the effects of brief, intense transcutaneous electrical stimulation at trigger points or acupuncture points on severe clinical pain. The data indicated that the procedure provides a powerful method for the control of several forms of pathological pain. The duration of relief frequently outlasted the twenty-minute period of stimulation by several hours, occasionally for days or weeks. Different patterns of the amount and duration of pain relief were observed. Daily stimulation carried out at home by the patient sometimes provided gradually increasing relief over periods of weeks or months. That these effects were not due to placebo phenomena was demonstrated in a double-blind study (Jeans, 1979).

Having established the effectiveness of brief periods of intense transcutaneous electrical stimulation, a study (Fox and Melzack, 1976) was then carried out to compare the relative effectiveness of transcutaneous stimulation and acupuncture on low back pain. The results showed that both forms of stimulation at the same points produce substantial decreases in pain intensity but neither procedure is statistically more effective than the other. Most patients were relieved of pain for several hours, and some for one or more days. Statistical analysis also failed to reveal any differences in the duration of pain relief between the two procedures. Interestingly, an almost identical study was carried out independently in Finland at the same time (Laitinen, 1976) and also found that the two procedures were equally effective in relieving low back pain.

These findings have important practical implications. The chief advantage of acupuncture is that the procedure is of short duration – at intense levels, stimulation may sometimes last only a few minutes. The method, however, is invasive, and requires licensed practitioners with specialized training. Transcutaneous electrical stimulation, on the other hand, is non-invasive, and once the appropriate points are located, it can be administered by paramedical personnel. Furthermore, once the procedure is found to be effective for a given patient, it can be self-administered by the patient with supervision by the physician.

Our understanding of hyperstimulation analgesia is further enhanced by studies which show that the distribution of acupuncture points is similar to that of trigger points (see p.249) and motor points (the points which produce maximal contraction of muscles and have been shown to lie above the area of highest density of innervating motor neurons on the muscle). When acupuncture needles are inserted into sites that reduce pain, they produce a deep, aching feeling when they are twirled manually or electrically stimulated. This is reminiscent of the deep, aching feeling reported by patients when a trigger point is stimulated by the pressure of a finger pushing on it. This similarity led Melzack, Stillwell and Fox (1977) to examine the correlation between trigger points and acupuncture points for pain. The results of their analysis showed that every trigger point reported in the western medical literature has a corresponding acupuncture point. Furthermore there is a close correspondence – 71% – between the pain syndromes associated with the two kinds of points. This close correlation suggests that trigger points and acupuncture points for pain, though discovered independently and labelled differently, represent the same phenomenon and can be explained in terms of similar underlying neural mechanisms.

A comparable study (Liu *et al.*, 1975) investigated the relationship between motor points and acupuncture loci and also found a remarkably high correspondence. This shows that there are sensitive sites on the body which produce a deep, aching feeling when they are palpated or needled, that they are intimately related to many common forms of chronic myofascial pains, and that many of these sites are related to the most densely innervated and most sensitive areas of muscles.

Ice massage

Ice packs and ice massage are standard methods of treatment in physical therapy. The reason why ice is effective, however, has until recently not been understood. Ice, of course, produces a local constriction of blood vessels and makes the area feel 'numb'. But ice must do much more because brief ice massage may relieve pain for long periods of time. Ice, moreover, has more than a numbing effect – it hurts. It produces aching, burning pain and therefore, conceivably, may act like acupuncture or intense transcutaneous electrical stimulation. Two recent studies suggest that this is the case.

In the first study (Melzack, Guité and Gonshor, 1980), patients suffering from acute dental pain were treated with ice massage of the back of the hand (at an area between the thumb and index finger) on the same side as the pain. The ice massage decreased the intensity of the dental pain by 50% or more in the majority of patients. Furthermore, the pain reductions produced by ice massage were significantly larger than those produced in control groups by tactile massage alone or with explicit suggestion. The results indicate that ice massage has pain-reducing effects comparable to those of transcutaneous electrical stimulation and acupuncture. These observations led to a second study (Melzack, Jeans, Stratford and Monks, 1980) which examined the relative effectiveness of ice massage and transcutaneous electrical stimulation (TES) for the relief of low back pain. Patients suffering chronic low back pain were treated with both ice massage and TES. The results showed that both methods are equally effective: about 65% of patients obtained pain relief greater than 33% with each method. The results showed that ice massage is an effective therapeutic tool, and even appears to be more effective than TES for some patients. It may also serve as an additional sensory-modulation method to alternate with TES to overcome adaptation effects. Taken together, the results of both studies point to neural mechanisms that are similar to those of acupuncture and intense transcutaneous electrical stimulation.

The 'needle effect'

The striking effectiveness of methods to relieve chronic pain by brief, intense sensory inputs has led several investigators to question whether their anaesthetic blocks relieve myofascial and back pains because of the anaesthetic agents or the insertion of the hypodermic needle. Astonishingly, the results are in favour of needling. Lewit (1979) has called this phenomenon the 'needle effect'.

In the 1950s, several investigators discovered, independently of one another, that the insertion of a hypodermic needle through the skin, without injecting an anaesthetic or injecting only normal saline (salt water), often produces a dramatic relief of myofascial pains associated with the musculoskeletal system. Travell and Rinzler, in a classic paper published in 1952, summarized the work they carried out over a period of years demonstrating that 'dry needling' of trigger points – simply moving a needle in and out of the area without injecting any substance – produced striking relief of myofascial pain. Similarly, Sola and Williams (1956) discovered that injection of normal saline was highly effective. In fact, Kibler (1958) reported that different kinds of anaesthetics have virtually identical effects which are barely influenced by the amount and concentration of the anaesthetic injected.

These observations led Frost, Jessen and Siggaard-Andersen (1980) to carry out a double-blind comparison of a local anaesthetic – mepivacaine – and saline injected into trigger points for myofascial pain. To their astonishment, the group that received saline tended to have significantly more relief of pain: 80% of patients with saline reported pain relief compared to 52% with mepivacaine. Furthermore, the average duration of relief was 3 hours for saline and 30 minutes for mepivacaine. Clearly, the pain relief could not be due to the anaesthetic but was more likely due to the insertion of the needle into the trigger point. The saline was more effective, they proposed, because it irritated tissues, which is the essential ingredient of the treatment, while the mepivacaine actually blocked the irritating effect of the needle.

These results are in agreement with Lewit's observations that the 'needle effect' is the crucial factor in relieving myofascial pain. The effectiveness of the treatment, he observes, bears little relationship to the agent injected, but is 'related to the intensity of pain produced at the trigger zone, and to the precision with which the site of maximal tenderness was located by the needle' (Lewit, 1979, p.83). The needle, in short, must penetrate at the point of maximum pain. While this sounds like torture, the brief shot of pain produced by the needle resulted in striking relief of pain in 86.8% of cases and persistent relief for months or even permanently in about 50% of the cases.

Physiological basis of hyperstimulation analgesia

There are three major properties of hyperstimulation analgesia: (1) a moderate-to-intense sensory input is applied to the body to alleviate pain; (2) the sensory input is sometimes applied to a site distant from the site of pain; and (3) the sensory input, which is usually of brief duration (ranging from a few seconds to 20 or 30 minutes) may relieve chronic pain for days, weeks, sometimes permanently.

The first property can be explained by the brainstem mechanisms, described in Chapter 7, that exert a descending inhibitory control over transmission through the dorsal horns as well as at

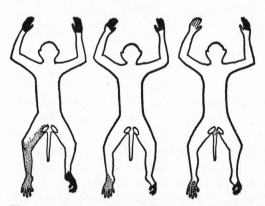

Figure 39. Excitatory and inhibitory receptive fields of dorsal horn cells in the monkey. The excitatory fields of three typical cells are indicated by the stippled areas. The inhibitory fields are shown in black. Large, medium, and small excitatory fields are illustrated from left to right. The inhibition of spontaneous or evoked activity was produced only by *intense* stimulation in the inhibitory fields, and persisted for as long as 1.2 seconds after stimulation was stopped. (from Wagman and Price, 1969, p.803)

higher levels in the somatic projection system. Intense somatic stimuli, of almost any kind, would produce pain but would also activate the brainstem mechanisms which could exert an inhibitory effect on the gate (Le Bars, Dickenson, and Besson, 1979a and b). However, this does not preclude direct inhibition at the level of the spinal cord. Wagman and Price (1969) found that the spontaneous or evoked activity of cells in lamina 5, whose receptive fields cover part or all of one of the legs, can be inhibited by intense stimulation of the opposite leg or even the hands (Figure 39). The short latencies of onset of the effect suggest that it may occur entirely by means of connections in the spinal cord. It is most likely, therefore, that both spinal and supraspinal mechanisms mediate the complex effects of intense stimulation on pain.

The same spinal and supraspinal mechanisms can also explain the second property – relief of pain by intense stimulation at a distant site. It is clear in Figure 39 that spinal cells excited by stimulation of a leg are inhibited by intense stimulation of areas as distant as the other leg or either hand. The brainstem mechanisms which exert a powerful descending inhibitory control provide an additional basis for inhibition of pain signals by intense stimulation at distant sites. These brainstem areas may be conceptualized as a 'central biasing mechanism' (Melzack, 1971, 1973) which acts as an inhibitory feedback system (Figure 40). Cells in the reticular formation and periaqueductal grey which respond to noxious stimuli exhibit a gross somatotopic organization characterized by large receptive fields (Groves, Miller, Parker and Rebec, 1973). Within the periaqueductal grey matter, Liebeskind and Mayer (1971) recorded responses evoked by noxious stimuli and found a somatotopic organization in which the face and forepaws are represented in the rostral portion whereas the hindpaws and tail are represented more caudally. Furthermore, when the periaqueductal area is electrically stimulated to produce analgesia, a complex somatotopic organization is revealed – there is a dorsoventral organization in which the face is represented dorsally and the more caudal parts of the body become analgesic as the electrode tip is moved ventrally (Soper, 1979). This basic organization exists throughout the rostrocaudal extent of the midbrain. It appears, then, that particular body areas project especially strongly to discrete regions of the peri-aqueductal grey which, in turn, exert an inhibitory control over pain signals from particular parts of the body.

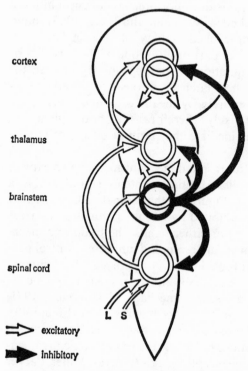

cortex

thalamus

brainstem

spinal cord

L S

⇒ excitatory

➡ inhibitory

Figure 40. Schematic diagram of the central biasing mechanism. Large and small fibres from a limb activate a neuron pool in the spinal cord, which excites neuron pools at successively higher levels. The central biasing mechanism, represented by the inhibitory projection system that originates in the brainstem reticular formation, modulates activity at all levels. Loss of inputs to the system would weaken the inhibition; increased sensory input or direct electrical stimulation would increase the inhibition. L, large fibres; S, small fibres. (from Melzack, 1971, p.409)

The final property – prolonged relief of pain by brief stimula-tion – can be understood if we recognize that pain may persist as a result of abnormal, memory-like activity. Intense stimulation could block this activity by direct spinal inhibition, or by means of inhibition through the structures that comprise the central biasing mechanism. The increased physical activity permitted by the relief of pain, as we noted earlier, would tend to prevent the recurrence of the abnormal neural activity and the pain it produces.

15
Psychological Control of Pain

The gate-control theory proposes that cognitive activities such as attention and suggestion can influence pain by acting at the earliest levels of sensory transmission. The degree of central control, however, would be determined, in part at least, by the temporal-spatial properties of the input patterns. Some of the most unbearable pains, such as cardiac pain, rise so rapidly in intensity that the patient is unable to achieve any control over them. On the other hand, more slowly rising temporal patterns are susceptible to central control and may allow the patient to 'think about something else' or use other stratagems to keep the pain under control.

The search for new approaches to pain therapy has profited by directing thinking towards the contributions of motivational and cognitive processes. Pain can be treated not only by trying to manipulate the sensory input, but also by influencing motivational and cognitive factors as well. In recent years, these methods have been shown to have considerable power in relieving pain.

Psychological procedures require effort and time on the part of the patient and the clinician. However, they provide an important approach to pain therapy, particularly for those pain states which cannot be brought under satisfactory control by local anaesthetics or any other techniques. Therapists have persistently sought methods to abolish pain in the way that telephone transmission can be abolished by cutting a wire. But no techniques have such clearcut results. Perhaps, then, we should not aim at totally abolishing pain, but, rather, at reducing it to bearable levels. Psychological methods, we now know, may decrease some kinds of pain from unbearable to bearable levels, an achievement which is gaining increasing recognition.

We have already reviewed the evidence (in Chapter 2) which shows unequivocally that psychological factors play an important role in pain perception and response. Distraction of attention, suggestion, evaluation of the meaning of the situation, and the feeling of control over potential injury are all capable of exerting a powerful influence on pain. In view of this evidence, then, it is not surprising that psychologists and psychiatrists have developed a variety of new methods to control pain. These methods utilize suggestion, distraction, relaxation, biofeedback, and other psychological techniques in the attempt to relieve pain. There are now so many of these techniques, in fact, that any newcomer to the field is immediately bewildered by the huge literature which attempts to evaluate them one at a time or several in combination. Claims are made for some techniques that lead patients to believe that the panacea for chronic pain has at last been found. Careful evaluation of the research, however, shows clearly that we are still a long way from perfect control of pain.

Many psychological approaches are known to produce some measure of pain relief. They include (1) the use of operant conditioning to diminish the frequency of pain-related behaviour patterns; (2) teaching patients to utilize feedback of electroencephalographic or other indices of physiological activity to develop a state of mind which allows them to cope with pain; (3) hypnotic suggestion techniques; (4) the use of stratagems to distract attention or change the meaning of the pain; (5) social modelling techniques; and (6) psychotherapeutic or pharmacological techniques to relieve depression. All of these approaches have value for the treatment of pain in some patients at least. They may not abolish pain entirely, but may decrease some kinds of pain from unbearable to bearable levels for variable periods of time.

A review of the literature reveals that a substantial amount of research is needed before it can be stated with certainty that any one of these methods is more effective than the others, or is more effective for one kind of pain than another. In fact, the widespread enthusiasm engendered by some of these new approaches is occasionally unwarranted.

Operant-conditioning techniques

Operant-conditioning methods are based on observations that

complex patterns of behaviour can be modified by the manipulation of rewards and punishments. Psychologists such as Wilbert
E. Fordyce (1976) assume that pain consists of 'behaviours' that
have been reinforced or rewarded, and the way to abolish 'pain
behaviours' is to stop all such rewards. Fordyce, like other fol-
lowers of the psychologist B. F. Skinner, is not concerned about
the 'experience of pain', which he believes to be private information and not suitable for scientific study. Rather, he is interested
in observable responses, stimuli, rewards and punishments.

What Fordyce says, in essence, is that people are often reinforced for having pain. When they complain of pain ('verbal pain
behaviour'), they get attention and sympathy from family, friends
and doctors; they don't do jobs they don't like; they can
avoid people they dislike; they get medicines with impressive-
sounding names; they may receive financial compensation without working; and they are often treated with a degree of respect
they never had when they were well. In this way, the pain and
other behaviour patterns associated with it (such as an abnormal
gait) are reinforced. The task of the behaviour therapist, then, is
to remove the reinforcements, to try to stop the patient from
complaining of pain, and to induce the patient to resume normal
behaviour patterns.

Fordyce (1976) has provided a thorough description of his
procedures to re-train the patient who suffers chronic pain. The
patient enters the hospital for a prolonged period (an average of
eight weeks) and all the usual 'crutches' are removed. Pain
behaviours such as complaints are ignored. All physical activity
is rewarded with smiles and praise. And, during this period,
medication is reduced to the barest minimum ('detoxification').
After the operant procedure, Fordyce reports, the patients are
more active, complain less, take fewer drugs, work, and generally
lead more normal lives. However, we are left with three vital
questions that need to be answered.

First, does the patient actually feel less pain as a result of the
training? That is, the patient is conditioned to diminish the frequency of certain 'pain behaviours'; but does that mean the
patient feels less pain or simply learns to complain less or walk
more in spite of the pain? Unfortunately, Fordyce dismisses the
whole question by implying that the problem is basically philoso-

phical and not one that an operant-conditioning psychologist need be concerned with. However, the problem is too important to be ignored; the failure to come to grips with it weakens the impact of the technique.

Second, how does the operant technique compare with other methods? Is it any better than a 'placebo' effect? It is hard to imagine a more powerful 'placebo' than the constant attention, encouragement, praise, and first-rate medical care that are an integral part of the complex operant procedure to diminish 'pain behaviours'. However, there have not been any controlled studies which compare Fordyce's operant technique to other therapeutic methods. The only attempt made to compare an operant-treatment group with a control group is so inadequate that no conclusions can be drawn. Roberts and Reinhardt (1980), in fact, used two so-called control groups: one consisted of patients who were rejected for treatment for reasons such as cardiac problems and severe mental disorders, and the other comprised patients who refused treatments. These are not control groups in any scientific sense. That is, they are not *matched* in any way to the experimental group to permit a comparison of the operant-conditioning treatment with a 'placebo' treatment or any other form of treatment.

Even in the absence of controlled data, the results are not impressive. In a study of a treatment programme essentially like Fordyce's, Anderson and his colleagues (1977) report that 74% of the patients who completed the programme reported 'leading normal lives without drugs' when they were contacted 6 months to 7 years after discharge. However, the patients comprised a highly selected group so that they were hardly 'typical' patients with chronic pain. Only 60 of 130 patients (46%) referred to the programme were accepted for treatment. Only 37 (29%) chose to enter, and 3 of these dropped out before the programme was completed. As Turk and Genest (1979, p.305) point out, 'when Anderson *et al.* report that 74% of the patients treated were "leading normal lives", they are actually speaking of only 26 (19%) of the original patients screened over a 7-year period'. It may be added that few conclusions can be drawn from a follow-up that ranges from 6 months to 7 years, without knowing how many patients were interviewed at each year after treatment.

The third question that concerns us is the cost of the 'operant-conditioning' programme. Even if the programme *did* work – and there is no evidence that it is better than a 'placebo' programme – it requires residence in a hospital for 4 to 8 weeks. The programme, then, is extremely expensive and requires a large amount of hospital space, time, and equipment. If this were the best of all possible worlds, this kind of treatment should be available to everyone. In fact, it is feasible for only a small number of patients, and well-to-do ones at that. Because of these limitations, it becomes important to determine the place of a technique such as this in societies that have limited funds for medical care.

These criticisms do not deny that patients in pain may use excessive amounts of drugs that actually harm rather than benefit them, that some patients may abuse a social system that pays financial compensation when people are disabled by pain, or that some people enjoy the sympathy, special attention and other 'rewards' of their pain. But Fordyce's programme is only one of many. Happily, there is evidence that simpler methods may produce effective results.

A recent study (Taylor *et al.*, 1980) has shown that patients with chronic abdominal or headache pain can be helped significantly by a relatively brief programme. The patients were first 'detoxified' – that is, all drugs were withdrawn on a schedule determined for each person. This procedure took 1 to 6 days, with an average of 3.7 days. The patients were then taught muscle-relaxation techniques and were given one or more brief supportive psychological therapy sessions. The average time spent in relaxation training was 1.5 hours and the time in supportive therapy was about 3 hours. The investigators found that this programme produced a significant reduction in pain in 71% of the patients. At a 6-month follow-up, all (100%) of the patients had less pain than before treatment, reported improvement in mood and increased activity, and were on significantly reduced medication. While these results are encouraging, they cannot be directly compared to those obtained in studies using 'operant-conditioning' methods since these patients had primarily chronic abdominal pain while the others had preponderantly back and neck pain. Furthermore, the study did not have any control groups. Nevertheless, the evidence suggests that the reduction or elimination of drug intake can be accomplished in relatively short periods of time, and that additional simple procedures such as relaxation and brief supportive therapy may be effective for some patients with chronic, moderate levels of pain.

However, for severe pain, these procedures are not as impressive. A recent study (Swanson *et al.*, 1979) investigated 200 patients with severe chronic pain problems, primarily of the back and neck. The mean duration of the pain was 7 years, and 'the average patient was hospitalized 6 times, had had two surgical procedures, and had received treatment with some combination of physical therapy, traction, body casts, (anaesthetic) blocks, neuroablative procedures, electrostimulation, acupuncture, hypnosis, biofeedback, and psychotherapy'. The treatment, which required an average length of hospitalization of 20 days, consisted of behaviour modification (similar to Fordyce's 'operant-conditioning' technique), physical rehabilitation measures, medication management, education group discussion, biofeedback-relaxation techniques, family member participation, and supportive psychological treatment. At the time of dismissal from the hospital, 59% of the patients had achieved moderate improvement or better. At a 3-month follow-up, 40% were still doing well, and after 1 year, only 25% continued to do well. Considering the severity of pain, this might be considered an achievement. But in the absence of any kind of control group, it is difficult to know whether 3 weeks of rest in the hospital with a daily programme of standard physiotherapy might not have done as well. Two conclusions can be drawn from studies such as this one: (1) complex, expensive programmes, in the long run, are disappointing in their effectiveness in relieving severe, chronic pain; and (2) no studies can lead to firm conclusions unless adequate, scientific, controlled procedures are used. Before we examine other psychological methods, therefore, we must first determine the criteria necessary to draw conclusions from clinical research on pain.

Need for controlled studies

The need for reliable, controlled, statistically valid studies applies equally to every psychological therapeutic procedure. For such research to provide meaningful data, it must meet the following essential criteria:

1 Carefully controlled studies, with patients suffering specific clinical problems, must demonstrate that the effect of the procedure is greater than the placebo effect that is part and parcel of every therapy – an effect known to be astonishingly powerful. Patients not only want to please the therapist, but suggestion, anticipation of relief, and diminished anxiety can all play a role in ameliorating any disease process.

2 The changes that the therapy produces must be of sufficient magnitude and duration to have clinical significance. If pain can only be reduced by ten per cent, or for periods that average 15 or 30 minutes per day, the therapy clearly has limited value, or perhaps none at all.

3 The procedure must be transferable from the laboratory or hospital milieu to the normal day-to-day environment. If a change that is demonstrated in the clinic cannot be reproduced in the home or office, the procedure has limited value.

4 Finally, it must be demonstrated that the psychological procedure, once acquired, will continue to be effective for many months or years. Even if a given procedure produces results that exceed the effect of a placebo, it must be able to produce those results for substantial periods of time. In short, follow-up studies are essential to show that the procedure continues to be effective long beyond the training period itself.

We will now examine a variety of clinical procedures to see how well they meet the above criteria.

Biofeedback

Few therapeutic procedures have created the enormous excitement and expectations of biofeedback. The discovery in the 1970s that it is possible to gain voluntary control over biological activities such as brain waves (EEG), blood pressure or heart rate was heralded by the news media as the panacea for a variety of illnesses. With the help of sensitive electronic equipment which monitors a person's EEG, heart rate, blood pressure, or muscle tension, it became possible to 'feed back' these biological signals to the person so that he knows, for example, that certain muscles are tense rather than relaxed. Then the person is taught to relax or use other stratagems to reduce muscle tension. The continuous feedback keeps the person apprised of how well he is doing in achieving control over these biological functions, some of which were previously thought to be 'autonomic' or beyond voluntary control. The expectations were enormous. People with high blood pressure could now learn to reduce it. People with abnormal heart activity could learn to control it.

Even pain, it was thought, could be controlled in this simple way – teach people to relax (for muscle-tension headache or backache) or to change their brainwaves to the 'alpha' pattern (steady 8–12 cycles per second) characteristic of relaxed meditational states, and the pain would vanish. Recent research on pain shows that biofeedback therapy is useful for relieving pain in some people. However, the pain relief is not achieved by biofeedback alone, but by the distraction, suggestion, relaxation, and sense of control that are all part of the biofeedback procedure.

Astonishingly, only a single study on biofeedback therapy for pain has so far provided definitive data that meet all of the criteria described above. Budzynski, Stoyva, and their colleagues (1973) have shown that tension headaches can be significantly reduced in about sixty-five per cent of people by teaching them to use feedback to relax the muscles of the forehead. The biofeedback training, moreover, was practised effectively in the home or office and continued to work in some cases that were followed for eighteen months. While these observations are exciting, tension headaches represent only one kind of pain.

The most enthusiastic claims for biofeedback were related to alpha brainwave activity (Kamiya, 1968). Some practitioners of yoga or transcendental meditation can produce large amounts of alpha brainwaves at will and simultaneously report feeling no pain when stuck with pins. Many observers, including writers for the mass media, quickly concluded that, by simply learning to increase alpha output, sufferers could banish pain. Given these suggestive data, as well as the massive advertising campaign by 'mind-control experts' who claimed they could teach people to abolish all kinds of clinical pain with only a few easy biofeedback lessons, Melzack and Perry (1975) carried out a study to test the claims. The patients they studied all suffered chronic pain due to a variety of injuries or diseases. Their main criterion in selecting patients was that they were in continuous pain of known physical origin as verified by the physicians who referred them to the study. Many of the patients had pain despite disc surgery, or the severing of pain pathways, and the pain was not substantially diminished by lying down or by drugs. In short, all the traditional pain-relieving procedures had failed.

A group of patients received alpha-biofeedback training to control their pain. Although the patients learned to produce significant increases in the amount of alpha rhythm in their brain-waves, they did not experience greater reductions in pain than those which occurred in 'placebo' baseline sessions. In these sessions, given prior to the alpha training, the patients were allowed to relax in a comfortable reclining chair, were distracted from their pain by being given a thorough description of the training procedures they would receive later, and were given strong anxiety-relieving assurances that the biofeedback would diminish their pain. This placebo condition, then, was just as effective as the elegant, extremely expensive electronic biofeedback equipment and procedure.

This conclusion is now supported by an impressive amount of research. Three major reviews of the literature on biofeedback have recently appeared. One of them (Silver and Blanchard, 1978) asks, in its title, 'are the machines really necessary?' Two of them deal specifically with biofeedback for pain problems (Turk *et al.*, 1979; Jessup, Newfield and Merskey, 1979), and one of these articles reviews a hundred papers that were published in the 1970s. The following summary (Turk *et al.*, 1979) is representative of the three articles:

The biofeedback literature for the regulation of pain is reviewed and found wanting on both conceptual and methodological grounds. In particular, studies on the use of biofeedback for the treatment of tension and migraine headaches and chronic pain indicate that biofeedback was not found to be superior to less expensive, less instrument-oriented treatments such as relaxation and coping skills training. The relative absence of needed control comparisons was noted, and the need for caution in promoting biofeedback was stressed.

It is evident, then, that we need to continue to examine bio-feedback therapy and separate the facts from the enthusiastic expectations. There is no evidence so far that biofeedback is the panacea promised by bestselling books. It is time to stop the exhilarating speculations and to carry out well-controlled research instead.

In fact, there has been an overreaction to the excesses of the early claims. As we shall soon see, the biofeedback procedure *does* add something important to psychological therapy for pain, and to deny it any value is to 'throw out the baby with the bathwater'. Biofeedback is a useful vehicle for distraction of attention, relaxation, suggestion, and providing the patient with a sense of control over his pain. Before considering this in detail, we will first look at other psychological approaches to the control of pain.

Hypnosis

Placebos are, without a doubt, the oldest form of pain therapy. Many of the herbs and medicines that have been used for thousands of years are now known to have no pharmacological value as analgesics, but their administration by doctors, medicine men or shamans has worked repeatedly. The results could only have been due to the powerful placebo effect. Hypnosis may be an equally ancient practice for the relief of pain. In primitive cultures, the rhythmic drumming and incantations that accompanied the medicines may well have had a hypnotic effect on the patient so that the strong suggestion that his pain would be relieved by the medicine would actually produce the desired effect. The use of repetitive incantations and music in the practice of medicine is as old as recorded history (Keele, 1957).

Modern hypnotic techniques, however, originated in the eighteenth century, and have been in continuous use as a powerful way to control pain as well as to 'cure' a variety of disorders (Hilgard and Hilgard, 1975; Sheehan and Perry, 1976). In the mid 1800s there was enormous excitement and interest in the use of hypnosis to produce analgesia for major surgery – an interest which declined after the discovery of the inhalant anaesthetics, but was revived in this century through the remarkable growth of psychology and psychiatry. Yet, despite a vast amount of excellent research on the effects of hypnosis on experimentally induced pain, there is virtually no reliable evidence from controlled clinical studies to show that it is effective for any form of chronic pain (Hilgard and Hilgard, 1975). That hypnosis has helped many individual patients is beyond dispute. But it remains to be shown that hypnotic suggestion is any better than a placebo pill or encouragement and moral support from the family physician or parish priest.

The number of people who are capable of undergoing major surgery solely with hypnotic analgesia is very small. It is sufficiently rare that the occasional operation performed under hypnosis without any drugs still merits newspaper headlines. This is not surprising because the proportion of people who are easily hypnotized – that is, are highly susceptible to hypnosis – is very small. Not more than fifteen per cent of the population falls into this category. The remainder can be hypnotized with varying degrees of ease or difficulty, and a substantial proportion cannot be hypnotized at all. There is no reason to doubt the reports that hypnosis can be used effectively to control a wide variety of pain problems such as phantom limb pain, cancer pain, and low back pain. But these studies generally consist of a small number of individual cases, and it is not known what proportion of patients suffering these pains can be helped by hypnosis, how long the effects last, or whether a placebo treatment would work equally well.

The mechanisms of hypnosis are extremely complex and, not surprisingly, are the source of heated debate (Sheehan and Perry, 1976). Some theorists maintain that hypnosis is a special, unique state of consciousness while others propose that it is nothing more than compliance to suggestions made by others and, therefore, determined largely by personal traits such as suggestibility and capacity for role-playing. Whatever the mechanisms may be, it is clear that hypnotic suggestion can be usefully employed to help patients achieve control over some kinds of chronic pain. Not all patients are helped, and the pain is rarely totally abolished. But the effect is sufficiently impressive to indicate that it is a valuable form of therapy.

Melzack and Perry (1975; 1980) recently examined the effects of hypnotic training on patients suffering chronic pain such as low back pain, arthritic pain and cancer pain. The hypnotic training was administered by means of tape-recorded instructions which were played to the patients while they were seated comfortably in a reclining chair.

The hypnotic-training instructions took about twenty minutes and began with techniques that focused attention on relaxing various muscle groups. The taped message also included 'ego-strengthening' suggestions in which the patients were told:

As a result of this deep relaxation – this deep hypnosis – you are going to feel physically stronger and fitter and healthier in every way. You will feel more alert – more wide awake – more energetic. You will become less easily tired – much less easily fatigued – much less easily discouraged. . . . Every day you will become stronger and steadier – your mind calmer and clearer – more composed – more placid – more tranquil. You will find that it takes a lot for things to worry you – it takes a lot for things to upset you even slightly. . . .

These patients reported an average pain reduction of 22%, which is not significantly greater than the 14% reduction they obtained in the placebo-baseline sessions, which provided them with a sympathetic hearing of their pain problem, strong suggestion that their pain would be relieved and an opportunity to relax in a comfortable clinical setting. However, the results are actually more impressive than is indicated by the relatively low *average* pain reduction for the group as a whole. Half of the patients – 50% – had their pain relieved by 33% or more as measured by the McGill Pain Questionnaire. During later practice sessions, in which the patients used the self-hypnosis according to the instructions they learned from the tape, 60% of the patients achieved 33% or more relief of pain. This is not only a substantial number of patients but also a substantial amount of pain relief for patients who had suffered severe chronic pain. The pain relief obtained by these patients, in fact, was statistically greater than the relief observed in a group of patients (described earlier) who received biofeedback training. Since biofeedback training represents an impressive 'control' procedure, it is evident that hypnotic training can be a valuable technique – for some patients at least – for the relief of chronic pain.

Relaxation

Generally, hypnosis begins with a period in which the patient is instructed to relax, followed by the hypnotic suggestions regarding pain, memory, or some other psychological function. Clearly, hypnosis is more than just relaxation (Sheehan and Perry, 1976). But the relaxation is a very important component of hypnosis, especially when hypnotic suggestion is used for the relief of pain. Relaxation, in fact, is an essential component in most forms of therapy for pain. Biofeedback training, for example, may be considered as a method in which electronic devices are used to aid relaxation. Autogenic training (Luthe, 1970), in which patients are taught to achieve feelings of heaviness and warmth in their limbs (usually a part of the subjective feelings of hypnosis), also emphasizes the importance of relaxation. So too transcendental meditation and yoga involve achievement of deep relaxation accompanied by subjective experiences of 'peace of mind, feeling at ease with the world, and a sense of well-being' (Benson *et al.*, 1977, p.441).

It is not surprising, therefore, that relaxation has been proposed to be the 'common denominator' of all such therapies, and that it decreases the activity of the sympathetic nervous system (Benson *et al.*, 1977). Most of us, in other words, are usually caught up in a state of tension and stress in a competitive world, so that we are constantly prepared for an emergency or 'fight-or-flight response'. This psychological stress produces muscle tension, as well as increased blood pressure, heart rate, respiratory rate, and adrenalin outflow. All of this activity feeds into the nervous system and produces feelings of tension and irritability, and may produce pain directly (such as tension headaches and backaches) or indirectly by facilitating activity in neuron pools that project pain signals to the brain.

Benson and his colleagues have proposed that the 'relaxation response' is the basis of all meditative practices. Relaxation, they suggest, induces the subjective experience of wellbeing which is often referred to as an 'altered state of consciousness'. In contrast to Jacobson's method of 'progressive relaxation', in which people are taught to relax individual muscle groups in progression throughout a therapy session, Benson *et al.*, (1977, p.442), have developed a simple technique based on a variety of historical religious practices. Their instructions for this non-cultic technique are the following:

1 Sit quietly in a comfortable position and close your eyes.

2 Deeply relax all your muscles, beginning at your feet and progressing up to your face. Keep them deeply relaxed.

3 Breathe through your nose. Become aware of your breathing. As you breathe out, say the word *one* silently to yourself. For example, breathe in . . . out, *one* ; in . . . out, *one*; etc. Continue for twenty minutes. You may open your eyes to check the time, but do not use an alarm. When you finish, sit quietly for several minutes at first with closed eyes and later with opened eyes.

4 Do not worry about whether you are successful in achieving a deep level of relaxation. Maintain a passive attitude and permit relaxation to occur at its own pace. Expect other thoughts. When these distracting thoughts occur, ignore them by thinking 'Oh well' and continue repeating 'one'. With practice, the response should come with little effort. Practise the technique once or twice daily, but not within two hours after any meal, since the digestive processes seem to interfere with the subjective changes.

This simple technique has now been shown (Benson *et al.,* 1977) to produce striking physiological changes characteristic of deep relaxation, such as decreased metabolism and lower blood pressure and respiration rate. So far, however, there is no evidence that the technique is any better or worse than progressive relaxation or autogenic training. All of these techniques are probably equally effective.

There is now convincing evidence that relaxation alone is as effective as biofeedback training. A study of tension headache (Cox *et al.,* 1975) showed that patients who were trained in either progressive relaxation *or* muscle-biofeedback achieved greater relief of their headaches than that produced by placebo medication. A similar study (Chesney and Shelton, 1976) found that muscle relaxation alone *or* a combination of muscle relaxation and muscle-biofeedback was more effective in relieving tension headaches than muscle-biofeedback alone. They concluded that relaxation training and practice, rather than biofeedback, are the essential component in the treatment of muscle-tension headaches. Yet another study (Blanchard *et al.,* 1978) found that muscle relaxation alone was better than biofeedback for a brief period during the training procedures, but in the long run both were equally effective.

It is evident from these data that relaxation is a simple, effective procedure for the treatment of muscle-tension headache. Unfortunately, there are, as yet, no comparable studies with patients suffering more severe kinds of pain such as low back pain or the neuralgias. We will soon see, however, that relaxation may be used as an adjunct to other procedures so that their effectiveness is enhanced to levels that are statistically greater than placebo or baseline control conditions.

Cognitive coping skills

Everyone, beginning at an early age, learns to cope with pain by using various strategies. The most common strategy is distraction of attention. For example, while sitting in a dental chair or waiting for an injection in the doctor's office, we often force ourselves to think about something else – such as a beautiful beach, a difficult chess problem, or some other absorbing thought. We may employ imagery by trying to conjure up the most vivid possible picture to distract our attention from the painful event. Alternatively, we may attend to the pain but give it a different quality by concentrating on the tingling, hot or pulsing qualities of the total pain experience rather than the unpleasant qualities.

In recent years, psychologists have devised a large number of ingenious methods that utilize different kinds of strategies or coping mechanisms. The following is a partial list of the strategies (Tan, 1980):

1 *Imaginative inattention.* The patient is trained to ignore the pain by evoking imagery which is incompatible with pain. For example, the patient is instructed to imagine himself at the beach, at a party, or in the country, depending on the image he can conjure up most vividly.

2 *Imaginative transformation of pain.* The patient is instructed to interpret the subjective experience in terms other than 'pain' (for example, transforming it into tingling or other purely sensory

qualities) or to minimize the experience as trivial or unreal.

3 Imaginative transformation of context. The patient is trained to acknowledge the pain but to transform the setting or context. For example, a patient with a sprained arm may picture himself as a fighter pilot who has been 'shot in the arm while being chased by an enemy plane.

4 Attention-diversion to external events. The patient focuses attention on environmental objects and may count ceiling tiles or concentrate on the weave of a piece of clothing.

5 Attention-diversion to internal events. The patient focuses attention on self-generated thoughts such as mental arithmetic or composing a limerick.

6 Somatization. The patient is trained to focus attention on the painful area but in a detached manner. For example, the patient may analyse the pain sensations as if preparing to write a magazine article about them.

These procedures are extremely clever. But are they effective for relieving pain? The evidence so far is encouraging but not conclusive. Of 27 studies carried out up to 1980, 15 indicated that these instructed coping strategies are superior to strategies generated spontaneously by subjects in control groups when laboratory pains are used (Tan, 1980). However, the fact that 12 of the studies failed to find significant differences indicates that the effect is not so robust that it always exceeds placebo effects. Nevertheless, it is evident that patients who are not instructed in particular strategies use their own strategies. In fact, even instructed patients may revert to strategies which they evolved themselves in the past and found useful. It is important, therefore, to have adequate control groups, and to examine the effects of the strategies on pain in real-life situations.

Two recent studies indicate that coping-strategy techniques are effective for clinical pain. The first (Horan, Layng and Pursell, 1976) investigated the effects of pleasant imagery guided by a tape on dental pain. The results showed that patients who utilized this strategy had significantly less discomfort than a control group which received no treatment instructions, and, more importantly, than a second control group instructed in 'neutral' imagery – that is, imagining numbers on a poster. The second study (Rybstein-Blinchik, 1979) examined patients who suffered severe pain due to amputation, rheumatoid arthritis, fractures, and other diseases or injuries. The results showed that patients who were trained in the coping strategy of imaginative transformation (or reinterpretation) of the pain had significantly less pain than patients who were taught two other strategies – diverting attention from the pain or concentrating on the pain (somatization). It is apparent, then, that particular procedures are effective for some patients, and for some kinds of pain. The approach is promising and may become more effective when patients' personalities are taken into account. For example, some people are less capable of generating imagery than others, and some people have a greater desire to cope personally with their pain than others, who may be more passive and prefer to have other people take full responsibility for its alleviation (Tan, 1980).

Multiple convergent therapy

It is evident, from our review so far, that several psychological procedures are capable of diminishing pain. No one of them helps all people or abolishes pain completely. But each produces some degree of pain relief so that life for the suffering patient becomes more bearable. Even a few hours of relief a day, or a decrease in pain so that a bedridden person is able to carry out some of life's day-to-day activities, is a substantial help in allowing people in continuous pain to live with some degree of dignity. Because each procedure may help a little, it is natural to try two or more procedures in combination to see whether the effects of each are additive. Happily, the evidence suggests that they are.

It has long been known that placebo effects enhance the power of any pain-relieving procedure. This has been substantiated beyond any doubt in the use of analgesic drugs (Beecher, 1959). A similar conclusion has been drawn from a study of the use of loud music and noise ('audio analgesia') for the relief of pain (Melzack, Weisz and Sprague, 1963). People were subjected to a laboratory pain (immersion of the hand in ice-water), and then given one of several procedures in the attempt to see whether any of them increased the amount of time they tolerated the pain. A group of subjects that received loud music and noise from an impressive-looking machine, but without explicit suggestion that it would relieve their pain, did not show increased tolerance to pain. Similarly, subjects who received strong suggestion that a gentle buzzing sound from the machine (a placebo control) would relieve their pain also failed to show increased pain tolerance. However, both the music-and-noise *and* the strong suggestion, when presented together, produced a significant increase in pain tolerance. This kind of additive effect has now been found in other studies in which patients suffering various kinds of chronic pain were presented with two different treatments.

Hypnosis and biofeedback

Melzack and Perry (1975) found that EEG biofeedback alone had no demonstrable effect on chronic pain compared to the level of pain relief obtained in 'placebo' baseline sessions. In contrast, they found that hypnotic training instructions produced substantial relief of pain – significantly greater than the effect of biofeedback. The subjects reported an average of 22% pain reduction, and 50% achieved pain decreases of 33% or more. Despite the magnitude of the effect, it was not statistically greater than that of the 'placebo' baseline sessions. However, when the hypnotic training instructions were presented *together* with biofeedback, the pain relief was significantly greater than that produced by the baseline placebo sessions. The average pain reduction was 36% and 58% of the patients reported pain decreases of 33% or more (Figure 41). This is especially impressive when the population of patients is considered: they had all suffered severe chronic pain for years, had received a variety of treatments including orthopaedic and neurological surgery, and were referred to the study because their physicians had exhausted all the conventional medical approaches.

The biofeedback clearly added something to the hypnotic training. The supposition that the 'something' is increased alpha activity in the EEG is not supported by the evidence, because all

three groups – biofeedback, hypnosis, and hypnosis-plus-bio-
feedback – showed the same degree of increased alpha activity

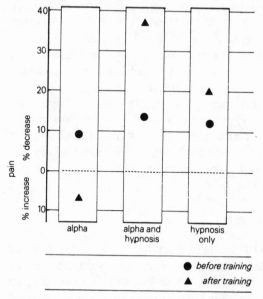

Figure 41. Average percentage decrease or increase in pain after placebo control
sessions, and after treatments with alpha biofeedback training, hypnosis, or a
combination of biofeedback and hypnosis. Only the combined treatment
produced statistically more relief than the placebo control sessions.

(indicating a relaxed state). However, although alpha activity is not
the critical factor, the biofeedback procedure could contribute to
the relief of pain by:

1 *Distracting attention from the painful area.* The patients distracted themselves by directing their attention to different inner
feelings and to a feedback signal which is attention-demanding.

2 *Providing still further strong suggestion that the pain would diminish.* This is in addition to that provided by the hypnotic training.

3 *Providing a period of relaxation in addition to that of the hypnotic
training.* The relaxation would produce a decrease in sensory
inputs, such as those from muscles and viscera, and thus would
reduce the general level of arousal. This would lower the patients'
anxiety levels, and thereby diminish the level of pain they felt.

4 Giving the sufferers a sense of control over pain. This is also known to reduce pain levels. The belief that one is able to do something about pain, which is inherent in the alpha-training procedure, can bring about a reduction in the anxiety associated with pain and, therefore, in the pain itself.

Similar results have recently been obtained with a procedure known as 'stress-inoculation training' (Meichenbaum and Turk, 1976) in which patients are (1) given information that provides them with an understanding of pain and the stresses that accompany it; (2) trained in a variety of coping strategies (such as relaxation, distraction and imagery techniques) and allowed to choose the ones they prefer; and (3) rehearsed in the use of the strategies while they conceptualize the pain and stress at each phase of the total pain experience. An investigation (Hartman and Ainsworth, 1980) of the effectiveness of stress-inoculation training in patients with severe, persistent pain found that the training by itself did not reduce pain significantly compared to pain-reductions that occurred during baseline control sessions in which the patients received only autogenic training (see p.344). However, when the stress-inoculation training was preceded by several sessions of alpha-biofeedback training, it produced significant reductions in pain compared to the baseline sessions. Once again, then, a *combination* of treatments was effective whereas a single procedure alone was not. The biofeedback sessions presumably facilitated the stress-inoculation training by providing the additional distraction, relaxation, suggestion and sense of control necessary to allow the patient to achieve a greater degree of pain relief.

It is interesting that stress–inoculation training failed to reduce pain caused by injection of substances into the tissues of the knee for a diagnostic procedure called an arthrogram (Tan, 1980). However, it is not known whether an additional procedure (such as biofeedback or hypnosis) would have produced significant reductions in pain or, as the experimenter noted, the arthrogram pain is too sudden, sharp and brief for coping strategies to be used effectively. It is important to keep in mind, in all studies such as these, that the temporal properties of the pain often determine the effectiveness or ineffectiveness of any procedure.

Sharp pains that rise rapidly to a peak are especially difficult to control by psychological procedures, while steady or slowly rising pains are easier to control by distraction, relaxation and other coping strategies.

Prepared childbirth training

The most famous of all psychological approaches to the control of pain is prepared childbirth training. We have seen earlier (Chapter 3) that labour pain is one of the most severe forms of pain, and several procedures have been developed to teach pregnant women how to cope with their pain when they are in labour. One of the methods, developed by Grantly Dick-Read (1944), is known as 'childbirth without fear'. More recently, Fernand Lamaze (1970) developed a programme for 'painless childbirth' which is widely known as 'Lamaze training'. Basically, these techniques include (1) providing detailed information on pregnancy and labour to the mother-to-be so that she knows what to expect and therefore experiences less anxiety; (2) relaxation training so that the woman can try to relax and calm herself when uterine contractions begin to increase in frequency, duration, and intensity; (3) coping strategies to distract attention from pain; and (4) breathing exercises which are useful to enhance relaxation, distract attention, as well as to aid in the process of giving birth.

Women in labour are subject to intense fears and anxieties related to their ability to bear the pain, to the possibility of medical complications, and to the baby's health. Prepared childbirth training, which is designed to reduce fear, anxiety and tension, should, therefore, also decrease pain. A recent study (Melzack *et al.*, 1981) demonstrates that it does, but the effects are not as great as people generally believe.

We observed earlier (Chapter 3) that some women report little pain during labour while others suffer severely. Several factors are significant predictors of labour pain. Women giving birth to their first baby (primiparas) generally have *less* pain if they (a) belong to higher socio-economic status groups, (b) do not have a history of menstrual difficulties, and (c) practised the procedures they learned in prepared childbirth training. Labour pain in multiparas (women who have given birth before) is influenced by the same factors, but it is especially important that the women feel that they have been adequately prepared for labour.

Table 6 shows the average pain scores (Pain Rating Index) of primiparas who received prepared childbirth training (PCT) and those who did not. The results for individual PCT instructors are also shown. PCT, in all cases, consisted of a series of classes that included instruction in obstetrical physiology, breathing exercises, and relaxation techniques. Clearly, there is considerable variability among different instructors' groups in the scores obtained during labour. Discussions held with some of the women suggested that this is due partly to differences in the instructors' enthusiasm about PCT.

Table 6 shows that PCT produces a significant decrease in total pain scores when compared to the scores of women who did not receive any training. Moreover, PCT does not merely diminish the affective dimension of pain, but also produces a significant decrease in the sensory dimension. A striking feature of Table 6, however, is that the average scores of women who received PCT are still very high. Instructor 1, for example, was clearly the most effective of all; yet the mean total pain scores of her patients are at about the same level as the average totals recorded for out-patients with chronic back pain and cancer (see Figure 5, p.67). Most significant is the fact that although this instructor strongly encouraged her patients to forgo epidural spinal blocks, five of the six women specifically requested an epidural block during the late stages of labour.

These observations should be interpreted in a positive sense (Melzack *et al.*, 1981). The fact that the current training procedures have statistically significant effects on pain is encouraging and indicates that psychological preparation is valuable. The additional fact that the average pain reduction is relatively small means that there is need for further development of these obviously useful procedures.

Conclusion

There is no longer any doubt that it is possible to reduce many kinds of clinical pain by means of different psychological therapies. It is important to keep in mind, however, that these

Mean PRI scores

Variable	Total	Sensory	Affective	Women given an epidural (%)
Women with no training, n = 26	37.2	22.6	4.0	82
Women with prepared childbirth training, n = 61	32.9	20.3	3.3	81
P values*	0.05	0.05	0.05	NS
Instructor no.				
1, n = 6	26.1	16.1	3.2	83
2, n = 3	27.3	18.6	1.3	100
3, n = 15	31.7	20.0	2.6	79
4, n = 12	32.3	18.4	3.2	89
5, n = 5	33.6	20.2	2.8	100
6, n = 20	37.0	23.0	3.5	79

*For significance of difference between means for women with and without training. NS = not significant.

Table 6. Effects of prepared childbirth training on pain in primiparas.

therapies rarely abolish pain entirely and are not equally effective for everyone. However, there are no perfect therapies of any kind. We have learned, as a result of literally hundreds of experiments, that there is a limit to the effectiveness of any given therapy; but, happily, the effects of two or more therapies given in combination are cumulative. Two therapies, each with slight effects that do not reach statistical significance, may produce significant reductions in pain when given together. For this reason, *multiple convergent therapy* is increasingly becoming the standard psychological approach to pain problems. Biofeedback, hypnosis and stress-inoculation training may each produce small effects. Two of the procedures together may have a large, significant effect. However, multiple convergent therapy does not refer only to psychological approaches. A psychological method may be used in combination with drugs or with sensory modulation procedures.

The data indicate that multiple convergent therapy using several psychological procedures is effective because each kind of therapy may have its predominant effect on a different mechanism. Relaxation, for example, may reduce muscle tension and generally reduce activity in the sympathetic nervous system. Hypnosis, however, may have its predominant effect by activating control processes that modulate the input as it is transmitted through the brain. Procedures which involve the diversion of attention (so that even spinal reflexes may fail to occur) may, conceivably, activate the descending systems of the brainstem so that inputs are modulated at spinal levels. It is evident, then, that different psychological procedures may each have different predominant effects, so that several procedures together work better because more modulating systems are activated. It is also possible, of course, that each system may be increasingly affected as more procedures are used.

Whatever the precise mechanisms may be, the evidence reviewed in this chapter shows convincingly that psychological approaches can have powerful effects on pain. However, there are limitations to the procedures, and it is important to recognize them. By doing so, we set the stage for new approaches, or the use of old approaches in different combinations. The field is young and growing rapidly. It holds great promise as an approach by itself or together with the powerful yet simple methods of sensory modulation that we are also just beginning to understand.

16
Pain Clinics and Hospices

While great strides have clearly been made in the control of pain, there are still many pain syndromes which are beyond our comprehension and our control. Back pains, especially of the lower back, are the most common kind of pain and literally millions of sufferers are continually seeking help. Sometimes they obtain temporary relief, but most continue to suffer. Migraine and tension headaches similarly plague millions of people. New drugs such as propranalol, and psychological techniques such as relaxation-training provide help for some, but the pains persist in the majority. Perhaps the most terrible of all pains are those suffered by some cancer patients in the terminal phases of the disease.

The inability to solve a patient's pain problem is deeply disturbing to both patients and therapists. At first, the patient respects the special knowledge of the various medical specialists, psychologists, physiotherapists, or other health professionals. But as the pain persists despite countless treatments, despite the claims often made in the media that sensational new pain cures have been found, and despite the best efforts by the therapists, the patient becomes understandably hostile. Respect is replaced by anger, hope by despair. This is clearly an intolerable situation. The presence of this alienation between the patient and those who take care of him has recently led to two crucial developments in the control of pain – the pain clinic and the hospice.

The pain clinic as a response to the challenge of the chronic pain patient

Presently, few hospitals are organized to cope with the more complex kinds of pain. People suffering severe pain may be transferred from one doctor to another (from neurologist to neurosurgeon and finally psychiatrist) with little or no help. They may cycle through these specialists several times without experiencing any significant pain relief. What is needed is a concerted effort in which new modes of therapy can be attempted and evaluated. In short, what is needed are *pain clinics* in which specialists can work together to deal specifically with pain problems. In such clinics, an interchange of ideas can occur and the conditions are conducive to novel, imaginative approaches. Pain, in such a clinic, is not merely a symptom which each specialist perceives from his point of view. Rather, it is the pain syndrome that is itself examined, and the integration of many specialities to treat it is more easily achieved.

The idea of a pain clinic can be traced quite clearly to the experience and ideas of Dr John J. Bonica of the University of Washington Medical School, who is an anaesthetist and author of several seminal books on the treatment of pain. The history of anaesthesia begins in the nineteenth century, with the discovery of the inhalant anaesthetics – nitrous oxide, ether and chloroform. These general anaesthetic agents were first treated as just another family of drugs which could be given by minimally trained nurses and medical students under the distant and distracted supervision of the surgeon who was operating. However, deaths caused by anaesthesia occurred sufficiently often that a group of specialists arose – anaesthetists (more commonly called anaesthesiologists in the United States). Since the 1940s they have done a remarkable job of making general anaesthesia a safe, controllable procedure so that deaths or serious side-effects attributable to anaesthesia are now down to very low levels, usually due to the accidents of human failure and poor training. Having solved most of their major initial problems, anaesthetists were given more and more responsibilities which strongly affected the treatment of pain in two ways. They took responsibility for the immediate recovery process after operation and in this phase inevitably had to face problems of control of post-operative pain. Secondly, they searched for more localized anaesthetics which would not produce a general anaesthesia but would simply numb one area.

In their search for ways to block nerves, anaesthetists developed extraordinary skills by which they could insert needles accurately into many deeply buried structures. While this skill was originally developed in order to apply a local, temporary anaesthetic, the same method could be used to inject fluids that destroy nerves, as we have seen in Chapter 13. These procedures allowed the anaesthetists to become neurosurgeons 'at a distance'. The classical neurosurgical method of operating on a structure was to expose it to direct vision and then to dissect it out or destroy it by electrocoagulation. This by itself is often a major operation with all its discomforts and threats; now the anaesthetists were able to achieve the same end results for a number of structures by aiming needles at the target, with the needle insertion as the only threat to the patient.

With these skills, anaesthetists such as Bonica found themselves receiving patients with particularly difficult pain problems. All too often, such patients would appear with a 'thick file', having already been examined and treated by a succession of specialists. Bonica felt that this position at the end of the line was totally unsatisfactory for all concerned and that it could be avoided by organization and education. He collected together a group of the traditional specialists who were particularly interested in the problems of pain. These, of course, included neurosurgeons, orthopaedic surgeons, neurologists, psychiatrists, psychologists, and so forth.

Let us follow the course of a single patient, such as the patient with low back pain described earlier (p.267), as if she had been treated at the pain clinic at the University of Washington Medical School. Ideally, she would have been referred to the clinic by the first physician she visited. Why would the doctor do such a thing rather than treating the patient himself? The answer is primarily a matter of education of physicians. Obviously, a very high percentage of patients who visit a doctor with a new complaint are completely within his field of expertise. However, he must learn the early signs of problem cases and be aware of those rare cases who are beyond his capability. Obviously, he must have good relations with the members of the pain clinic and have confidence in them. We must, of necessity, mention here the role of the financial structure of the medical system which may encourage doctors to treat and overtreat patients to the patients' detriment and the doctors' profit. Each society has to study its nature to be certain that it does not allow or even require doctors to carry out unnecessary, time-wasting, money-wasting and potentially harmful examinations and therapies.

The patient arrives for her first visit to the pain clinic and meets a single doctor who will from then on be responsible for her care and follow up. He takes a history and carries out an examination and makes all the necessary tests. This doctor might come from any of the traditional specialties but has a particular interest in pain problems and is especially experienced with them. So far, this may appear to the reader like the development of yet another specialty, and the movement certainly contains that danger. However, this doctor has access to consultations with all the relevant specialties and in this lies the crucial innovation of the pain clinic. The patient may be presented to a meeting of specialists, each of whom has received a detailed summary of the patient's condition. At these meetings, the combined experience of the specialists can be brought together and a cautious step-by-step plan of treatment can be initiated. It is seen that this cooperative approach can have great advantages for the patient, but runs counter to a hallowed tradition of medicine, in which one doctor establishes a relationship with one patient and 'does his thing'. The patient of the pain clinic has her single doctor but he takes on the role of her collator and interpreter rather than the classical role of all-powerful controller.

The system brings with it three important advantages. The first is educational – the professionals can learn not only from a special group of patients but also from each other. In the best of these clinics, basic scientists are also present so that they too can experience the real nature of the problems rather than learn them second-hand. The second advantage to grouping together many pain patients and many concerned professionals is that it allows the development of new therapies. This has been particularly crucial for the beginning of psychological treatments directed at patients with chronic intractable pain. Clearly, the patients must be carefully selected in cooperation with the traditional specialists – who must themselves remain in close collaboration with the psychologists and their patients. Two of the most important psychologists in this initiative have been W. E. Fordyce (1976) and R. S. Sternbach (1974) who have pioneered the application of the methods of experimental psychology in the attempt to control the behaviour of pain patients The third advantage of pain clinics is that they allow the accumulation of data – such as the relative effectiveness of different therapeutic procedures – that are often lost as the patient visits each specialist in his own clinic. The pain clinic allows the development of a battery of techniques to control pain. The pharmacological, sensory, and psychological methods of pain control do not exclude each other. A combination of several methods – such as electrical stimulation of nerves and appropriate drugs – may be necessary to provide satisfactory relief. The effective combination may differ for each type of pain, and possibly for each individual, depending on such factors as the patient's earlier medical history, pattern of spread of trigger zones, and the duration of the pain. But it is only in a clinic, where many cases are seen and complete data files are kept, that sufficient experience and knowledge can be acquired to allow the best judgement in each case.

The idea of pain clinics has spread during the past ten years. There is at least one in every major city of the western world. Obviously, each one differs depending on the personality and training of the professionals involved and on the forces at work in society. Some areas have developed specialized headache clinics, for example. In some regions, the old specialists have formed themselves into particularly aggressive guilds where they may lay claim to some disease state, and dismiss the concept of pain clinics as unnecessary to the practice of 'proper medicine'. These internecine medical struggles may trap the patient in the bonds of one specialty.

The success of the idea of the pain clinic has inevitably led to the usual venal abuses of a good idea. Some specialists have simply re-labelled their old restricted services without enlarging the scope of their concepts or specialties in order to solve the patients' problems. It is true that knowledge about pain is rapidly expanding – as is the number of therapies – but it would be a great pity if this led simply to the development of yet another specialty with its restrictive practices and contrived ways of thinking. A greater danger is already apparent in the appearance of the quack who possesses a single untested approach and re-labels his artifice wth the modern, trendy title of 'pain clinic' and attracts the desperate, driven patient who has received little relief from the more serious sources of help.

The hospice as a response
to the challenge of the dying patient

There are few problems that are more challenging than the relief of pain in people with cancer – people whose lives are coming to an end. Many of us do not fear death but rather fear the pain that may precede it. Patients in the last stages of cancer have often come to terms with the knowledge that the end is near. Their worry is that they may not have the courage to bear the pain of their final weeks with the dignity they fought so hard to achieve in daily life. There is no merit to this suffering, no lesson to be learned.

The proportion of people who develop cancer is frighteningly high. Although it strikes primarily at older people, some forms of cancer occur in children and adolescents. Each year, in the United States, about 700,000 new cases of cancer are diagnosed and about 400,000 people die from it (Bonica, 1980). Because tumours grow very slowly at first, cancer is rarely painful at its onset or during its early phases. In a large number of patients, however, cancer cells break away from the primary site and migrate to other tissues where they grow (metastasize) rapidly. Patients with metastatic cancer usually develop pain which increases in severity until it becomes relentless suffering. Furthermore, some patients develop pain directly or indirectly as a result of therapy. Bonica (1980) estimates that moderate to severe pain is experienced by about forty per cent of patients with intermediate stages of the disease, and by sixty to eighty per cent of patients with advanced cancer.

A major challenge that confronts physicians who treat terminally ill people is the judicious use of drugs. At present, this decision depends largely on the individual physician. One physician may seek any means, even major surgical operations, to avoid administering morphine, presumably out of fear of turning the terminal patient into an addict. Another may decide that a person's final weeks should be spent in tranquillity, and provide drugs such as morphine whenever they are requested by the patient. These are complex social issues and they may be handled best by a group of physicians and scientists who have gained familiarity with the ravages of prolonged severe pain on the human mind. As a result of this need in society, there has recently been a remarkable development – the hospice, whose sole aim is to provide care to terminally ill patients so that they can live the remainder of their days free of pain and other distressing symptoms. The concept of the hospice is best understood in historical perspective.

Up to the nineteenth century, the medical hospital was a place for care, for feeding and for isolation. Treatment played only a minor role. The patient lay in bed, awaiting the outcome of his disease, praying to his god for recovery or redemption, expecting few curative miracles from the surgeons and physicians. Quite obviously, a tremendous revolution has taken place in the actions of hospital doctors and in the expectations of the patients. Attention is now focused on active diagnosis and treatment. The enormous cost of occupation of hospital beds, largely because complex equipment and specialized services are extremely expensive, almost forbids the possibility of long stays in the modern hospital. Yet the need persists for a place for those beyond cure. In response to this need, a small number of hospices have continued in the medieval tradition, almost bypassed by the nineteenth and twentieth centuries. They are most commonly maintained by religious orders and have been virtually ignored by the mainstream of modern medicine. Until very recently, medical students received no lectures about the care of the dying and never visited a hospice as part of their training. Local doctors would sometimes schedule visits to a hospice as part of their busy general duties in the community. So the enormous responsibility of care for the patients has rested on the staff, and all honour is due to these people for their loving care and dedication to their patients. But we must face the fact that they were essentially untrained for their task – beyond the general principles of nursing – because no training existed for responding to the special needs of these patients. By experience, by inspiration and by dedication, the hospice staff did the best they could.

There are three social forces which maintain and increase the need for institutions for the care of the dying. First, the very success of medicine and public health has produced an aging population in all developed countries. This, by itself, brings larger numbers of people into older age where there is a greater likelihood of developing cancer. Second, the aging of the population combined with the shattering of the old family patterns leaves more and more lonely, sick people who can no longer count on the care of the traditional extended family. Lastly, the movement of academic medical interest towards cure rather than care has left both patients and hospices to look after themselves.

A revolution is now taking place to meet the special needs of the terminally ill, and Cicely Saunders is the key figure in the revolution. Her personal history is of special relevance to the problem we are discussing. When World War II broke out in 1939, she was a student of philosophy. Questioning the role of philosophy in the dramatic times which were beginning, she became a nurse. However, she soon suffered a back injury in the course of nursing which forced her to take a more sedentary job. She became a hospital 'almoner', which would now be called a social worker. This occupation, especially at that time, had an aspect of handling those problems with which the physicians could no longer cope.

Saunders inevitably became concerned with the incurable and terminally sick patients, and was deeply dissatisfied with what she saw. The patients, who were so deserving of loving personal attention in the last days of their life, were instead abandoned in isolated wards – in despair, depressed and facing death in utter loneliness. Her attitude was a totally different one and coloured all of her subsequent actions to help the dying patient: 'You matter because you are you. You matter to the last moment of your life, and we will do all we can to help you not only to die peacefully, but also to live until you die' (Saunders, 1976, p.6).

Saunders became aware that her training as philosopher-nurse-social worker did not provide her either professionally or politically with the power to find a solution to the problems which worried her. Therefore, well into her thirties, she started from the beginning and completed a full medical training, never losing sight of her goal which was to improve the lot of the abandoned ones. She worked first in existing hospices and then with a team of powerful associates. Together, they collected money and built an extraordinary institution, St Christopher's Hospice in London. It opened in 1967 and has become a gathering point for those who wish to learn how to care for incurable people in the best possible way. It is important to add that she and many of her closest associates are deeply committed Christians. This is important because a commitment to religion, to the concept that death is a transition from this world to a more glorious one, greatly helps these people to work constantly with dying human beings and to cope with their own pain when their patients die.

Gerard Manley Hopkins, who was a priest, wrote a poem about the death of a blacksmith, 'Felix Randal'. In it, he expresses a certain sense of satisfaction for both the helper and the sufferer in having completed a good job of life and death. The line, 'This seeing the sick endears them to us, us too it endears', epitomizes the approach pattern of the caring person rather than the withdrawal shown by many of those who face a sick person. The poem expresses a very different sentiment from that of the traditional doctor, who used to believe that his duty ended when he diagnosed his patient's illness as incurable.

There is another, almost political, aspect of the importance of religion for this group of people who set out to change the face of death. Their aim was to use every possible means to enhance the quality of their patients' lives until they died. In place of the lonely misery of dying in a large impersonal hospital, patients were encouraged to have contact with friends and relatives, and the medical emphasis was on relief of symptoms – especially pain – rather than cure, which was out of the question for these patients. Yet failure to try to cure has the inherent danger of being accused of 'killing the patient' by withholding treatment. Such an accusation is inconceivable against the group at St Christopher's, with their religious insistence on respect for life and their total rejection of mercy killing or euthanasia. Murder is an intentional act. However, excessive efforts to prolong the patient's life while adding to his misery, suffering, isolation and loss of dignity may equally be considered an assault on the patient. The key to the philosophy at St Christopher's is to allow the patient to die with the greatest possible dignity, not to prolong suffering and misery. There is a time in life when nature may be considered to have run its course. To try to prolong life in such a person now becomes unnatural and grotesque.

Let us follow the course of a patient entering the hospice. There are two initial rules which are strictly followed. Firstly, the patient must come from a relatively small geographical area around the hospice. In the dense packing of London, this area contains up to one million people. The reasons for this geographical restriction are twofold: relatives and friends can visit with ease and, more importantly, the patients have almost always already been in close contact with the hospice before admission. This is done partly by out-patient visits to the hospice but also, in a much more original way, by the provision of a 'flying team' which works in close collaboration with the family doctor. One should mention here that in Britain the National Health Service has promoted and emphasized the general practitioner or family doctor; every citizen has chosen a doctor and has the right to unlimited service (which has been paid by his taxes); all patients also have rights to home care as well as hospital care. St Christopher's has established close contact with the doctors in the area and with the home nursing and help services. The specialized team from the hospice – which includes doctors, nurses and social workers – has thereby established as much contact as is necessary with the aim of keeping the patient at home and as comfortable as possible. Therefore, it is rare for a patient to arrive at St Christopher's unknown and unexpected. All of this has the added advantage that the patient is somewhat familiar with the hospice and some of its staff and is, consequently, not in terror of an unfamiliar environment in addition to the miseries of his disease and his impending death.

The second rule is that the patient's admission is decided on by a hospice committee made up of nurses, doctors and other responsible people. Their job is to consider all aspects of the patient's case and to decide if it is time for admission to St Christopher's, or perhaps to another hospital with specialized facilities, or possibly to bring more aid to the patient's home. The procedure has the advantage of bringing out in discussion all possible solutions; it also has the important side effect of insulating individual staff members from the enormous personal pressures for admission which patients, and especially their relatives, can generate. In this way, patients in real need are admitted when alternatives fail. Need is the only criterion; the patient's religion or lack of it is irrelevant, as is his financial position, since the hospice is maintained partly by charitable contributions and partly by the National Health Service. The majority of patients are in the terminal stages of cancer, but some may be admitted who suffer from diseases characterized by slowly progressing paralysis until they are beyond any self-care. The average period from admission to death is twelve days, which indicates the careful and successful selection of patients who have been treated comfortably at home until that time. The average figure, however, hides a very broad range, from a few who die very soon after admission to others who are not desperately ill but who have had some serious episode such as the onset of severe pain or paralysis.

On entering the hospice, the patient enters an atmosphere of intensive caring. An absolute promise is made that he will from now on never be alone unless he wishes. This promise is kept absolutely so that a vigil is maintained even if the patient sinks into a state of terminal, final unconsciousness. There is to be no question in the staff's mind of alternation between approach and withdrawal. From now on, approach, care and compassion are the constant features of living and dying. This is an important matter for friends and relatives as well as for the patient, because, now that continuous professional care is assured, they too can learn to approach. The staff become as skilled in helping the relatives in this matter as they do in teaching the patient to accept and expect communication and togetherness. With the exception of a few patients selected to be in single rooms for various personal reasons, the patients live in open wards with many beds rather than in the usual isolation cubicles. The effect is that patients become concerned with each other. A man within a few hours of death was asked how he felt and said, 'I'm feeling good but I'm worried about Jack in the bed over there.' A great deal of the fear of death is not so much a fear of the death itself but the idea of the indignity and agony of the period immediately before death. These patients witness other patients slipping calmly and quietly away and this itself is a tremendous relief to their own fears and fantasies.

None of this careful setting of the scene would have much meaning if the patient suffered symptoms which precluded a sense of dignity. People in agonizing pain, for example, scream out, weep, and want only to be alone in their misery. In those dying of cancer, there are many miserable symptoms, of which pain is the most common:

Pain	66%
Loss of appetite	62%
Cough	49%
Breathlessness	41%
Vomiting and nausea	41%
Insomnia	24%
Weakness	21%
Difficulty in swallowing	16%
Drowsiness	10%

Table 7. Main symptoms felt by 607 patients admitted to St Christopher's Hospice with terminal cancer in 1976.

In a remarkable short book, the staff of St Christopher's have summarized their general approach and specifically their knowledge of symptom control (Saunders, 1978). In their treatment of pain, they have turned especially to the use of narcotic drugs. We have discussed these in detail in Chapter 12, but it is interesting to trace the history of the way this team approached the use of narcotics. The Brompton Hospital in London, which treated large numbers of terminal cancer patients in the nineteenth century, developed a mixture of drugs which has come to be known as the 'Brompton Cocktail'. More officially, it was called 'mist euphorians': the euphoria-producing mixture. It contained honey, gin, cocaine and heroin with some flavouring. It was given to suffering patients in the terminal stages of painful cancer and, not surprisingly, they were considerably relieved of their miseries. This effective mixture contains two signs of old-fashioned medicine. The doctors had looked at the patients, selected a series of drugs which they believed would counteract the various symptoms and added them all together in a single mixture. This approach is called 'polypharmacy' and has the economy of giving the patient a single medicine. However, a drawback is that if the patient's symptoms require an increased dose of one drug, the patient receives an increase of all the components. Furthermore, it is impossible to unravel which part of the mixture of powerful drugs is actually helping the patient and which parts may be ineffective or even harming him. The second old-fashioned aspect was that the nineteenth-century doctors were not yet sensitive to the growing social awareness, which has become acute and nearly hysterical in the twentieth century, of the danger of alcohol, cocaine and powerful narcotics such as heroin or morphine.

In those days, and extending well into this century, gin or brandy was such a common first treatment for all ailments, especially painful ones, that many patients were drunk much of the time. The reason, of course, is that alcohol is an excellent analgesic. Not far from the Brompton Hospital, a Temperance Hospital was set up in the 1880s which provided all the contemporary medicine and surgery except alcohol, and the physicians believed that their patients were doing better sober than those intoxicated in the surrounding hospitals. Cocaine was becoming a popular drug and was freely available for sale to anyone, without fear or anticipation of danger. Similarly, narcotics were used widely by the middle classes and there were none of the contemporary severe restrictions and fear.

The immensely useful Brompton Mixture survived into this century as an old-fashioned recipe used in the old-fashioned way. By the turn of the century, however, the medical profession had begun to think otherwise. Doctors came to be impressed with the addiction problems of giving narcotics and specifically with the belief that once a patient was started on a narcotic, he developed 'tolerance' to the drug: that is, there was an increase in the amount needed to produce the required effect. It was thought that this tolerance rose so rapidly that the drug eventually became ineffective. Therefore, it was believed that narcotics must be saved for desperate circumstances and given as late as possible, in minimal doses spaced as widely apart as possible. This attitude has led to a pattern of medical *under-use* of these drugs and needless suffering (Bonica, 1980).

In recent years, however, due largely to the courage and determination of the St Christopher's team (including the outstanding pharmacologist Robert Twycross), the Brompton Mixture has achieved recognized medical status. It has now been shown beyond any doubt that the mixture is effective for the large majority of patients who have pain in the terminal stages of cancer. Just as importantly, it has been found that dependence (addiction) and tolerance are not problems in the treatment of pain in terminally ill patients. Once an effective dose has been found, it maintains its effectiveness for months. If the dose suddenly becomes insufficient to control pain, it is most likely due to a change in the patient's medical status (that is, spread or growth of the tumour) rather than to tolerance. In fact, it has been shown that the amount of morphine can be *reduced* without any ill effects when therapy (such as radiation therapy) produces a shrinkage of the tumour and a reduction of pain. The reduction of the amount of morphine is not accompanied by any evidence of withdrawal or other signs of addiction. Twycross has also demonstrated two other important facts: the narcotic is the essential ingredient of the mixture and – to everyone's surprise – morphine is as effective as heroin, possibly even more effective.

A general belief had arisen that heroin was superior to other narcotics, particularly in its freedom from side effects. An interesting political battle had been fought by doctors in Britain to retain their right to prescribe what they believed to be a valuable drug. In many countries, including the United States, doctors gave in to social pressure from police forces. They said that heroin was producing such havoc that it should be totally banned since, according to claims, a substantial amount of illegal heroin came from medical sources. It is sadly obvious that this surrender by American doctors to political and social pressure had little effect on the availability of heroin on the streets but did remove it from suffering patients. Finally, Twycross (1978) organized a proper study of the supposed superiority of heroin over other narcotics. The method of test involves giving one drug and observing its effect and then substituting an equivalent dose of another drug in such a way that the patient and the person who gives the drug and records the effect do not know which drug is given. This is given the technical jargon name of a 'double-blind crossover study'; double-blind meaning that neither patient nor observer is told which drug is given, and crossover meaning that after one has been studied, the patient is then tested with the other one.

When the code was broken in the Twycross study, it was discovered to everyone's astonishment that neither the patients nor the observers could tell the difference between equivalent doses of heroin or morphine. In fact, a careful analysis of the data showed that in males (but not females), morphine was more effective than the equivalent dose of heroin: the men on heroin had more pain and were more depressed. (Twycross attributes the increased depression to the presence of greater levels of pain.) The St Christopher's team, which had been active in the defence of heroin, have consequently dropped the drug from general use, retaining it only for one special circumstance. Heroin is more powerful milligram for milligram than morphine by a ratio of .5 to 1, and it is also much more soluble. Therefore, if a patient reaches a stage where he needs very large amounts of narcotic by injection, he receives a much smaller, more concentrated dose of heroin solution which hurts less after injection than the much larger volume needed to inject the equivalent dose of morphine. After all the controversy and the anecdotes surrounding heroin, careful experimentation now allows us to state calmly and concretely the merits and demerits of heroin.

As a result of a series of excellent studies, the Brompton Mixture was recognized by the 'British Pharmaceutical Codex' in 1973 as a legitimate elixir for the treatment of severe pain. The standard mixture contains a variable amount of morphine ('titrated' to meet the patient's needs), 10mg of cocaine, 2.5ml of ethyl alcohol (ninety-eight per cent), 5 ml of flavouring syrup, and a variable amount of chloroform water, for a total of 20ml. As we shall soon see, morphine alone in water is as effective as the elaborate Brompton Mixture, and the much simpler morphine solution is now used increasingly because it is so easy for hospital pharmacies to prepare. These mixtures have the tendency to produce nausea, and are therefore given with drugs known as phenothiazines which enhance the analgesic properties of morphine *and* block the nausea. The mixture or solution is taken every four hours (or every three in some cases) and the dose of the narcotic is carefully adjusted ('titrated') over a period of days until a dose is found that not only takes the pain away but *keeps* it away; that is, each dose is taken *before* the pain returns. The pain, and the terror of its return, are gone. Yet the patient is lucid, able –

indeed, often eager – to talk, to see relatives and friends, to clear up financial problems and even to reassure the soon-to-be bereaved.

We have taken the example of St Christopher's investigation of the Brompton Mixture as an example of their attitude and revolutionary form of care. Each patient is an individual with unique psychological and physical needs and while the hospice workers have built up tremendous experience with these patients, there are no 'types'. Patients are not 'breast cancers' or 'lung cancers', they are individuals whose particular disease may or may not have certain characteristics in common with other individuals with that class of cancer. While the St Christopher's team are rightly proud of what they have done and are anxious to teach others, the fact that some of their patients still die in pain despite all the available therapies requires an intensification of their search and questioning. This hospice need not necessarily be duplicated in all details because each society has its own requirements, depending on the nature of the staff, the patients and the society itself.

One of the first attempts to translate their ideas to another setting began with the work of Dr Balfour Mount, at the Royal Victoria Hospital in Montreal, Canada, who set up a special ward within a large general hospital rather than build a separate hospice. We shall examine the work of Dr Mount in the next section. Another example of translating the St Christopher's concept into a totally different environment is being built up at St Thomas's Hospital in London where, instead of creating a special ward, a specialized team is available for patients who remain in whatever ward is best suited to their needs. Whatever may be the particular solution, the general idea of the new hospice movement and consideration of problems of the dying are now increasingly accepted.

While the idea of a hospice like St Christopher's is one of the great humanitarian advances of our century, it unfortunately represents an unachievable aim for all poor societies and even many rich ones. Given the fact that a society has only a certain amount of money for health and welfare, there is a genuine debate, even in the most enlightened societies, whether a substantial portion of public funds should go towards care of the healthy or of the dying. Should a large sum of money given to health care be directed toward acquiring, let us say, a machine for a new and better kind of X-ray for a general hospital, or should it go into the development of a hospice? This problem has been confronted and debated by decent, well-intentioned people, and has often ended in stalemate. Few countries are as daring as Britain, or have a Cicely Saunders to champion and pioneer a great cause in the face of established medical practice.

Palliative care service

Several people in Canada and the United States have found an answer to the dilemma. The best known and most influential of them – mentioned briefly before – is Balfour Mount of Montreal's Royal Victoria Hospital, a teaching hospital of McGill University. Dr Mount, trained as a urological surgeon, became interested early in his career in the circumstances of dying in western society and found the same dismal conditions that appalled Cicely Saunders.

During his search for a solution to care for the dying patient, he soon discovered St Christopher's Hospice and became one of its most ardent and compelling proponents. He encountered resistance from many of his colleagues, however, who felt that the limited funds of society are better directed at care of the healthy than of the dying. Mount felt otherwise, for many important reasons. Because it is not possible to cure cancer after it has progressed to a certain stage, the only concern must be to make the patient as comfortable as possible. It is important, then, to provide physicians with skills aimed specifically at palliation of symptoms such as pain, nausea, or constipation. This is why pain relief is so essential. It is absurd to talk about the 'quality of life' when a person is in agony or constantly vomiting.

There is another important reason for providing special care: in our western societies, a very large proportion (seventy per cent in Canada) of people die in hospitals or related institutions. As a result the patient is removed from familiar surroundings and encounters isolation and depersonalization. Mount was disturbed by the number of dying patients who lie in some isolated ward, away from the people they love and with whom they would like to spend their last days or hours. As death approaches, interactions between staff and patients become strained. As a result, physicians visit less often and nursing care decreases. For example, it takes longer for a nurse to answer the bell rung by a dying patient than by a patient who will recover. In the absence of special training, all members of health care teams are subject to the fears and anxieties that are part of our death-denying, cure-oriented society. Death is a fact that threatens us, and we tend to deny, avoid, or have as little contact with it as possible.

Because few societies can afford a hospice like St Christopher's, Dr Mount took the next logical step: to integrate a specialized Palliative Care Unit (PCU) within a large general hospital. The concept is simple: a ward of ten or twelve beds is set aside in the hospital and is devoted solely to the care of terminally ill patients who have severe pain and special problems. Like St Christopher's, the staff is an astonishingly devoted group. To spend all one's working time caring for dying patients is a difficult task, and the team requires frequent opportunities for group discussions and to obtain help when they confront their own psychological problems. Once the unit functions well, however, its services are magnificent. Terminally ill patients receive constant care and attention, with pain and other problems continually monitored and ministered to. Volunteers of all ages become friends with the patients – talk to them, comb their hair, hold their hands, weep and laugh with them. The team helps bring the family together and assuage the feelings of guilt that trouble exhausted spouses, children or parents who must leave to get some sleep or food. The staff guide the bereavement process of all members of the dying person's family. Clergy of all denominations are also present to provide religious comfort when (and only when) it is requested.

At the same time, the unit is attractively decorated, and patients' friends and family are always welcome. In contrast to the rigid visiting hours in most large hospitals, people can visit whenever they wish. Family members may stay overnight and, if the patient wishes it, may even share the bed in a private room. Children and pets are especially welcome. If a patient has a favourite dish, and the physician feels it can be digested without problem, then food may be brought in.

A marvellous feature of the PCU, which is described in detail by Ajemian and Mount (1980), is the fact that patients are able to go home when their condition stabilizes and for as long as is reasonable. The PCU, therefore, has been extended to form a Palliative Care Service beyond the confines of the hospital. The patients are given a bottle of the Brompton Mixture and instructions on how much to take and how often. A special home-care nurse visits often, or phones, and keeps close track of the patient. Any increase in pain or other change in the patient's condition results in a rapid return to the unit and the necessary attention to the problem. But while at home the patients are with people they love and in surroundings that are familiar and comforting. They are 'special' at home, and these days are precious.

The enormous success of the Palliative Care Unit and its auxil-iary services is evident from the manifest gratitude of the patients and those close to them, and from the fact that similar units have been (or are being) developed throughout the world. Two im-portant questions arise: is the PCU financially feasible, and is it really effective in allowing people to die with the dignity that is the right of every human being? The answers to both are un-equivocally affirmative.

A cost analysis of the PCU shows that society actually saves money by providing such a service. Unnecessary operations, X-rays, blood tests, and various treatments are not carried out. Feelings of guilt are understood and dealt with appropriately. The team effort means that services are provided efficiently. Time that the stabilized patient spends at home is time away from the hospital and therefore a saving of hospital funds. A well-run Palliative Care Service, then, is not only humanitarian but rep-resents the most efficient way for a humane society to treat people who are terminally ill.

A further saving is now permitted by the finding that a solution of morphine in water is as effective as the Brompton Mixture (Melzack, Mount and Gordon, 1979). A small amount of alcohol is added as an anti-bacterial and anti-fungal agent. The morphine solution, because it is simple, is much cheaper and saves the time of the busy hospital pharmacist. By eliminating all the un-necessary ingredients, it is now possible to add new substances on a rational basis. Thus, studies are now under way to see whether anti-depressant drugs augment the effects of the morphine solution, and thereby not only produce a better mood and outlook but also decrease pain still further. An important observation in all of these studies is that none of the patients has abused the availability of morphine. The patients, whether in the hospital or at home, took the prescribed dose of the drug on schedule, and some even asked to have the dose decreased when their pain diminished (Mount, Ajemian and Scott, 1976).

A special study was carried out to answer the second major question: whether the PCU environment plays a role in the control of pain. In particular, the purpose of the study was to determine the effects of different psychological environments on the analgesic properties of the Brompton Mixture. Patients in two standard hospital environments – the wards and private rooms – served as 'controls'. Patients in the Palliative Care Unit comprised the 'experimental group'. The results showed clearly that the patients in the PCU had significantly less pain than those in the wards and in private rooms. None of the patients in the PCU had pain at distressing/horrible/excruciating levels, but 10% of the private patients and 13% of the ward patients had pain at these levels. Since the dosages of morphine and other ingredients were comparable for the three groups, the significantly greater effectiveness of the Brompton Mixture in the PCU can only be due to the psychological impact of the unit itself. The presence of a highly concerned staff, and the help of volunteers who provide comfort and good cheer, as well as all the other amenities of the unit must undoubtedly have had a strong psychological effect on the pain (Melzack, Ofiesh and Mount, 1976).

However, the Brompton Mixture (or morphine solution) is not the answer to every cancer patient's pain – unfortunately. About 10% of the patients seen at the PCU in the above study had to be excluded immediately because the Brompton Mixture, even with high doses of morphine, did not control their pain: 1 had severe bladder spasms, 2 had sharp nerve-root pain that radiated into the legs, and 5 complained of severe pain, a major component of which was their despair and anguish at their impending death. These patients were treated with additional or other methods in the attempt to achieve physical and psychological comfort. The final results of the study showed that the Brompton Mixture was effective in controlling pain in 90% of patients in the PCU and 75 to 80% of patients in wards or private rooms. Clearly, the patients whose pain is uncontrolled represent a major challenge to clinical ingenuity. Other methods are necessary for those patients still in pain, and we have discussed a variety of pain-control methods in previous chapters.

This brings us to the final value of a hospice or palliative care service: when a team of experts from different disciplines pool their knowledge, the pain due to cancer can be controlled in the vast majority of patients. Using all the techniques available in a carefully planned way, St Christopher's Hospice was able to achieve effective control of pain in all but 7 patients out of 349 in a typical year. This is a remarkable achievement in which pharmacological, psychological, and other methods were used together to the great advantage of the suffering patient.

The nature of the clinical breakthrough

The development of pain clinics and hospices represent a breakthrough of the highest importance in the clinical control of pain. They are radical, new approaches to old problems. The gate-control theory of pain has provided, in large part, the conceptual background – the foundation – for new approaches to pain. The theory argues that pain does not have a single cause and is not even a single entity. There are multiple, interacting physiological and psychological mechanisms, and a rational approach to pain control requires multiple approaches that converge to produce a reduction in pain. Within this framework, the multi-disciplinary approach that is the hallmark of the pain clinic and the hospice takes on special significance. But still more, the pain clinic and the hospice represent an understanding that chronic pain and terminal pain each require a whole new set of challenges and skills. Acute pain, which is the basis of the traditional training of physicians, is wonderfully controlled by our modern-day drugs. Chronic pain, however, requires a new set of rules, and we are still novices in these new approaches to pain. Chronic pain and terminal pain are major challenges to the scientist and clinician. But the giant step has been the recognition that they are special problems. The challenges before us are clear: to conquer pain and suffering in all their forms.

17
The Future of Pain Control

So far, we have described many of the exciting recent advances in pain research and therapy. Yet despite all the recently acquired knowledge of pain mechanisms and the successes of new therapies, pain still presents an enormous challenge to the scientists who try to understand it, to the therapists who try to treat it, to the patients who try to cope with it, and to society at large which must provide the encouragement and financial resources for research and treatment to put an end to suffering.

Although we have tried to cover the field as broadly as possible, some aspects of it have not yet been discussed. For example, new pain syndromes are still being discovered. In 1971, Spillane, Nathan, Kelly and Marsden described the syndrome of 'painful legs and moving toes', in which patients suffer terrible pain in the leg and foot, and show spontaneous movements of the toes that are beyond their voluntary control. The syndrome appears to be due to nerve-root lesions that generate nerve impulses that spread in the spinal cord and produce the continual motor outflow that evokes the incessant movements (Nathan, 1978). The most baffling syndromes, however, are the most common ones which plague tens of millions of people: low back pain and headache. We will discuss the special problem of low back pain later in this chapter because it provides a measure of how far we are from understanding pain. The 'low back pain syndrome' is, in fact, not a syndrome but a complex set of symptoms common to many syndromes that still need to be unravelled (Grahame, 1980).

There are also many kinds of headaches, although two types are most common: tension headache and migraine (Dalessio, 1980; Hunter and Philips, 1981). An analysis of migraine headaches provides us with an idea of the complexity of the mechanisms involved (Dalessio, 1974). As a result of stress or some other triggering event, a branch of a major artery to the brain undergoes sudden constriction. Consequently, less blood flows to the brain and a sequence of events occurs which is similar to an inflammation reaction. The initial constriction leads to increased metabolic demands by brain cells which elicit a dilation of the blood vessels in the brain and even of the cranial arteries outside the skull. These arterial changes provoke the release of histamine, prostaglandins, serotonin, adrenalin, noradrenalin, and brady-kinen in addition to a variety of other substances. The release of these substances and the dilation of blood vessels produce oedema, a lowering of pain threshold, and the eventual pounding headache. Since the initial arterial constriction which started the entire sequence may have occurred on one side, it is possible that all of the above events may result in a headache on only one side of the head.

It is clear from this analysis, which is greatly simplified (see Dalessio, 1974, 1980), that the approach to migraine control is necessarily complex. The initial stressor or other causal event may be treated in many ways, including psychological approaches (Adams, Feuerstein and Fowler, 1980). Control of blood-vessel diameter may also be attempted by use of specific drugs such as ergotamine. If this fails, propranalol or other blockers may be tried. The release of prostaglandins also means that aspirin and other anti-inflammatory agents may be used. When all these treatments fail – as they do in some unfortunate patients –then we are confronted with a greater challenge than ever. Consequently, an active search is in progress for antagonists for the many chemical substances that are released during the inflammatory process as well as for psychological methods to decrease stress.

Our purpose in this chapter is not to make predictions on where the breakthroughs in pain control will occur. Part of the excitement of science lies in the fact that they usually occur unexpectedly, and often as a result of a chance observation. We, like our colleagues, receive enormous pleasure as we watch scientific progress taking place – sometimes gradually, sometimes with breathtaking speed. However, we are aware of problems and challenges that will inevitably be part of the story of pain research and therapy in the future.

The pattern of new discoveries

A major challenge in future research is to develop a proper perspective toward new therapeutic discoveries. The discovery of some new drug or technological advance in treatment is generally announced with great fanfare. Yet, as we have seen, only two major classes of analgesic drugs have so far been shown beyond doubt to be effective: salicylates and opiates. Great claims are made for one brand name of a drug over another, but basically they all fit into the same two classes. New kinds of drugs have been discovered – such as zomepirac sodium and nefopam-hydrochloride – but they have yet to stand the test of time. We also know now that some non-steroid, anti-inflammatory drugs, which inhibit prostaglandin synthesis, are powerful analgesics for some kinds of pain. But these too need a great deal of clinical research before their place is established firmly in the pharmacopoeia of analgesics.

Scientists have long been aware that the 'coming out' of new

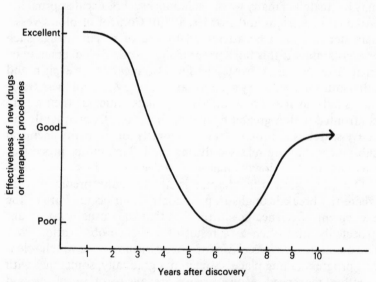

Figure 42. Diagram of the pattern of effectiveness after discovery of most new drugs or therapeutic procedures to control pain. Excellent results obtained in the first few years give way to poor results, followed by a period in which the drug or procedure is found to be another 'good' form of therapy for pain.

therapeutic agents and techniques follows a characteristic sequence (Figure 42). In the first few years, the research data are exciting and the new discovery assumes Nobel-prize-winning proportions. Then there is a period of scepticism in which the drugs sometimes appear to be even less effective than the old ones. Finally, the research usually shows that a good – not great, but good – new analgesic drug or treatment has been found that can respectably take its place along with the others. In the course of all of this, it is evident that progress has been made, but not a major breakthrough. We must always keep this sequence in mind; there are no panaceas – not yet anyway. Even the endorphins and enkephalins, which were believed after their discovery to be the key to the whole puzzle of pain and the guideposts to the perfect analgesics, are now seen in perspective. They are, without a doubt, scientifically important steps to understanding pain and analgesia. A host of new opioid and other pain-related substances were discovered in an incredibly short time. But their roles in pain and analgesia are poorly understood and their practical implications for pain therapy are uncertain.

Multiple convergent therapies

The gate-control theory has provided a conceptual framework for the multiple contributions to pain. In contrast to specificity theory which proposes that pain intensity is proportional to the severity of injury, the gate theory holds instead that pain intensity is determined by multiple factors, including descending controls from the brain, converging visceral inputs, and so forth. These multiple contributions are summarized in Figure 43. (Melzack and Loeser, 1978).

The concept of multiple influences on the transmission (T) cells in the central nervous system has important therapeutic implications. Therapy at present is often predicated on a one-cause–one-effect relationship. In contrast, Figure 43 indicates that multiple interactions determine the nature of the pattern which is generated by the T cells. Attempts can therefore be made to change the pattern by *simultaneous* use of several procedures. Thus, it is plausible to provide patients with an anti-depressant drug, electrical stimulation at trigger points *and* relaxation procedures all at the same time. Therapeutic procedures in combination are often more effective than the mere additive effects of each presented by itself (Melzack, Weisz and Sprague, 1963; Melzack and Perry, 1975). This kind of approach is reasonable in

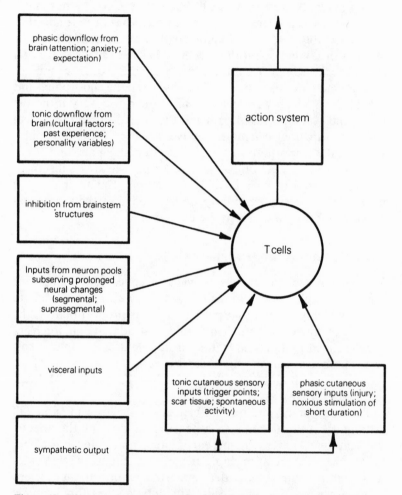

Figure 43. Diagram of the concept of multiple influences on the transmission (T) cells in the central nervous system. The concept suggests that attempts can be made to change the pattern of output of the T cells by simultaneous use of several therapeutic procedures.

terms of multiple interacting influences on the neural mechanisms that produce chronic pain, and is being used increasingly in the treatment of pain. The difficulties encountered in treating chronic low back pain, for example, underscore the need for multiple convergent approaches in its treatment.

Low back pain

Low back pain is one of the most common types of pain, yet is poorly understood. It illustrates the complexity of interactions among different contributing factors and the need for multiple approaches in treatment.

The only definite causes of low back pain are herniation of discs and arthritis of vertebral joints. However, these conditions are not always found in patients with low back pain. As many as 60–78% of patients who suffer low back pain have no apparent physical signs. That is, despite X-rays and thorough orthopaedic examination, there is no evidence of disc disease, arthritis, or any other symptoms that can be considered the cause of the pain (Loeser, 1980).

Even when there are clearcut physical and neurological signs of disc herniation (in which the disc pushes out of its space and presses against nerve roots), complete relief of back pain and related sciatic pain by surgery occurs in only about 60% of cases. The rate of success in different reports ranges from 50% to 95%. Removal of a disc is most likely to be effective in patients with clear evidence of nerve-root compression. However, in all cases, the evidence points to the great value of rest. In fact, over half of the patients who suffer an episode of low back pain become symptom-free in a month or so without any health care intervention other than prolonged rest (Loeser, 1980).

There have been many promising therapies which have later turned out to be less exciting than the original expectation. The injection of papain, an enzyme, to dissolve the disc seemed at first to be a major advance but now turns out, in experimental studies, to be no more effective than an injection of an inert liquid (Schwetschenau *et al.*, 1976). Fusion of several vertebrae makes intuitive sense as a way to provide structural support to unstable vertebrae in people who suffer low back pain with evidence of a herniated lumbar disc, but the results fail to show that fusion is beneficial. In fact it may be deleterious. Loeser (1980) and Sweet (1980) urge strongly against continuation of the procedure in cases of disc protrusion.

In short, even when physical causes are clearly present, low back pain remains a problem after surgery for a substantial number of patients. And we are still confronted with the high proportion of people who have no obvious physical signs and still suffer agony.

Low back pain usually has a particularly unpleasant quality. It is deep, aching and burning and sometimes immobilizes the patient who is terrified of moving and triggering a severe bout of pain. Often the pains radiate down the leg and are called sciatic pain because they follow the innervation pattern of the sciatic nerve. For patients with minor physical signs such as curvature of the spine, or 'normal' disc disease that occurs with aging, surgery is rarely effective. Such patients, then, in the desperate search for relief of their pain, sometimes prevail on surgeons to carry out successive operations. After orthopaedic operations fail, these patients may undergo section of sensory roots (rhizotomy), of the spinal cord (cordotomy) and other operations; few of them help.

A variety of forms of physical therapy may help low back pain. The most effective is a regimen of special exercises that develop the back muscles. Transcutaneous electrical stimulation, ice massage, and acupuncture may all help some patients. Injections of trigger points may be effective as well. Recently, it has been shown (Brena *et al.*, 1980) that injection of a long-lasting anaesthetic (bupivacaine) into the sympathetic ganglia relieves pain in a substantial number of people. But so does injection of saline, indicating that the mere hyperstimulation of the ganglia can bring about changes in the nervous system.

It is possible that the major culprit in many cases of low back pain is abnormal activity in nerve-root fibres due to minor changes in the surrounding vertebrae and tissues. The roots may be affected by compression caused by degenerated disc material (which commonly occurs during normal aging), interference with the blood supply, stress on ligaments and joints that surround the nerve, and so forth. These 'minor' irritations may be cumulative and eventually produce symptoms of 'low back sprain' (Gunn and Milbrandt, 1978). This can be the beginning of a 'vicious circle', because later pain would enhance the autonomic effects, produce spasm, pain, and progressive deterioration of a situation that began 'harmlessly' with normal aging processes (or possibly due to relatively minor physical trauma in younger people). Whatever the reason, the ensuing mechanisms are complex.

The actual neural mechanisms that are involved in back pain, even when disc herniation has occurred, are not clear. Evidently, either an increase or a decrease in input may be the basis of pain. Howe, Loeser, and Calvin (1977) found that chronically scarred axons tend to fire repetitively after mechanical compression and thereby produce an abnormal, high-frequency input through the dorsal roots, which could be the basis of low back pain and sciatica. On the other hand, prolonged compression of a nerve root may have the opposite effect – it may produce a marked decrease (rather than the expected increase) in firing in the root fibres (Wall, Waxman and Basbaum, 1974). The decrease could, of course, remove inhibitory influences and produce hyperactive spinal cells, which would tend to 'open the gate' and produce more pain.

As a result of the persistence of low back pain despite ortho-paedic surgery, neurosurgery and countless drugs – most fail to work and some, such as tranquillizers, increase depression – it is not surprising that psychological therapy has become an important new approach to the problem. Indeed, anti-depressants (such as the tricyclic drugs) are sometimes remarkably effective in relieving the pain as well as the patient's depression. The various kinds of therapy that are effective are behaviour modification, progressive relaxation, hypnosis in its various modes of use, biofeedback to help learn to relax muscles, and so forth. All of these, it has been shown, help *some* patients. But no one of them is more effective than the others. In fact, clinics that employ several procedures at the same time get the best results. One group (Swanson *et al.*, 1976) found that patients with several syndromes, but mostly low back pain, were helped by a combination of techniques; about 80% of patients received marked to moderate improvement after treatment, and 50% claimed they were still improved 3 to 6 months later. Interestingly, most patients reported that the pain was unchanged but they were able to work, to live with their pain, and lead more normal lives. Another study, specifically on chronic low back pain (Gottlieb *et al.*, 1977), also used a battery of techniques and found that about 60% of patients were able to resume a normal life style. The therapy in this study, it should be noted, required an average hospitalization period of 45 days. At 6 months after the programme, about 80% of the successful patients contacted still reported that they were living a normal life style.

The multiplicity of causes and treatments

The evidence on low back pain permits two important conclusions: (1) low back pain is not a single syndrome produced by a single causal agent; and (2) the most effective approach to pain relief and return to a normal life style is to use multiple convergent procedures.

It has been seen that disc disease and vertebral arthritis play a role in only a relatively small proportion of patients. However, other physical factors may play a role. Many patients with low back pain have tense muscles and many have clearcut trigger points which evoke severe pain when they are mechanically activated. Furthermore, many patients become depressed by their disability, lose their self-esteem, become obsessed with their health and are anxious. Finally, it has become clear that in a proportion of patients, low back pain is referred as a result of disease in another part of the body, especially in the pelvis (Loeser, 1980). Pain may be referred to the lower back as a result of a variety of visceral diseases that have gone undetected. Jones (1938), in a remarkable study, showed that inflating a balloon at various levels of the digestive system sometimes produces pain felt in the back. In other people, the pain is felt at the site of a scar of an earlier operation. Surgery of the back, then, can leave a scar that may potentially become the site of referred pain.

Therapists must look for trigger points, evidence of excessive sympathetic and muscle activity, and other physical contributions which can be helped by any one of the variety of sensory-modulation procedures. In addition, psychological assessment is essential to determine the psychological contributions – tension, anxiety, fear, and especially depression. The psychological methods described above can all potentially help to some degree. Finally, the patient, who has been terrorized by the pain and sometimes victimized unintentionally by health care professionals who do not understand the complexity of the problem, must be guided back to a normal life style. Behaviour modification methods, particularly those that recognize the patients' capacity to understand the problem and their need for satisfactory coping strategies, appear to be useful. The studies which report impressive relief of low back pain (Swanson *et al.*, 1976; Gottlieb *et al.*, 1977) have utilized virtually all of the above procedures at the same time.

The puzzle of pain, as we have seen, is far from solved. Increased research on pain is clearly needed. The number of scientists who work on the problem is small in comparison with the magnitude of its importance. We have a remarkable capacity to forget pains that we have suffered in the past, and it is often difficult to comprehend the suffering of another person. Research time and money are devoted to many problems of obvious clinical significance, but pain, often considered the symptom and not the disease, receives far less attention. Yet, there are few problems more worthy of human endeavour than the relief of pain and suffering.

But even when we acknowledge the priority of the problem and provide the funds for research, new problems arise that are the concern of all humane people – the ethics of research on pain.

The ethics of research with humans and animals

In recent years, there has been a rising tide of disquiet about the use of animals or people in experiments. This problem is especially serious for scientists involved in research on pain.

Experiments on healthy human subjects
Let us first consider the question of experiments on people, since most societies and individuals have debated this issue thoroughly and have reached fairly definite conclusions. The horrible experiments carried out on innocent people (who were considered

'inferior') by German physicians in the World War II are well known. This intentional destruction of some human beings for the presumed benefit of others produced a worldwide revulsion, which led doctors all over the world to examine not only the so-called experiments in concentration camps but also their own actions. In particular, it led to the Helsinki Convention of the World Health Organization, which stressed that experiments could take place only with the genuine voluntary, informed agreement of the subjects. It was felt that prisoners could never be considered free to volunteer because of the danger of implied prolongation of the prison term if they did not volunteer. Even students were felt not to be genuinely free to volunteer for their own professor's experiments because of the considerable, if hidden, power the professor has over students. This type of consideration has led to a very general practice, often required by law, for the examination of all experiments on people by ethics committees. These groups consider the social need and likely benefit of the work, the potential dangers, the skill of the experimenters and above all, the freedom of the subject to give his consent when he is in possession of all the facts.

Experiments on human patients

Patients place themselves in the hands of the doctor and, in some way, take part in an unwritten contract that they will submit to the doctor's orders believing that these are for their benefit. Temporarily, each patient voluntarily gives up some of his natural freedoms. The classical response of doctors to this situation is that absolutely nothing may be done to the patient which is not specifically directed to that patient's benefit. Some doctors adhere to this principle without any deviation, but we must see where such strictness leads. Suppose that the examination of a small blood sample from a particular patient may help doctors understand the course and nature of a disease. Taking the blood has no conceivable benefit to the particular patient and would therefore be forbidden by the old rules but it might help future patients with that disease. Here it may be reasonable to consider the patient as a 'normal' human subject, and to propose the test to the hospital's ethics committee and ask the patient's consent. But, is the patient free? He might reasonably say to the doctor, 'I am suffering enough. No more needles, thank you.' Or he might also reasonably say to himself, 'I am dependent on this doctor's good will and interest and if he wants a guinea pig, I had better agree.' Even if the doctor has a sufficiently good rapport with the patient to overcome this questioning by him, the consent must be informed consent in which the patient understands what the problems might be. How honest will the doctor be? Will he think it relevant to mention that one in a thousand punctures of a vein to take blood results in a fairly painful bruise and one in a million produces infection? Probably not, the excuse being that such facts would unnecessarily disturb the patient and, needless to say, decrease the number of volunteers. More seriously, some patients may have such limited knowledge about their bodies or be of such low intelligence that it is difficult and time consuming to teach them the facts they would need to understand before they could consent. Obviously, there are considerable dangers hidden under this innocent phrase of 'informed consent' but there are also considerable opportunities for the experimenter to develop a closer relationship with his subjects.

Experiments on patients in pain
It is obvious that if a new drug or procedure has passed all reasonable tests on animals as an effective anti-pain method, it must eventually be tried out on people. In the case of a new drug, the effective dose must be established since there is a variable conversion factor between man and animals depending on the type of drug. Narcotics, for example, are about ten times less effective on rats, mice, cats and dogs than they are on man. On the other hand, aspirin-like compounds are quite similar in their bodyweight/dose relationship in humans and animals. More important, anti-pain procedures which seem excellent in animals may be quite unacceptable in man, especially because of subtle side effects on ways of thinking and feeling which are not apparent in animals. For example, the powerful psychotrophic drug d-lysergic acid (LSD) has been given to cancer patients and many appeared pain-free and comfortable during the prolonged action of the drug but, on being offered a second dose, almost all patients refused to repeat the experience because they disliked the disturbing psychological effects. Similarly, certain types of surgery,

especially of the brain, may produce such unpleasant long-term reactions that the patients eventually feel worse.

Perhaps, the most serious problem in testing a new procedure on patients is the existence of the placebo response discussed earlier (p.41). The ethical problem is that the test may involve deliberately giving the patient a placebo injection or tablet which the tester believes will not affect the pain. In these studies, the worst that may happen is that the patient may be in pain for a period of three to four hours until the next regular drug dose is due. Furthermore, if the pain becomes intolerable, the test can be abandoned and a known effective medicine can be given. All this may not seem very serious and most patients agree to take the risk, for the benefit of mankind, of suffering discomfort or pain to discover if a new drug is superior to an old one or to a placebo. The patient and the experimenters are usually even more willing to try a new procedure if there is no known adequate control for the kind of pain under investigation.

However, the situation becomes much more serious in the case of procedures such as surgery. Finneson, in *Diagnosis and Management of Pain Symptoms,* writes:

Probably surgery has the most potent placebo effect that can be exercised in medicine. The detailed preliminaries, the rendering unconscious via anaesthesia, and the removal or manipulation of vital organs within the body all create an almost mystic and profound emotional effect on the patient. This effect of course varies greatly from patient to patient, but in evaluating the results of any large series of surgical procedures this placebo effect must certainly be considered. A well-known physician, an outstanding pioneer in the field of neurosurgery, when faced with a problem case of low back pain that he believed to be non-organic in etiology occasionally resorted to having the patient prepared and anaesthetized for laminectomy (surgery of the spine) and merely made the skin incision which he then promptly sutured. Although several cases were reportedly 'cured' by this method, I would guess that the long-term results were not uniformly happy (Finneson, 1969, p.30).

After this remarkable statement, Finneson goes on to describe many of the procedures used by neurosurgeons without once again referring to the powerful placebo effects of surgery.

In animal experiments, it is a commonly accepted practice to match an operation which has an intended effect with a mock or 'sham' operation in which an animal is anaesthetized, part of the brain is exposed, but the ultimate lesion is not made. It is inconceivable that such a procedure should be carried out on people. Yet such operations have been done by accident. A woman with severe low back pain radiating into one leg was diagnosed as having a herniated intervertebral disc and was being operated on. As the surgeon was approaching the region of the disc, the patient developed cardiovascular problems and it was decided to terminate the operation, quickly sew her up and to start the necessary resuscitation procedures. When the patient recovered consciousness, she no longer complained of her pain and this relief persisted for at least one year.

Other examples relate to trigeminal neuralgia, which occurs on one side and which may be treated by surgically cutting the sensory nerve supply to that side of the face. In White and Sweet's (1969) classic textbook, *Pain and the Neurosurgeon*, two cases are reported where surgeons by mistake operated on the wrong side. Both patients' pains disappeared while the other side of their face was numb. Finally, there is a recent report of a double-blind trial in neurosurgery (Schwetschenau *et al.*, 1976). It was proposed that instead of surgically removing herniated discs, it might be possible to achieve the same end by injecting the proteolytic (protein-destroying) enzyme, papain, into the disc to dissolve it. It was apparently used successfully on dogs who, like people, also suffer from disc herniations. Then, in a world-famous military hospital, patients with verified disc protrusions had their intervertebral spaces injected either with the enzyme or with the same volume of an inert solution without the enzyme. There was no difference in the recovery rate of the two groups of patients. This was taken as evidence that the enzyme was ineffective. But what was a surprise was the very high percentage of the 'control' cases who recovered. It is not our intention here to suggest that most surgery has only a placebo effect or that the effects may be due to hyperstimulation of tissues by needle injection, but to point to the practical and ethical problems which make it progressively more difficult – or even impossible – to carry out a definitive trial of the effectiveness of complex procedures.

Differences between real and experimental pain

There are major differences between the type of pain which a patient complains of and the type of pain induced in healthy volunteer subjects. Henry K. Beecher wrote a magnificent book on *Measurement of Subjective Responses* in 1959 in which he showed that drugs such as the narcotics, which clearly help patients in pain, have no effect at all on the pain thresholds measured by many different types of experimental tests. These tests include the use of electric shocks, rapid heating with a hot lamp or rapid cooling with ice water. Since that time, Beecher himself discovered a test in which narcotics produced a raised threshold in normal subjects. A blood-pressure cuff is placed around the upper arm and is pumped up until no blood flows through the lower arm and hand. The subject then opens and closes his hand at a fixed rate. Slowly, over a period of minutes, a very unpleasant cramp-like pain develops in the arm and grows in intensity. This pain can be interrupted in seconds by releasing the blood-pressure cuff and allowing the blood to circulate again. The time taken for the pain to become intolerable is prolonged by giving the normal subject a narcotic. Other tests, one using cool rather than ice-cold water, have now also been shown to respond to narcotics in normal subjects. The difference between these new tests which are affected by narcotics and the old ones which are not is that the new tests may generate a steady barrage of nerve impulses, which more closely imitate the situation in disease, rather than the brief volley generated by the momentary stimuli used in the old tests. We have already seen (Chapter 11) that both kinds of tests demonstrate strikingly different effects in rats by the use of narcotics and other drugs. For this reason, many new drugs are tested on patients after a definable injury such as a tooth extraction or some other surgical operation, or who are suffering some continuous painful condition such as arthritis.

We have seen that the most useful pain tests, in normal subjects, for studying the effectiveness of narcotics are those which most closely imitate the condition of a real patient with real pain. However, there are some terrible types of clinical pain which do not have an experimental analogue in normal people. These include the dysaesthesias in which patients have peculiarly unpleasant, unusual sensations following nerve injury. Another example is the horrible, continuous pain which occurs when nerve cells in the brain or spinal cord lose their input. These dreadful pains are quite unlike any which a normal person will volunteer to receive.

A final reason why we must turn to patients already in pain rather than using healthy people without pain is that there is evidence that prolonged pain, which no normal person would volunteer to accept, produces terrible psychological effects (Sternbach, 1974). This state, with its depression, lethargy and obsession, is a specially urgent challenge, and the only way we can examine this unique situation is to study the patients themselves. Therefore, it appears that 'the proper study of man in pain is on man in pain'.

Experiments on animals

Just as most societies have decided that war is a legal, acceptable way to sacrifice people for the benefit of society, most societies have also formalized the sacrifice of animals. Most of this killing is for food but growing numbers of animals are killed for knowledge, especially for medical health purposes. For millennia, there have been groups who opposed this decision. The Brahmins of India, who respect all forms of animal life, are strict vegetarians and walk carefully to avoid stepping on insects. Some of the modern groups who support extensions of these basic feelings are highly consistent, not only as vegetarians but by refusing to wear leather or to keep household pets since this itself represents an imprisonment of free creatures. These serious considerations by ecological movements, such as Greenpeace, question man's disturbance of nature and his tendency to domesticate, trap, cage, or kill living creatures. These organized groups of highly considerate people are not to be dismissed or confused with the older, often sentimental anti-vivisectionist movements directed at saving cats and dogs yet supported predominantly by rich women wearing fur coats and carrying crocodile-skin handbags, and caring nothing for wild animals or for rats, mice or frogs. It is also evident that some aspects of the new anti-vivisectionist movement are fuelled by a general anti-intellectual wave in which science is a particular target.

There are serious people in these movements and it important is for all of us to consider and react to their arguments. Miss A. Walder, a full-time campaigner against animal experiments, has written the following:

There is little doubt that attempts to raise the standard of humanity observed in animal experimentation continue to be frustrated by the stark opposition which characterizes the viewpoints of 'anti-vivisectionists' on the one hand and 'interested' experimenters on the other ... It must surely be a matter of universal regret that such polarization of views may help to sustain a large amount of pain and distress which could be reduced. And if critics of animal experimentation are sometimes guilty of ignorance, this is maintained by the secrecy and silence which commonly screens animal experimentation ... It will go some way to improving the social image of science if scientists can provide cogent evidence of *their* humane concern and motivation by showing that they abjure the infliction of pain or distress on animals and that this is *their* ethic. The present polarization into pro- and anti-vivisection will only be resolved by the fostering of constructive dialogue and joint *action* between scientists involved in animal experimentation and those who seek to improve the welfare of animals in our society (Walder, 1980, p.1).

If we start with the majority opinion that animals may be raised and killed for man's benefit partly as food and partly as a source of knowledge to help mankind in sickness, we must still consider the permissible range within which we can operate without brutalizing ourselves with our own cruelty. First, we can start with the attitude of the sensitive farmer or pet owner who wants the animal in his care to be healthy, to grow, to have a proper animal social life and, when the time comes, to die swiftly and painlessly. Governments often legislate about these matters but they need to be continually vigilant. The problem for the scientist and his society arises when he begins to manipulate the animal. First, we need a clear concept of what constitutes pain and suffering in an animal. This is easy when an injured animal is howling or thrashing about, and clearly such episodes should be avoided or brought to a rapid end. However, animals (like people) may not show such obvious signs, and we must be especially sensitive to subtle cues of pain and suffering.

The crucial question, however, is whether we *ever* have the right to inflict suffering on an animal. Everyone must reach his own decision on this. Clearly, there are two conflicting questions. How great is our need as humans for the answer to the question, provided at the expense of an animal's suffering? How great is the animal's suffering which is needed to provide the answer? Let us take the specific example of the pain of arthritis which cripples millions of us. We do not know its origin or how to cure it. We can experimentally produce an acute arthritis in rats which appears to have many features of a type of arthritis commonly seen in people. For about two months, these animals show definite signs of pain. They develop swollen joints, their movement is restricted, they squeal when a joint is pressed gently, and they often keep their paws lifted in the air, favouring them as any animal or human does when a hand or arm has been hurt. The animals are in pain, but the pain is evidently bearable because the rats continue to eat normally, do not lose weight, and maintain their normal cleanliness. (Those rats that develop severe reactions can be killed quickly and humanely.) Given these facts, should scientists continue or discontinue such experiments on arthritis, with the hope of finding a treatment or cure and thereby alleviating the pain? The experiments are not designed merely to imitate a human disease in animals but to understand the disease and to test procedures to abolish the pain without further damage to the joint.

Each person must examine each experiment and decide if the gains of knowledge and the loss of dignity which comes from inflicting suffering justify the work. Regarding the experiment on arthritic pain just described, each reader must reach his own decision. There are no rigid rules, nor should there be. Each person must make the decision within the framework of his own moral system and his personal priorities. What is urgently needed is more dialogue between understanding people who are ready to see each other's point of view, debate the questions that are raised, and reach what seems to be the most reasonable conclusion under the circumstances at the time. At stake in this debate is the discovery of ways to relieve the terrible pain and suffering – due to cancer, arthritis, strokes, and a multitude of other causes – that continue to plague a large proportion of mankind.

The future: a summary of the challenge of pain

While we always hope for unexpected discoveries, there are certain areas to which we can look for advances. A summary of these key areas in the prediction, prevention and treatment of pain also summarizes this book.

Prediction

It is usually difficult, if not impossible, to predict that chronic pain will result from a particular injury or disease. However, it may be possible to predict the occurrence of low back pain in some patients. Because low back pain is so prevalent, it is clearly desirable to seek ways of predicting who is susceptible to such pain. The difficulty of prediction is fully recognized by physicians who see patients with severe back pain but have little or no apparent physical abnormality, as well as patients with major physical abnormalities of the spine yet who have no pain. Obviously, the many other factors we discussed earlier influence the effect of the input on central cells. Personality and the patient's general level of stress and tension play a major role. Gunn and Milbrandt (1978) observed subtle indices of abnormal sympathetic activity in the painful areas of patients with 'low back sprain' but also found them in some of their control patients who had no pain at all. Thermographic studies (Karpman *et al.*, 1970) which found hot areas that corresponded to the painful region in patients with back pain also found such areas in control patients with no pain. Do these signs of abnormal sympathetic activity mean that these 'control' patients will have pain at a later time, perhaps triggered by a minor physical or psychological trauma? Studies to answer this question are feasible but expensive. However, if it is indeed possible to predict that certain people will develop back pain, it may also be possible to prevent it. The enormous cost of low back pain to the patient and to society (in terms of days away from work and health care services) warrant such studies.

Related to the prediction of susceptibility to back pain is the prediction of the efficacy of treatment for particular patients. We have seen that it is now possible to distinguish between patients with organic symptoms and those without them on the basis of the McGill Pain Questionnaire (Leavitt and Garron, 1979). It is conceivable, then, that the constellation of words chosen by patients may, together with information obtained with personality questionnaires, suggest the most effective type of treatment for a particular patient and the probability of a successful outcome. These attempts at prediction are just beginning, but hold great promise for the ultimate prevention and treatment of pain.

Prevention
Ideas for the prevention of pain range widely in feasibility. The number of people who suffer chronic pain as a result of injury in car accidents could clearly be decreased by the better design of cars as well as by laws that lower the maximum speed. In the United States, the lowering of the maximum speed from 70 to 55 miles per hour resulted in about 10,000 fewer deaths each year and, accordingly, many fewer injuries of the head, neck, back and peripheral nerves and their associated chronic, crippling pains. Similarly, many working situations which inflict repeated small injuries are ignored while others have achieved a good safety record. The gnarled, scarred arthritic hands of the deep-sea fisherman on a trawler hasten the end of his active life at sea. They are unnecessarily accepted as a fact of life. In many cases of low back pain, small tears of muscle and ligaments during excessive contraction are suspected as a common cause. If true, then it is reasonable to expect that a combination of physical exercise and improved work habits could reduce this nearly universal condition with its pain and economic loss.

War is yet another cause of frightful suffering. New weapons produce horrible injuries and, at the same time, improved medical procedures have raised the survival rate. All politicians should, on a regular basis, visit veterans' hospitals to see the gruesome nature of the injuries and the effect of the chronic suffering on those men. Perhaps such a procedure might contribute to the abolition of war and the inevitable pain and suffering it inflicts on countless people.

At a more feasible level, there are many ways to decrease the probability of suffering. Surgical incisions, tooth extractions, even episiotomies are necessary, but a proportion of them produce prolonged pain and discomfort, particularly when nerves are injured. With study and modification of technique, many of these pains could be avoided. The more extensive the surgery the more likely the chronic pain, and yet these 'side effects' are often neglected while patient and doctor concentrate on the original reason for the operation. Ignorance may turn out to be the ultimate incurable disease in doctors and patients, but ignorance *is* curable by cooperation and education. We have discussed the pressures which desperate patients can exert on doctors to overtreat with drugs and repeated surgery. Hopefully, pain clinics will play a role in preventing iatrogenic pain – the pain caused accidentally or through ignorance by medical treatment.

Obviously we must continue to make every effort must continue to cure the fundamental origin of disease but, at the same time, we need to look at the possibility of pain prevention before it occurs. Painful diseases follow damage to nerves by injury, by surgeons, by infection and by poisons. We have discussed injury by accidents, war and surgery, but virus infection remains a problem. Shingles (herpes zoster) is followed in a proportion of cases by post-herpetic neuralgia – a prolonged, continuous pain of such intensity that it ruins the lives of some older people. The disease is normally a short but painful virus infection of peripheral nerves but it is rational to treat the disease with great vigour because of the danger of prolonged pain. A new, clever treatment destroys the ability of the virus to duplicate by changing one of its components, uridine, which is part of the virus's DNA molecule. It is claimed that this speeds up recovery and reduces the frequency of post-herpetic neuralgia. Another treatment, which consists simply of an injection of local anaesthetic around the affected nerve, produces more rapid healing of the diseased tissues and the prevention of post-herpetic pain (Colding, 1969. This treatment may work because it shortens the period of continuous bombardment of the nervous system during the acute phase or, more intriguingly, because it blocks the transport of chemical substances along nerves, which is another effect of local anaesthetics. Two common medical conditions – alcoholism and diabetes – are sometimes associated with severe pain due to the destruction of nerves. We need to understand what it is about alcohol and diabetes that destroys nerves in order to prevent that destruction. We have also noted that pain related to cancer is usually prevented from reaching intolerable levels by the intelligent administration of morphine. Unfortunately, the pain remains out of control in a small proportion of patients. The most common cause of these intractable pains is the erosion of nerves and roots by cancer, and the prevention of this erosion needs early diagnosis and special control. The future, we hope, will bring an increasing recognition of all of these problems as well as steps that will lead to their solution.

Because low back pain is the most common of all pains, it merits special consideration. Exercise is by far the best way to prevent low back pain. It should be carried out by people who have periodic episodes of pain as well as by people without pain because we know that a high proportion of people are certain to develop this crippling pain problem. Ways to teach people to practise preventive procedures is one of the major problems that confronts the health professions in the future.

Treatment

Enormous advances have been made in the treatment of pain during the past decade, partly because of our increased knowledge about pain mechanisms and partly because new theoretical concepts have opened up a field that lay conceptually stagnant for centuries. The field has come alive – full of new controversy and renewed fascination. New questions are constantly being raised that are sure to challenge the young investigator and lead to new understanding and new treatments.

Pharmacological control. The field with the greatest potential is neurochemistry and pharmacology, which touches on every aspect of pain. Damaged tissue releases chemicals which directly and indirectly excite nerve fibres. Some of these chemicals are known or suspected but in some situations, such as ischaemic muscle or heart tissue, we know nothing and yet we could. The huge array of aspirin-like compounds and the steroids prevent the release of some of the chemicals and therefore stop pain. To identify the pain-producing chemicals and to develop antagonists will produce new forms of analgesics that act on the source.

We observed earlier that when a nerve fibre is transected, it emits sprouts which have new properties not shared by the normal parent fibre. The sprout membrane generates nerve impulses in a novel way – spontaneously, during gentle pressure, and when normally ineffective chemicals are applied. One of these novel chemical sensitivities is to the transmitter emitted by the sympathetic nervous system, and this is why some of these pains respond so well to drugs or surgery which affect the sympathetic system. The special sensitivities of these cut nerves offer the possibility that drugs and other manipulations will affect only the damaged area without influencing normal tissue.

Nerves carry not only nerve impulses but also chemicals which are needed for the normal function of the cells on which they end. When a nerve is cut or chemically treated in the periphery, cells in the spinal cord increase their excitability and there is even a change in the routing of the normal flow of impulses. The very small unmyelinated peripheral fibres and the peptides they contain are suspected of being particularly important in carrying this signal of injury. The identification of these chemical messengers and the discovery of how to manipulate them will have important therapeutic implications both for nerves and for the central nervous system since local changes induce distant reactions.

The neurochemical transactions in the spinal cord provide yet a further challenge to the neurochemist and pharmacologist. The cord is the site of interaction and transmission of arriving nerve impulses. These major interactions continue with second-by-second changes. There is growing evidence that the small cells of substantia gelatinosa play a role in these interactions but we know little of the details and nothing of the chemicals involved. In addition, powerful inhibitory systems descend from the brain and particularly affect the transmission to the brain of injury signals. A beginning has been made in identifying the origins of these systems as well as their pathways and chemical transmitters. Recent practical consequences include the use of drugs to encourage descending inhibition and with the surgical implantation of electrodes in the midbrain to activate descending inhibitory systems. Elucidation of these systems is an exciting future target but we need, above all, to understand the natural circumstances under which these systems operate.

Slowly acting systems control the distribution of cord excitability. We are only just beginning to realize that slow, long-term actions set the background on which the rapid controls (described above) operate. The site of these slow controls seems likely to include the substantia gelatinosa and a new area only recently located in the core of the spinal cord. It is tempting to propose that the peptides play a role in this system. Eleven such peptides, including the enkephalins, have been located in these areas. The central core appears part of a continuous system which runs the entire length of the neuraxis from the hypothalamus to the lower end of the spinal cord. Thus we have signs of long-acting, slowly shifting control systems side-by-side with the rapid control systems, and this has obvious implications for the future of pain control.

Sensory control. This approach has made extraordinary progress in recent years. The original procedure of electrically stimulating the skin or nerves (Wall and Sweet, 1967) has led to new forms of stimulation and the recognition that intense stimulation is often particularly effective in relieving many forms of pain (Melzack, 1975b). Our understanding of the delicate balance among the facilitatory and inhibitory controls from peripheral fibres and from the brain has led to stimulation of the dorsal columns, the periaqueductal grey matter, the sensory thalamus, and other areas. Recent research of the use of heat, cold and vibration suggests that we shall, in the future, see more ingenious ways of modulating the sensory input.

Psychological control. Pain associated with injury or disease is felt by a human being in a particular situation with a personal history, culture and genetic background. As in all complex behaviour in man, we have no clear evidence of genetic effects, but studies in the rat indicate that there is a strong genetic influence on the effect of nerve lesions on pain responses (Inbal *et al.*, 1980). Furthermore, in people in pain, there is often a divergence between public display and private suffering, which is determined by complex personal and cultural factors which we are just beginning to comprehend.

We need to understand not only the details of tissue damage but also the nature of the brain which processes the messages. A particular patient at the end of his life with a painful terminal disease may appear depressed. Is this his nature, is it a rational reaction to impending death, or is it caused by the pain? If we treat his depression with any of the anti-depressant drugs, what happens to his pain? These are legitimate scientific questions from which we shall learn much about pain while helping patients. We already have some fascinating hints to the answer. In the case of post-herpetic neuralgia, the pain appears to be helped by anti-depressants independently of their effect on the depression. Clearly we need to unravel which aspects of personality are affected by pain, which aspects of pain affect the expression of personality, and which of these can be manipulated to the patient's benefit. Many factors are involved and therefore multiple manipulations of expectation, anxiety, understanding, control, relaxation and coping may help.

It is an astonishing fact that a total of sixty-eight treatments for phantom limb pain can be found in the modern literature (Sherman *et al.*, 1980). The physician or other health professional confronted with a patient in severe chronic pain is understandably in a quandary: which of all of these therapies is the most appropriate? Many of the therapies to which patients are subjected have hardly been assessed at all. Treatment must be given but we must also insist that it be properly evaluated. In a case such as this, pain clinics can play an important role so that each specialty does not work in isolation. We have stressed in this book the multiple factors which interact to produce a particular individual's pain. This indicates multiple causes and therefore the possibility that multiple therapies are required. This adds to the complexity of assessment and to the ethical and economic difficulties of carrying out the necessary tests.

Our natural resources in the brain
We have evolved to react to the multiple circumstances of injury in multiple, subtle ways. Injury does not occur in isolation and neither does pain. Injury, which may or may not produce pain, is usually followed by a phase of adjustments to minimize the destructive effects of the injury, followed by a phase of recovery in which behaviour is characterized by rest and recuperation. To these three we must add the special circumstances of people who may perceive death as an end to suffering or as a desperate crisis to be resisted. We have within us the resources to control each of

these phases and the study of humans shows that we continually bring these resources into action to increase or decrease pain. We are just learning how to help people mobilize these resources for their own benefit.

Ultimately, the greatest challenge of pain continues to be the patient who has received every known treatment yet continues to suffer. No matter how splendid the progress in recent years in pain research and treatment, there are still large numbers of people who fail to respond to the best efforts of all the best therapists. These people – with excruciating cancer, post-herpetic neuralgia, low back pain – are the true measures of our knowledge and capability. Until we have learned to control this suffering the challenge of pain is as great as ever.

Glossary

Definitions with an asterisk (*) are reproduced from Merskey *et al.* (1979).

ablation The removal by surgery of any part of the body. In neurosurgery, refers to removal of part of the brain.

afferent fibre Nerve fibre which conducts nerve impulses from a sense organ to the central nervous system, or from lower to higher levels in sensory projection systems in the spinal cord and brain.

anaesthesia Total loss of sensation in all or part of the body.

anaesthesia dolorosa* Pain in an area or region which is anaesthetic.

anaesthetic As an adjective, refers to an area that has lost all sensitivity. As a noun, refers to drugs that induce the total loss of sensitivity either in a localized area or in the whole body after loss of consciousness.

analgesia Loss of sensitivity to pain without loss of other sensory qualities or of consciousness.

analgesic As an adjective, refers to an area that is insensitive to pain. As a noun, refers to any pain-relieving drug.

antidromic Propagation of a nerve impulse along an axon in a direction that is the reverse of the normal direction of transmission.

arthrogram A procedure to obtain an X-ray of a joint after injection of a special dye that facilitates visualization of the structures of the joint.

asymbolia Loss of the ability to appreciate some aspect of the sensory world. *Pain asymbolia*: inability to appreciate pain – that is, feel it in the normal way or grasp its implications.

axon The part of a nerve cell (neuron) which is the essential conducting portion. Often called simply the 'nerve fibre'.

brachial plexus The nerves to and from the arm at the level of the shoulder before they connect with the spinal cord.

brainstem The part of the brain that lies between the spinal cord and the cerebral cortex. Generally refers to those parts of the brain called the medulla oblongata, pons, and midbrain. Sometimes it is used to include the thalamus.

causalgia* A syndrome of sustained burning pain after a traumatic nerve lesion combined with vasomotor and sudomotor dysfunction and later trophic changes.

central nervous system In mammals, refers to the spinal cord and brain.

central pain* Pain associated with a lesion of the central nervous system.

clonic From the word 'clonus' referring to rapid alternate contraction and relaxation of a muscle.

commissural fibres A tract of neurons that connects two areas on opposite sides of the brain or spinal cord.

contralateral On the opposite side.

conversion hysteria Transformation of an emotional disturbance into a physical manifestation such as paralysis, anaesthesia of part of the body, or pain.

cortex The outer layer of an organ. Thus, *cerebral cortex*: the layers of nerve cells at the outer part of the brain.

cutaneous Relating to the skin.

decompression The relief of pressure within an organ by means of an operation to release excessive fluid. Thus, *subtemporal decompression*: the release of cerebrospinal fluid or blood through a burr-hole near the temporal (or lower side) part of the skull.

dendrite The part of a nerve cell (neuron) which conducts nerve impulses toward the cell body.

dermatome The area of skin innervated by a single sensory root of the spinal cord.

dysaesthesia* An unpleasant abnormal sensation.

ecchymosis Bruise; bleeding under the skin, usually after injury.

efferent fibre Neuron which conducts nerve impulses away from the central nervous system (to muscles or glands), or from higher to lower areas in the nervous system (such as a neuron that transmits from the brain to the spinal cord).

electroencephalogram (EEG) A recording of electrical activity of the brain, usually through electrodes placed on the scalp.

encephalon The brain. Thus, *encephalopathy*: any disease of the brain.

ephapse An artificial synapse (junction) between two conducting fibres that may occur after injury.

evisceration Removal of viscera (abdominal and thoracic organs).

ganglion An aggregate of nerve cell bodies. Thus, *sympathetic ganglion*: nerve cell bodies associated with the sympathetic nervous system.

herniation (of a disc) Protrusion of the intervertebral disc so that it presses against nerve roots and usually produces pain in addition to other symptoms.

hyperaesthetic Excessively sensitive, so that even non-noxious stimuli (such as a light touch) evoke pain.

hyperalgesia* Increased sensitivity to noxious stimulation.

hyperpathia* A painful syndrome, characterized by delay, overreaction and after-sensation to a stimulus, especially a repetitive stimulus.

hypoaesthesia Decreased sensitivity to all somatic stimulation.

hypoalgesia* Diminished sensitivity to noxious stimulation.

iatrogenic Pain or other medical problems produced inadvertently as a result of medical treatment.

introspection The analysis, by a person, of the sensory, emotional and other qualities of conscious experience.

ipsilateral On the same side.

jactitations Jerking, paroxysmal movements.

lumbar The part of the back and sides of the body between the lowest pair of ribs and the top of the pelvis.

median nerve One of the three major nerves that supply the hand. The other two are the radial and ulnar nerves. The sensory area innervated by the median nerve is complex but may be described roughly as the middle portion of the hand, particularly the middle and index fingers and the adjacent portions of the thumb and ring fingers.

metastases Secondary tumours that have spread from the initial primary site.

myelin A fatty substance surrounding nerve fibres, thereby forming an insulating sheath. *Myelinated*: covered by a myelin sheath.

neuralgia* Pain in the distribution of a nerve or nerves.

neuraxis The central nervous system from lowest to highest levels.

neuritis* Inflammation of a nerve or nerves.

neuroma A nodule in a cut nerve where regeneration fails.

neuron The structural unit of the nervous system, consisting of a nerve cell and its conducting dendrites and axon.

neuropathy A disturbance of function or pathological change in a nerve.

nociceptor* A receptor preferentially sensitive to a noxious or potentially noxious stimulus.

noxious A noxious stimulus is one which produces or is potentially capable of producing tissue damage.

orthodromic Propagation of a nerve impulse in the normal direction; in axons, away from the cell body.

pain threshold* The least stimulus intensity at which a subject perceives pain.

pain tolerance level* The greatest stimulus intensity causing pain that a subject is prepared to tolerate.

peripheral nerves Bundles of nerve fibres that connect sensory or motor organs to the central nervous system.

pinna The external part of the ear.

placebo Latin word that means 'I will please'. Usually a pill or injectable solution of sugar or salt given in place of an analgesic agent.

polysurgical addiction Refers to patients who appear to have a compelling need for surgical operations.

post-tetanic potentiation From 'tetanus', which refers to the continued contraction of a muscle, which can be produced by a rapid succession of electrically excited nerve impulses. Post-tetanic potentiation refers to the enhancement (potentiation) of muscle contractions or of nerve signals in motor neurons after prolonged, intense stimulation of the related sensory root.

proprioceptive Sensory signals from muscles, tendons and joints.

psychophysics Study of the relationship between stimulus intensity and the intensity of the resultant sensory experience.

roentgenography The use of X-rays to reveal internal structure. The name is derived from Wilhelm Roentgen, the discoverer of X-rays.

sacrum The continuation of the backbone below the lumbar vertebrae, consisting of several vertebrae joined together and making up the central bone of the pelvis. Thus, *sacral*: relating to the sacrum.

soma Greek word for 'body'. Somatic (or 'somatosensory') input refers to sensory signals from all tissues of the body, including skin, viscera, muscles or joints.

somaesthesis Sensory experience derived from the body.

subtemporal decompression See *decompression*.

sudomotor Activity of the sweat glands.

sympathetic nervous system One part of the autonomic nervous system, consisting of a chain of ganglia lying outside and parallel to the spinal cord, and nerve fibres that conduct to viscera, blood vessels and glands.

synapse The relay junction between two neurons. The axon terminals of a neuron release a chemical transmitter that flows across the synapse and influences the dendrites or cell body of an adjacent neuron. The transmitter may excite the cell (or facilitate its excitation by other neurons) or it may inhibit the cell and prevent it from firing (or decrease its firing rate).

thalamus One of the major relay stations of the central nervous system, lying at the top of the brainstem and between the cerebral hemispheres. It relays information projected by the sensory systems to the cortex and by the cortex to motor systems or to other brain areas.

trigeminal nerve The fifth nerve of the head. It carries sensory signals from the skin of the face, parts of the eyes, and a large part of the inner structures and membranes of the mouth and nose.

trophic Relative to nutrition, such as changes in the nutrition of skin tissue after a nerve injury.

vasomotor Activity of the blood vessels.

viscera The specialized internal organs of the abdomen and chest. Singular: *viscus*.

References

ABBOTT, F. V., 'Studies on morphine analgesia in an animal model of tonic pain', McGill University (Ph.D. thesis), Montreal, 1980.

ABBOTT, F. V., and MELZACK, R., 'Analgesia produced by stimulation of limbic structures and its relation to epileptiform after-discharges', *Exper. Neurol.*, 62(1978) 720–34.

ADAMS, H. E., FEUERSTEIN, M., and FOWLER, J. L., 'Migraine headache: review of parameters, etiology, and intervention', *Psychol. Bull.*, 87(1980) 217–37.

ADAMS, J. E., HOSOBUCHI, Y., and FIELDS, H. L., 'Thalamic syndrome and electrical stimulation of internal capsule', *J. Neurosurg.*, 41(1974) 740–44.

AJEMIAN, I., and MOUNT, B. M. (eds.), *The R.V.H. Manual on Palliative/Hospice Care,* Arno Press, New York, 1980.

ANDERSON, D. G., JAMIESON, J. L., and MAN, S. C., 'Analgesic effects of acupuncture on the pain of ice-water: a double-blind study', *Canad. J. Psychol.,* 28(1974) 239–44.

ANDERSON, T. P., COLE, T. M., GULLICKSON, G., HUDGENS, A., and ROBERTS, A. H., 'Behavior modification of chronic pain: a treatment program by a multidisciplinary team', *J. clin. Orthop.*, 129(1977) 96–100.

ANGAUT-PETIT, D., 'The dorsal column system. I. Existence of long ascending post-synaptic fibres in the cat's funiculus gracilis', *Exper. Brain Res.*, 22(1975a) 457–70.

ANGAUT-PETIT, D., 'The dorsal column system. II. Functional properties and bulbar relay of the post-synaptic fibres of the cat's fasciculus gracilis', *Exper. Brain Res.*, 22(1975b) 471–93.

AWAD, E. A., 'Interstitial myofibrositis: Hypothesis of the mechanism', *Arch. Phys. Med.*, 54(1973) 449–53.

BAILEY, A. A., and MOERSCH, F. P., 'Phantom limb', *Canad. Med. Assn J.*, 45(1941) 37–42.

BALAGURA, S., and RALPH, T., 'The analgesic effect of electrical stimulation of the diencephalon and mesencephalon', *Brain Res.*, 60(1973) 369–81.

BARBER, J., 'Utilizing hypnosis in the treatment of pain'; in OBORNE, D. J., GRUNEBERG, M. M., and EISER, J. R. (eds.), *Research in Psychology and Medicine,* Vol. 1, Academic Press, London, 1979, pp. 35–40.

BARBUT, D., POLAK, J. M., and WALL, P. D., 'Substance P in spinal cord dorsal horn decreases following peripheral nerve injury', *Brain Res.*, 205(1981) 289–98.

BARON, R. A., BYRNE, D., and KANTROWITZ, B. H., *Psychology, Understanding Behavior*, Saunders, Philadelphia, 1977.

BASBAUM, A. I., 'Conduction of the effects of noxious stimulation by short-fiber multisynaptic systems of the spinal cord in the rat', *Exp. Neurol.*, 40(1973) 699–716.

BASBAUM, A. I., and FIELDS, H. L., 'Endogenous pain control mechanisms: review and hypothesis', *Ann. Neurol.*, 4(1978) 451–62.

BASBAUM, A. I., and FIELDS, H. L., 'The origin of descending pathways in the dorsolateral funiculus of the spinal cord of the cat and rat', *J. Comp. Neurol.*, 187(1979) 513–32.

BASBAUM, A. I., MARLEY, N. J. E., O'KEEFE, J., and CLANTON, C. H., 'Reversal of morphine and stimulus produced analgesia by subtotal spinal cord lesions', *Pain*, 3(1977) 43–56.

BAXTER, D. W., and OLSZEWSKI, J., 'Congenital insensitivity to pain', *Brain*, 83(1960) 381–93.

BECKER, D. P., GLUCK, H., NULSEN, F. E., and JANE, J. A., 'An inquiry into the neurophysiological basis for pain', *J. Neurosurg.*, 30(1969) 1–13.

BEECHER, H. K., *Measurement of Subjective Responses*, Oxford University Press, New York, 1959.

BELL, C., SIERRA, G., BUENDIA, N., and SEGUNDO, J. P., 'Sensory properties of neurons in the mesencephalic reticular formation', *J. Neurophysiol.*, 27(1964) 961–87.

BENSON, H., and EPSTEIN, M. D., 'The placebo effect: a neglected asset in the care of patients', *J. Amer. Med. Assn*, 232(1975) 1225–7.

BENSON, H., KOTCH, J. B., CRASSWELLER, K. D., and GREENWOOD, M. M., 'Historical and clinical considerations of the relaxation response', *Amer. Scientist*, 65(1977) 441–5.

BISHOP, G. H., 'Neural mechanisms of cutaneous sense', *Physiol. Rev.* 26(1946) 77–102.

BISHOP, G. H., 'The relation between nerve fiber size and sensory modality: phylogenetic implications of the afferent innervation of the cortex', *J. Nerv. ment. Dis.*, 128(1959) 89–114.

BLANCHARD, E., THEOBALD, D., WILLIAMSON, D., SILVER, B., and BROWN, D., 'Temperature biofeedback in the treatment of migraine headaches', *Arch. gen. Psychiat.*, 35(1978) 581–8.

BOIVIE, J., 'The termination of the spinothalamic tract in the cat', *Exper. Brain Res.*, 12(1971) 331–53.

BONICA, J. J., *The Management of Pain*, Lea and Febiger, Philadelphia, 1953.

BONICA, J. J., 'Management of myofascial pain syndromes in general practice', *J. Amer. Med. Assn*, 164(1957) 732–8.

BONICA, J. J., 'Anesthesiology in the People's Republic of China', *Anesthesiology*, 40(1974) 175–86.

BONICA, J. J., 'Organization and function of a pain clinic'; in J. J. BONICA (ed.), *Advances in Neurology*, Vol. 4, Raven Press, New York, 1974, pp. 433–43.

BONICA, J. J., 'Cancer pain'; in J. J. BONICA (ed.), *Pain*, Raven Press, New York, 1980, pp. 335–62.

BORING, E. G., *Sensation and Perception in the History of Experimental Psychology*, Appleton-Century-Crofts, New York, 1942.

BOTTERELL, E. H., CALLAGHAN, J. C., and JOUSSE, A. T., 'Pain in paraplegia: clinical management and surgical treatment', *Proc. Roy. Soc. Med.*, 47(1954) 281–8.

BOWERS, K. S., 'Pain, anxiety, and perceived control', *J. consult. clin. Psychol.*, 32(1968) 596–602.

BOWSHER, D., and ALBE-FESSARD, D., 'The anatomophysiological basis of somatosensory discrimination', *Int. Rev. Neurobiol.*, 8(1965) 35–75.

BRENA, S. F., WOLF, S. L., CHAPMAN, S. L., and HAMMONDS, W. D., 'Chronic back pain: electromyographic, motion and behavioral assessments following sympathetic nerve blocks and placebos', *Pain*, 8(1980) 1–10.

BRENDSTRUP, P., JESPERSEN, K., and ASBOC-HANSEN, G., 'Morphological and chemical connective tissue changes in fibrositic muscles', *Ann. Rheum. Dis.*, 16(1957) 438–40.

BROCKBANK, W., *Ancient Therapeutic Arts*, Heinemann, London, 1954.

BROMAGE, P. R., CAMPORESI, E., and LESLIE, J., 'Epidural narcotics in volunteers: sensitivity to pain and to carbon dioxide', *Pain*, 9(1980) 145–60.

BROMAGE, P. R., and MELZACK, R., 'Phantom limbs and the body schema', *Canad. Anaesth. Soc. J.*, 21(1974) 267–74.

BROWDER, E. J., and GALLAGHER, J. P., 'Dorsal cordotomy for painful phantom limb', *Ann. Surg.*, 128(1948) 456–69.

BROWN, A. G., 'Effects of descending impulses on transmission through the spino-cervical tract', *J. Physiol.* (Lond.), 219(1971) 103–25.

BROWN, A. G., ROSE, P. K., and SNOW, P. S., 'Morphology and organization of axon collaterals from afferent fibers of slowly adapting Type I units in cat spinal cord', *J. Physiol.*, 277(1978) 15–27.

BUDZYNSKI, T. H., STOYVA, J. M., ADLER, C. S., and MULLANEY, D. J., 'EMG biofeedback and tension headache: a controlled outcome study', *Psychosom. Med.*, 35(1973) 484–96.

CALVIN, W. H., LOESER, J. D., and HOWE, J. F., 'A neurophysiological theory for the pain mechanism in tic douloureux', *Pain*, 3(1977) 147–54.

CAMPBELL, J. N., MEYER, R. A., and LAMOTTE, R. H., 'Sensitization of myelinated nociceptive afferents that innervate monkey hand', *J. Neurophysiol.*, 42(1979) 1669–80.

CARLEN, P. L., WALL, P. D., NADVORNA, H., and STEINBACH, T., 'Phantom limbs and related phenomena in recent traumatic amputations', *Neurology*, 28(1978) 211–17.

CASEY, K. L., 'Nociceptive mechanisms in the thalamus of awake squirrel monkey', *J. Neurophysiol.*, 29(1966) 727–50.

CASEY, K. L., 'Somatosensory responses of bulboreticular units in awake cat: relation to escape-producing stimuli', *Science*, 173(1971a) 77–80.

CASEY, K. L., 'Responses of bulboreticular units to somatic stimuli eliciting escape behavior in the cat', *Int. J. Neurosci.*, 2(1971b) 15–28.

CASEY, K. L., 'Reticular formation and pain: toward a unifying concept'; in J. J. BONICA (ed.), *Pain*, Raven Press, New York, 1980, pp. 93–105.

CASEY, K. L. KEENE, J. J., and MORROW, T., 'Bulboreticular and medial thalamic unit activity in relation to aversive behavior and pain'; in J. J. BONICA (ed.), *Pain, Advances in Neurology*, Vol. 4, Raven Press, New York, 1974, pp. 197–205.

CASSINARI, V., and PAGNI, C. A., *Central Pain: A Neurosurgical Study*, Harvard University Press, Cambridge, Mass., 1969.

CERVERO, F., IGGO, A., and OGAWA, H., 'Nociceptor driven dorsal horn cells in the lumbar spinal cord of the cat', *Pain*, 2(1976) 5–24.

CHAPMAN, C. R., COLPITTS, Y. M., BENEDETTI, C., KITAEFF, R., and GEHRIG, J. D., 'Evoked potential assessment of acupunctural analgesia: attempted reversal with naloxone', *Pain*, 9(1980) 183–97.

CHAPMAN, C. R., WILSON, M. E., and GEHRIG, J. D., 'Comparative effects of acupuncture and transcutaneous stimulation on the perception of painful dental stimuli', *Pain*, 2(1976) 265–83.

CHERRY, L., 'Solving the mysteries of pain', *New York Times Magazine*, Jan. 30(1977) 12–13; 50–53.

CHESNEY, M. A., and SHELTON, J. L., 'A comparison of muscle relaxation and electromyogram biofeedback treatments for muscle contraction headache', *J. behav. exper. Psychiat.*, 7(1976) 221–5.

CLARK, W. C., and CLARK, S. B., 'Pain responses in Nepalese porters', *Science*, 209 (1980) 410–12.

CO, L. L., SCHMITZ, T. H., HAVDALA, H., REYES, A., and WESTERMAN, M. P., 'Acupuncture: an evaluation in the painful crises of sickle cell anaemia', *Pain*, 7(1979) 181–5.

COGHILL, G. E., *Anatomy and the Problem of Behaviour*, Cambridge University Press, Cambridge, 1929.

COHEN, H., 'The mechanism of visceral pain', *Trans. Med. Soc. London*, 64(1944) 65–99.

COLDING, A., 'The effect of regional sympathetic blocks in the treatment of herpes zoster: a survey of 300 cases', *Acta anaesth. Scand.*, 13(1969) 133–40.

COMINGS, D. E., and AMROMIN, G. D., 'Autosomal dominant insensitivity to pain with hyperplastic myelinopathy and autosomal dominant indifference to pain', *Neurology*, 24(1974) 838–48.

CORSSEN, G., HOLCOMB, M. C., MOUSTAPHA, I., LANGFORD, K., VITEK, J. J., and CEBALLOS, R., 'Alcohol-induced adenolysis of the pituitary gland: a new approach to control of intractable cancer pain', *Anesthes. Analges.*, 56(1977) 414–21.

COULTER, J. D., FOREMAN, R. D., BEALL, J. E., and WILLIS, W. D., 'Cerebral cortical modulation of primate spinothalamic neurons'; in J. J. BONICA and D. ALBE-FESSARD (eds.), *Advances in Pain Research and Therapy*, Vol. 1, Raven Press, New York, 1976, pp.271–7.

COULTER, J. D., MAUNZ, R. A., and WILLIS, W. D., 'Effects of stimulation of sensorimotor cortex on primate spinothalamic neurons', *Brain Res.*, 65(1974) 351–6.

COX, D. J., FREUNDLICH, A., and MEYER, R. C., 'Differential effectiveness of electromyographic feedback, verbal relaxation instructions, and medication placebo with tension headaches', *J. consult. clin. Psychol.*, 43(1975) 892–8.

COX, V. C., and VALENSTEIN, E. S., 'Attenuation of aversive properties of peripheral shock by hypothalamic stimulation', *Science*, 149(1965) 323–5.

CRONHOLM, B., 'Phantom limbs in amputees', *Acta Psychiat. Neurol. Scand.*, Suppl. 72(1951) 1–310.

CSILLIK, B., and KNYIHAR, E., 'Biodynamic plasticity in the rolando substance', *Progr. Neurobiol.*, 10(1978) 208–30.

DALESSIO, D. J., 'Vascular permeability and vasoactive substances: their relationship to migraine'; in J. J. BONICA (ed.), *Advances in Neurology*, Vol. 4, Raven Press, New York, 1974, pp.395–401.

DALESSIO, D. J. (ed.), *Wolff's Headache and Other Head Pain*, Oxford University Press, New York, 1980.

DALLENBACH, K. M., 'The temperature spots and end-organs', *Amer. J. Psychol.*, 39(1927) 402–27.

DALLENBACH, K. M., 'Pain: history and present status', *Amer. J. Psychol.*, 52(1939) 331-47.

DAVIS, L., and MARTIN, J., 'Studies upon spinal cord injuries. II. The nature and treatment of pain', *J. Neurosurg.*, 4(1947) 483–91.

DELGADO, J. M. R., 'Cerebral structures involved in transmission and elaboration of noxious stimulation', *J. Neurophysiol.*, 18(1955) 261–75.

DELGADO, J. M. R., ROSVOLD, H. E., and LOONEY, E., 'Evoking conditioned fear by electrical stimulation of subcortical structures in the monkey brain', *J. comp. physiol. Psychol.*, 49(1956) 373–80.

DENNIS, S. G., CHOINIÈRE, M., and MELZACK, R., 'Stimulation-produced analgesia in rats: assessment by two pain tests and correlation with self-stimulation', *Exper. Neurol.*, 68(1980) 295–309.

DENNIS, S. G., and MELZACK, R., 'Pain-signalling systems in the dorsal and ventral spinal cord', *Pain*, 4(1977) 97–132.

DENNIS, S. G., and MELZACK, R., 'Self-mutilation after dorsal rhizotomy in rats: effects of prior pain and pattern of root lesions', *Exper. Neurol.*, 65(1979) 412–21.

DENNIS, S. G., and MELZACK, R., 'Pain modulation by 5-hydroxytryptaminergic agents and morphine as measured by three pain tests', *Exper. Neurol.*, 69(1980) 260–70.

DENNIS, S. G., MELZACK, R., GUTMAN, S., and BOUCHER, F., 'Pain modulation by adrenergic agents and morphine as measured by three pain tests', *Life Sci.*, 26(1980) 1247–59.

DENNIS, S. G., YEOMANS, J. S., and DEUTSCH, J. A., 'Adaption of aversive brain stimulation. III. Excitability characteristics of behaviorally relevant neural substrates', *Behav. Biol.*, 18(1976) 531–44.

DENNY-BROWN, D., KIRK, E. J., and YANAGISAWA, N., 'The tract of

Lissauer in relation to sensory transmission in the dorsal horn of spinal cord in the macaque', *J. Comp. Neurol.*, 151(1973) 175–200.

DESCARTES, R., *L'homme* (1664); translated by M. FOSTER, *Lectures on the History of Physiology during the 16th, 17th and 18th Centuries*, Cambridge University Press, Cambridge, 1901.

DEVOR, M., and CLAMAN, D., 'Mapping and plasticity of acid phosphatase afferents in the rat dorsal horn', *Brain Res.*, 190(1980) 17–28.

DEVOR, M., MERRILL, E. G., and WALL, P. D., 'Dorsal horn cells that respond to stimulation of distant dorsal roots', *J. Physiol.*, 270(1977) 519–31.

DEVOR, M., and WALL, P. D., 'Reorganization of spinal cord sensory map after peripheral nerve injury', *Nature*, 275(1978) 75–6.

DEVOR, M., and WALL, P. D., 'Effect of peripheral nerve injury on receptive fields of cells in cat spinal cord', *J. Comp. Neurol.*, 199(1981a) 277–91.

DEVOR, M., and WALL, P. D., 'Plasticity in the spinal cord sensory map following peripheral nerve injury in rats', *J. Neurosci.*, 1(1981b) 679–84.

DICK-READ, G., *Childbirth without Fear*, Harper, New York, 1944.

DIMITRIJEVIC, M. R., and NATHAN, P. W., 'Studies of spasticity in man. 4. Changes in flexion reflex with repetitive cutaneous stimulation', *Brain*, 93(1970) 743–68.

DONALDSON, H. H., 'On the temperature sense', *Mind*, 10(1885) 399–416.

DOSTROVSKY, J. O., MILLAR, J., and WALL, P. D., 'The immediate shift of afferent drive of dorsal column nucleus cells following deafferentation: a comparison of acute and chronic deafferentation in gracile nucleus and spinal cord', *Exper. Neurol.*, 52(1976) 480–95.

DRAKE, C. G., and MCKENZIE, K. G., 'Mesencephalic tractotomy for pain', *J. Neurosurg.*, 10(1953) 457–62.

DUBUISSON, D., and DENNIS, S. G., 'The formalin test: a quantitative study of the analgesic effects of morphine, meperidine, and brain stem stimulation in rats and cats', *Pain*, 4(1977) 161–74.

DUBUISSON, D., and MELZACK, R., 'Classification of clinical pain descriptions by multiple group discriminant analysis', *Exper. Neurol.*, 51(1976) 480–87.

DUBUISSON, D., and WALL, P. D., 'Descending influences on receptive fields and activity of single units recorded in laminae 1, 2 and 3 of cat spinal cord', *Brain Res.*, 199(1980) 283–98.

DUGGAN, A. W., HALL, J. G., and HEADLEY, P. M., 'Morphine, enkephalin and the substantia gelatinosa', *Nature*, 264(1976) 456–8.

DYCK, P. J., LAMBERT, E. H., and O'BRIEN, P. C., 'Pain in peripheral neuropathy related to rate and kind of fiber degeneration', *Neurology*, 22(1976) 466–71.

DYKES, R. W., 'Nociception', *Brain Res.*, 99(1975) 229–45.

ECHLIN, F., OWENS, F. M., and WELLS, W. L., 'Observations on "major" and "minor" causalgia', *Arch. Neurol. Psychiat.*, 62(1949) 183–203.

EDINGER, L., 'Vergleichend-entwicklungsgeschichtliche und anatomische studien im Bereiche des centralnervensystems', *Anat. Anz.*, 4(1889) 121–8.

EGBERT, L. D., BATTIT, G. E., WELCH, C. D., and BARTLETT, M. K., 'Reduction of post-operative pain by encouragement and instruction of patients', *New Eng. J. Med.*, 270(1964) 825–7.

ELLIOTT, F. A., 'Acupuncture and other forms of counter-irritation', *Trans. Studies Coll. Phys. Phil.*, 30(1962) 81–4.

ELTON, D., STUART, G. V., and BURROWS, G. D., 'Self-esteem and chronic pain', *J. Psychosom. Res.*, 22(1978) 25–30.

ERIKSSON, M. B. E., SJOLUND, B. H., and NIELZEN, S., 'Long term results of peripheral conditioning stimulation as an analgesic measure in chronic pain', *Pain*, 6(1979) 335–47.

EVANS, F. J., 'The placebo response in pain reduction'; in J. J. BONICA (ed.), *Advances in Neurology*, Vol. 4, Raven Press, New York, 1974, pp.289–96.

EWALT, J. R., RANDALL, G. C., and MORRIS, H., 'The phantom limb', *Psychosom. Med.*, 9(1947) 118–23.

FEINSTEIN, B., LUCE, J. C., and LANGTON, J. N. K., 'The influence of phantom limbs'; in P. KLOPSTEG and P. WILSON (eds.), *Human Limbs and Their Substitutes*, McGraw-Hill, New York, 1954, pp.79–138.

FETZ, E. E., 'Pyramidal tract effects on interneurons in cat lumbar dorsal horn', *J. Neurophysiol.*, 31(1968) 68–80.

FINNESON, B., *Diagnosis and Management of Pain Syndromes*, Saunders, Philadelphia, 1969.

FITZGERALD, M., 'The sensitization of cutaneous nociceptors by spread from a nearby injury', *J. Physiol.*, 278(1978) 44–5.

FITZGERALD, M., and WALL, P. D., 'The laminar organization of dorsal horn cells responding to peripheral C fibre stimulation', *Exper. Brain Res.*, 41(1980) 36–44.

FITZGERALD, M., and WOOLF, C. J., 'The stereospecific effect of naloxone on rat dorsal horn neurons', *Pain*, 9(1980) 293–306.

FOLTZ, E. L., and WHITE, L. E., 'Pain "relief" by frontal cingulumotomy', *J. Neurosurg.*, 19(1962) 89–100.

FORDYCE, W. E., *Behavioral Methods for Chronic Pain and Illness*, C. V. Mosby, St Louis, Mo., 1976.

FOX, E. J., and MELZACK, R., 'Transcutaneous electrical stimulation and acupuncture: comparison of treatment for low back pain', *Pain*, 2(1976) 141–8.

FRANÇOIS-FRANCK, C. E., 'Signification physiologique de la résection du sympathique', *Bull. Acad. Nat. Med.* (Paris), 41(1899) 565–94.

FREEMAN, W., and WATTS, J. W., *Psychosurgery in the Treatment of Mental Disorders and Intractable Pain*, C. C. Thomas, Springfield, Ill. 1950.

FREY, M. VON, 'Beitrage zur Sinnesphysiologie der Haut', *Ber. d. kgl. sächs. Ges. d. Wiss., math.-phys. Kl.*, 47(1895) 166–84.

FROST, F. A., JESSEN, B., and SIGGAARD-ANDERSEN, J., 'A control, double-blind comparison of mepivacaine injection versus saline injection for myofascial pain', *Lancet*, 8 March(1980) 499–501.

GARDNER, W. J., and LICKLIDER, J. C. R., 'Auditory analgesia in dental operations', *J. Amer. Dent. Assn*, 59(1959) 1144–9.

GARFIELD, E., 'Most cited articles of the 1960s. 3. Preclinical basic research', *Current Contents*, 23(5) (1980) 5–13.

GAW, A. C., CHANG, L. W., and SHAW, L. C., 'Efficacy of acupuncture on osteoarthritic pain', *New Eng. J. Med.*, 293(1975) 375–8.

GERARD, R. W., 'The physiology of pain: abnormal neuron states in causalgia and related phenomena', *Anesthesiology*, 12(1951) 1–13.

GHIA, J. N., MAO, W., TOOMEY, T. C., and GREGG, J. M., 'Acupuncture and chronic pain mechanisms', *Pain*, 2(1976) 285–99.

GIBSON, S. J., POLAK, J. M., BLOOM, S. R., and WALL, P. D., 'The distribution of nine peptides in rat spinal cord', *J. Comp. Neurol.*, 201(1981) 65–79.

GLOOR, P., 'Inputs and outputs of the amygdala: what the amygdala is trying to tell the rest of the brain'; in K. E. LIVINGSTON and D. HORNYKIEWICZ(eds.), *Limbic Mechanisms*, Plenum Press, New York, 1978, pp. 189–209.

GLYN, J. H., 'Rheumatic pains: some concepts and hypotheses', *Proc. Roy. Soc. Med.*, 64(1971) 354–60.

GOBEL, S., 'Neural circuitry in the substantia gelatinosa rolando'; in J. J. BONICA, D. ALBE-FESSARD, and J. C. LIEBESKIND (eds.), *Advances in Pain Research and Therapy*, Vol. 3, Raven Press, New York, 1979, pp. 175–95.

GOLDSCHEIDER, A., 'Histologische untersuchungen uber die Endingungsweise der Hautsinnesnerven beim Menschen', *Arch. Physiol. Leipzig, Suppl. Bd.*(1886) 191–231.

GOLDSCHEIDER, A., *Ueber den Schmerz in Physiologischer und Klinischer Hinsicht*, Hirschwald, Berlin, 1894.

GOODMAN, L. S., and GILMAN, A., *The Pharmacological Basis of Therapeutics*, Macmillan, New York, 1980.

GOTTLIEB, H., STRITE, L. C., KOLLER, R., MADORSKY, A., HOCKERSMITH, V., KLEEMAN, M., and WAGNER, J., 'Comprehensive rehabilitation of patients having chronic low back pain', *Arch. Phys. Med. Rehabil.*, 58(1977) 101–8.

GRACELY, R. H., 'Psychophysical asessment of human pain'; in J. J. BONICA, J. C. LIEBESKIND, and D. G. ALBE-FESSARD (eds.), *Advances in Pain Research and Therapy*, Vol. 3, Raven Press, New York, 1979, pp. 805–24.

GRAHAM, C., BOND, S. S., GERKOVICH, M. M., and COOK, M. R., 'Use of the McGill Pain Questionnaire in the assessment of cancer pain: replicability and consistency', *Pain*, 8(1980) 377–87.

GRAHAME, R.(ed.), *Clinics in Rheumatic Diseases, Low Back Pain*, Saunders, Philadelphia, 1980.

GROSS, Y., and MELZACK, R.,'Body image; dissociation of real and perceived limbs by pressure-cuff ischemia', *Exper. Neurol.*, 61(1978) 680–88.

GROVES, P. M., MILLER, S. W., PARKER, M. V., and REBEC, G. V.,

'Organization by sensory modality in the reticular formation of the rat', *Brain Res.*, 54(1973) 207–12.

GUNN, C. C., and MILBRANDT, W. E., 'Early and subtle signs in low back sprain', *Spine*, 3(1978) 267–81.

HAGBARTH, K. E., and KERR, D. I. B., 'Central influences on spinal afferent conduction', *J. Neurophysiol.*, 17(1954) 295–307.

HALL, K. R. L., and STRIDE, E., 'The varying response to pain in psychiatric disorders: a study in abnormal psychology', *Brit. J. Med. Psychol.*, 27(1954) 48–60.

HALLIDAY, A. M., and MINGAY, R., 'Retroactive raising of a sensory threshold by a contralateral stimulus', *Quart. J. exper. Psychol.*, 13(1961) 1–11.

HAMMOND, D. L., LEVY, R. A., and PROUDFIT, H. K., 'Hypoalgesia following microinjection of noradrenergic antagonists in the nucleus raphe magnus', *Pain*, 9(1980) 85–101.

HANDWERKER, O., IGGO, A., and ZIMMERMANN, M., 'Segmental and supraspinal action on dorsal horn neurons responding to noxious and non-noxious skin stimuli', *Pain*, 1(1975) 147–66.

HANNINGTON-KIFF, J. G., *Pain Relief*, Heinemann, London, 1974.

HARDY, J. D., WOLFF, H. G., and GOODELL, H., *Pain Sensations and Reactions*, Williams and Wilkins, Baltimore, 1952.

HARTMAN, L. M., and AINSWORTH, K. D., 'Self-regulation of chronic pain', *Canad. J. Psychiat.*, 25(1980) 38–43.

HAYES, M. H., 'A study of cutaneous after-sensations', *Psych. Monogr.*, 14(1912) 1–89.

HEAD, H., *Studies in Neurology*, Kegan Paul, London, 1920.

HEBB, D. O., *The Organization of Behavior*, Wiley, New York, 1949.

HEBB, D. O., 'Science and the world of imagination', *Canad. Psychol. Rev.*, 16(1975) 4–11.

HENDERSON, W. R., and SMYTH, G. E., 'Phantom limbs', *J. Neurol. Neurosurg. Psychiat.*, 11(1948) 88–112.

HERZ, A., ALBUS, K., METYS, J., SCHUBERT, P., and TESCHEMACHER, H., 'On the sites for the anti-nociceptive action of morphine and fentanyl', *Neuropharmacol.*, 9(1970) 539–51.

HILGARD, E. R., 'A neodissociation interpretation of pain reduction by hypnosis', *Psychol. Rev.*, 80(1973) 396–411.

HILGARD, E. R., and HILGARD, J., *Hypnosis in the Relief of Pain*, William Kaufmann, Los Altos, Cal., 1975.

HILL, H. E., KORNETSKY, C. H., FLANARY, H. G., and WIKLER, A., 'Effects of anxiety and morphine on discrimination of intensities of painful stimuli', *J. Clin. Invest.*, 31(1952a) 473–80.

HILL, H. E., KORNETSKY, C. H., FLANARY, H. G., and WIKLER, A., 'Studies of anxiety associated with anticipation of pain. I. Effects of morphine', *Arch. Neurol. Psychiat.*, 67(1952b) 612–19.

HILLMAN, P., and WALL, P. D., 'Inhibitory and excitatory factors influencing the receptive fields of lamina 5 spinal cord cells', *Exper. Brain Res.*, 9(1969) 284–306.

HOKANSON, J. E., DEGOOD, D. E., FORREST, M. S., and BRITTAIN, T. M., 'Availability of avoidance behaviors in modulating vascular-stress responses', *J. personality soc. Psychol.*, 19(1971) 60–68.

HONGO, T., JANKOWSKA, E., and LUNDBERG, A., 'Post synaptic excitation and inhibition from primary afferents in neurons of the spinocervical tract', *J. Physiol.*, 199(1968) 569–92.

HORAN, J. J., LAYNG, F. C., and PURSELL, C. H., 'Preliminary study of effects of "in vivo" emotive imagery in dental discomfort', *Percept. Motor Skills*, 42(1976) 105–6.

HOSOBUCHI, Y., ADAMS, J. E., and LINCHITZ, R., 'Pain relief by electrical stimulation of the central gray matter in humans and its reversal by naloxone', *Science*, 177(1977) 183–6.

HOSOBUCHI, Y., ADAMS, J. E., and RUTKIN, B., 'Chronic thalamic stimulation for the control of facial anesthesia dolorosa', *Arch. Neurol.*, 29(1973) 158–61.

HOWE, J. F., LOESER, J. D., and CALVIN, W. H., 'Mechanosensitivity of dorsal root ganglia and chronically injured axons: a physiological basis for the radicular pain of nerve root compression', *Pain*, 3(1977) 25–41.

HUGHES, J., and KOSTERLITZ, H. W., 'Opioid peptides', *Brit. Med. Bull.*, 33(1977) 157–61.

HUNT, S. P., KELLY, J. S., and EMSON, P. C., 'The electron microscope localization of methionine enkephalin within the superficial layers of the spinal cord', *Neuroscience*, 5(1980) 1871–90.

HUNTER, M., and PHILIPS, C., 'The experience of headache – an assessment of the qualities of tension headache pain', *Pain*, 10(1981) 209–19.

HUTCHINS, H. C., and REYNOLDS, O. E., 'Experimental investigation of the referred pain of aerodontalgia', *J. dent. Res.*, 26(1947) 3–8.

HUXLEY, A., *The Devils of Loudon*, Harper, New York, 1952.

IGGO, A., 'Critical remarks on the gate control theory'; in R. JANZEN *et al.* (eds.), *Pain*, Churchill Livingstone, London, 1972, pp. 127–8.

INBAL, R., DEVOR, M., TUCHENDLER, O., and LIEBLICH, I., 'Autotomy following nerve injury: genetic factors in the development of chronic pain', *Pain*, 9(1980) 327–37.

JANCSO, N., JANCSO-GABOR, A., and SZOLCSANYI, J., 'Direct evidence for neurogenic inflammation and its prevention by denervation and by pre-treatment with capsaicin', *Brit. J. Pharmacol. Chemother.*, 31(1967) 138–51.

JEANS, M. E., 'Relief of chronic pain by brief, intense transcutaneous electrical stimulation – a double-blind study'; in J. J. BONICA, J. C. LIEBESKIND, and D. G. ALBE-FESSARD (eds.), *Advances in Pain Research and Therapy*, Vol. 3, Raven Press, New York, 1979, pp. 601–6.

JESSELL, T. W., and IVERSEN, L. L., 'Opiate analgesics inhibit substance P release from rat spinal trigeminal nucleus', *Nature*, 268(1977) 549–51.

JESSUP, B. A., NEWFIELD, R. W. J., and MERSKEY, H., 'Biofeedback therapy for headache and other pain: an evaluative review', *Pain*, 7(1979) 225–70.

JONES, C. M., *Digestive Tract Pain: Diagnosis and Treatment; Experimental Observations*, Macmillan, New York, 1938.

KALLIO, K. E., 'Permanency of the results obtained by sympathetic surgery in the treatment of phantom pain', *Acta Orthop. Scand.*, 19(1950) 391–7.

KAMIYA, J., 'Conscious control of brain waves', *Psychol. Today*, 1(1968) 56–60.

KAO, F. F., *Acupuncture Therapeutics*, Eastern Press, New Haven, Conn., 1973.

KARPMAN, H. L., KNEBEL, A., SEMEL, C. J., and COOPER, J., 'Clinical studies in thermography', *Arch. Environ. Health*, 20(1970) 412–17.

KATZ, J., and LEVIN, A. B., 'Treatment of diffuse metastatic cancer pain by instillation of alcohol into the sella turcica', *Anesthesiology*, 46(1977) 115–21.

KEEGAN, J. J., and GARRETT, F. D., 'The segmental distribution of the cutaneous nerves in the limbs of man', *Anat. Rec.*, 102(1948) 409–37.

KEELE, K. D., *Anatomies of Pain*, Oxford University Press, London, 1957.

KEELE, C. A., and ARMSTRONG, D., *Substances Producing Pain and Itch*, Arnold, London, 1964.

KEERI-SZANTO, M., 'Drugs or drums: what relieves post-operative pain?', *Pain*, 6(1979) 217–30.

KENNARD, M. A., and HAUGEN, F. P., 'The relation of subcutaneous focal sensitivity to referred pain of cardiac origin', *Anesthesiology*, 16(1955) 297–311.

KERR, D. I. B., HAUGEN, F. P., and MELZACK, R., 'Responses evoked in the brainstem by tooth stimulation', *Amer. J. Physiol.*, 183(1955) 253–8.

KERR, F. W. L., and LIPPMANN, H. H., 'The primate spinothalamic tract as demonstrated by anterolateral cordotomy and commissural myelotomy'; in J. J. BONICA (ed.), *Pain, Advances in Neurology*, Vol. 4, Raven Press, New York, 1974, pp. 147–56.

KERR, F. W. L., WILSON, P. R., and NIJENSOHN, D. E., 'Acupuncture reduces the trigeminal evoked response in decerebrate cats', *Exper. Neurol.*, 61(1978) 84–95.

KIBLER, M., *Das storungsfeld bei Gelenkserkrankungen und inneren Krankheiten*, Hippokrates, Stuttgart, 1958.

KIBLER, R. F., and NATHAN, P. W., 'Relief of pain and paraesthesiae by nerve block distal to a lesion', *J. Neurol. Neurosurg. Psychiat.*, 23(1960) 91–8.

KING, H. E., CLAUSEN, J., and SCARFF, J. E., 'Cutaneous thresholds for pain before and after unilateral prefrontal lobotomy', *J. nerv. ment. Dis.*, 112(1950) 93–6.

KIRK, E. J., and DENNY-BROWN, D., 'Functional variation of dermatome in the macaque monkey following dorsal root lesions', *J. Comp. Neurol.*, 139(1970) 307–20.

KOLB, L. C., *The Painful Phantom: Psychology, Physiology and Treatment*, C. C. Thomas, Springfield, Ill., 1954.

KOPELL, H. P., and THOMPSON, W. A. L., *Peripheral Entrapment Neuropathies*, Robert E. Krieger, Huntington, New York, 1976.

KORR, I. M., THOMAS, P. E., and WRIGHT, H. M., 'Symposium on the functional implications of segmental facilitation', *J. Amer. Osteopath. Assn*, 54(1955) 1–18.

KOSAMBI, D. D., 'Living prehistory in India', *Sci. Amer.*, 216(2) (1967) 105–14.

KRAINICK, J. U., THODEN, U., and REICHERT, T., 'Pain reduction in amputees by long term spinal cord stimulation', *J. Neurosurg.*, 52(1980) 346–50.

KUGELBERG, E., and LINDBLOM, U., 'The mechanism of pain in trigeminal neuralgia', *J. Neurol. Neurosurg. Psychiat.*, 22(1959) 36–43.

LAITINEN, J., 'Acupuncture and transcutaneous electric stimulation in the treatment of chronic sacrolumbalgia and ischialgia', *Amer. J. Chinese Med.*, 4(1976) 169–75.

LAMAZE, F., *Painless Childbirth: Psychoprophylactic Method*, Regnery, Chicago, 1970.

LAMBERT, W. E., LIBMAN, E., and POSER, E. G., 'Effect of increased salience of membership group on pain tolerance', *J. Personality*, 28(1960) 350–57.

LANGER, E., JANIS, I. L., and WOLFER, J. A., 'Reduction of psychological stress in surgical patients', *J. exper. soc. Psychol.*, 11(1975) 155–65.

LARSELL, O., *Anatomy of the Nervous System*, Appleton-Century, New York, 1951.

LASAGNA, L., MOSTELLER, F., VON FELSINGER, J. M., and BEECHER, H. K., 'A study of the placebo response', *Amer. J. Med.*, 16(1954) 770–79.

LEAVITT, F., and GARRON, D. C., 'The detection of psychological disturbance in patients with low back pain', *J. Psychosom. Res.*, 23(1979) 149–54.

LEAVITT, F., GARRON, D. C., 'Validity of a back-pain classification scale for detecting psychological disturbance as measured by the MMPI', *J. clin. psych.*, 36(1980) 186–9.

LE BARS, D., DICKENSON, A. H., and BESSON, J.-M., 'Diffuse noxious inhibitory controls (DNIC). I. Effects on dorsal horn convergent neurones in the rat', *Pain*, 6(1979a) 283–304.

LE BARS, D., DICKENSON, A. H., and BESSON, J.-M., 'Diffuse noxious inhibitory controls (DNIC). II. Lack of effect on non-convergent neurones, supraspinal involvement and theoretical implications', *Pain*, 6(1979b) 305–27.

LERICHE, R., *The Surgery of Pain*, Williams and Wilkins, Baltimore, 1939.

LEVITT, M., and LEVITT, J., 'Sensory hindlimb representation in the SmI cortex of the cat after spinal tractotomies', *Exper. Neurol.*, 22(1968) 276–302.

LEWIS, T., *Pain*, Macmillan, New York, 1942.

LEWIT, K., 'The needle effect in the relief of myofascial pain', *Pain*, 6(1979) 83–90.

LICHSTEIN, L., and SACKETT, G. P., 'Reactions by differentially raised Rhesus monkeys to noxious stimulation', *Dev. Psychobiol.*, 4(1971) 339–52.

LIEBESKIND, J. C., and MAYER, D. J., 'Somatosensory evoked responses in the mesencephalic central gray matter of the rat', *Brain Res.* 27(1971) 133–51.

LIEBESKIND, J. C., and PAUL, L. A., 'Psychological and physiological mechanisms of pain', *Ann. Rev. Psychol.*, 28(1977) 41–60.

LINDBLOM, U., and MEYERSON, B. A., 'Influence on touch, vibration and cutaneous pain of dorsal column stimulation in man', *Pain*, 1(1975) 257–70.

LINDBLOM, U., and TEGNER, R., 'Are the endorphins active in clinical pain states? Narcotic antagonism in chronic pain patients', *Pain*, 7(1979) 65–8.

LIPTON, S., MILES, J. B., and WILLIAMS, N. E., 'Pituitary injection of alcohol for inoperable and intractable cancer pain'; in J. J. BONICA, J. C. LIEBESKIND, and D. G. ALBE-FESSARD (eds.), *Advances in Pain Research and Therapy*, Vol. 3, Raven Press, New York, 1979, pp. 905–9.

LIU, Y. K., VARELA, M., and OSWALD, R., 'The correspondence between some motor points and acupuncture loci', *Amer. J. Chinese Med.*, 3(1975) 347–58.

LIVINGSTON, W. K., *Pain Mechanisms*, Macmillan, New York, 1943.

LIVINGSTON, W. K., 'The vicious circle in causalgia', *Ann. N.Y. Acad. Sci.*, 50(1948) 247–58.

LIVINGSTON, W. K., 'What is pain?', *Sci. Amer.*, 196(3) (1953) 59–66.

LOESER, J. D., 'The management of tic douloureux', *Pain*, 3(1977) 155–62.

LOESER, J. D., 'Low back pain'; in J. J. BONICA (ed.), *Pain*, Raven Press, New York, 1980, pp. 363–77.

LOESER, J. D., and WARD, A. A., 'Some effects of deafferentation on neurons of the cat spinal cord', *Arch. Neurol.*, 17(1967) 629–36.

LOESER, J. D., WARD, A. A., and WHITE, L. E., 'Chronic deafferentation of human spinal cord neurons', *J. Neurosurg.*, 29(1968) 48–50.

LOH, L., NATHAN, P. W., SCHOTT, G. D., and WILSON, P. G., 'Effects of regional guanethidine infusion in certain painful states', *J. Neurol., Neurosurg. Psychiat.*, 43(1980) 446–51.

LOH, L., NATHAN, P. W. and SCHOTT, G. D., 'Pain due to lesions of central nervous system removed by sympathetic block'. *Brit. Med. J.*, 282(1981) 1026–8.

LUTHE, W., *Autogenic Therapy*, Vol. 4: *Research and Theory*, Grune and Stratton, New York, 1970.

LYNN, B., 'Cutaneous hyperalgesia', *Brit. Med. Bull.*, 33(1977) 103–8.

MACCARTY, C. S., and DRAKE, R. L., 'Neurosurgical procedures for the control of pain', *Proc. Staff Meetings Mayo Clin.*, 31(1956) 208–14.

MACLEAN, P., 'Psychosomatics', *Hdbk Physiol.*, 3(1958) 1723–44.

MANNHEIMER, C., and CARLSSON, C. A., 'The analgesic effect of transcutaneous electrical nerve stimulation (TNS) in patients with rheumatoid arthritis. A comparative study of different pulse patterns', *Pain*, 6(1979) 329–34.

MANNHEIMER, C., LUND, S., and CARLSSON, C. A., 'The effect of transcutaneous electrical nerve stimulation (TNS) on joint pain in patients with rheumatoid arthritis', *Scand. J. Rheumatol.*, 7(1978) 13–16.

MARK, V. H., ERVIN, F. R., and YAKOVLEV, P. E., 'Stereotactic thalamotomy', *Arch. Neurol.*, 8(1963) 528–38.

MARSHALL, H. R., *Pain, Pleasure, and Aesthetics*, Macmillan, London, 1894.

MARTINEZ-URRUTIA, A., 'Anxiety and pain in surgical patients', *J. consult. clin. Psychol.*, 43(1975) 437–42.

MAYER, D. J., PRICE, D. D., and BECKER, D. P., 'Neurophysiological characterization of the anterolateral spinal cord neurons contributing to pain in man', *Pain*, 1(1975) 51–8.

MAYER, D. J., and WATKINS, L. R., 'The role of endorphins in endogenous pain control systems; in H. M. EMRICH (ed.), *Modern Problems in Pharmacopsychiatry: The Role of Endorphins in Neuropsychiatry*, S. Karger, Basel, 1981.

MAYER, D. J., WOLFLE, T. L., AKIL, H., CARDER, B., and LIEBESKIND, J. C., 'Analgesia from electrical stimulation in the brainstem of the rat', *Science*, 174(1971) 1351–4.

MAZARS, G. J., MERIENNE, L., and CIOLOCA, C., 'Contribution of thalamic stimulation to the pathophysiology of pain'; in J. J. BONICA and D. ALBE-FESSARD (eds.), *Advances in Pain Research and Therapy*, Vol. 1, Raven Press, New York, 1976, pp. 483–5.

McGIVERN, R. F., and BERNTSON, G. G., 'Mediation of diurnal fluctuations in pain sensitivity in the rat by food intake patterns: reversal by naloxone', *Science*, 210(1980) 210–11.

McGLASHAN, T. H., EVANS, F. J., and ORNE, M. T., 'The nature of hypnotic analgesia and placebo response to experimental pain', *Psychosom. Med.*, 31(1969) 227–46.

McMURRAY, G. A., 'Experimental study of a case of insensitivity to pain', *Arch. Neurol. Psychiat.*, 64(1950) 650–67.

MEHLER, W. R., 'The anatomy of the so-called "pain tract" in man'; in J. D. FRENCH and R. W. PORTER (eds.), *Basic Research in Paraplegia*, Thomas, Springfield, 1962, pp. 26–55.

MEICHENBAUM, D., and TURK, D., 'The cognitive-behavioral management of anxiety, anger, and pain'; in P. O. DAVIDSON (ed.), *The Behavioral Management of Anxiety, Depression, and Pain*, Brunner Mazel, New York, 1976, pp. 1–34.

MELZACK, R., 'The perception of pain', *Sci. Amer.* 204(2) (1961) 41–9.

MELZACK, R., 'Effects of early experience on behavior: experimental and conceptual considerations'; in P. HOCH and J. ZUBIN (eds.), *Psychopathology of Perception*, Grune and Stratton, New York, 1965, pp. 271–99.

MELZACK, R., 'The role of early experience in emotional arousal', *Ann. N.Y. Acad. Sci.*, 159(1969) 721–30.

MELZACK, R., 'Phantom limb pain: implications for treatment of pathological pain', *Anesthesiology*, 35(1971) 409–19.

MELZACK, R., *The Puzzle of Pain*, Basic Books, New York, 1973.

MELZACK, R., 'The McGill Pain Questionnaire: major properties and scoring methods', *Pain*, 1(1975a) 277–99.

MELZACK, R., 'Prolonged relief of pain by brief, intense transcutaneous somatic stimulation', *Pain*, 1(1975b) 357–73.

MELZACK, R., and BROMAGE, P. R., 'Experimental phantom limbs', *Exper. Neurol.*, 39(1973) 261–9.

MELZACK, R., and CASEY, K. L., 'Sensory, motivational, and central control determinants of pain: a new conceptual model'; in D. KENSHALO (ed.), *The Skin Senses*, Thomas, Springfield, Ill., 1968, pp. 423–43.

MELZACK, R., and EISENBERG, H., 'Skin sensory afterglows', *Science*, 159(1968) 445–7.

MELZACK, R., GUITÉ, S., and GONSHOR, A., 'Relief of dental pain by ice massage of the hand', *Canad. Med. Assn J.*, 122(1980) 189–91.

MELZACK, R., JEANS, M. E., STRATFORD, J. G., and MONKS, R. C., 'Ice massage and transcutaneous electrical stimulation: comparison of treatment for low back pain', *Pain*, 9(1980) 209–17.

MELZACK, R., and LOESER, J. D., 'Phantom body pain in paraplegics: evidence for a central "pattern generating mechanism" for pain', *Pain*, 4(1978) 195–210.

MELZACK, R., and MELINKOFF, D. F., 'Analgesia produced by brain stimulation: evidence of a prolonged onset period', *Exper. Neurol.*, 43(1974) 369–74.

MELZACK, R., MOUNT, B. M., and GORDON, J.M., 'The Brompton Mixture versus morphine solution given orally: effects on pain', *Canad. Med. Assn J.*, 120(1979) 435–8.

MELZACK, R., OFIESH, J. G., and MOUNT, B. M., 'The Brompton Mixture: effects on pain in cancer patients', *Canad. Med. Assn J.*, 115(1976) 125–9.

MELZACK, R., and PERRY, C., 'Self-regulation of pain: the use of alpha-feedback and hypnotic training for the control of chronic pain', *Exper. Neurol.*, 46(1975) 452–69.

MELZACK, R., and PERRY, C., *Psychological Control of Pain*, BMA Audio Cassettes, New York, 1980.

MELZACK, R., ROSE, G., and MCGINTY, D., 'Skin sensitivity to thermal stimuli', *Exper. Neurol.*, 6(1962) 300–314.

MELZACK, R., and SCHECTER, B., 'Itch and vibration', *Science*, 147(1965) 1047–8.

MELZACK, R., and SCOTT, T. H., 'The effects of early experience on the response to pain', *J. comp. physiol. Psychol.*, 50(1957) 155–61.

MELZACK, R., STILLWELL, D. M., and FOX, E. J., 'Trigger points and acupuncture points for pain: correlations and implications', *Pain*, 3(1977) 3–23.

MELZACK, R., STOTLER, W. A., and LIVINGSTON, W. K., 'Effects of discrete brainstem lesions in cats on perception of noxious stimulation', *J. Neurophysiol.*, 21(1958) 353–67.

MELZACK, R., TAENZER, P., FELDMAN, P., and KINCH, R. A., 'Labour is still painful after prepared childbirth training', *Canad. Med. Assn J.*, 125(1981) 357–63.

MELZACK, R., and TORGERSON, W. S. 'On the language of pain', *Anesthesiology*, 34(1971) 50–59.

MELZACK, R., and WALL, P. D., 'On the nature of cutaneous sensory mechanisms', *Brain*, 85(1962) 331–56.

MELZACK, R., and WALL, P. D., 'Pain mechanisms: a new theory', *Science*, 150(1965) 971–9.

MELZACK, R., and WALL, P. D., 'Psychophysiology of pain', *Int. Anesthesiol. Clinics*, 8(1970) 3–34.

MELZACK, R., WALL, P. D., and TY, T .C., 'Acute pain in an emergency clinic: latency of onset and descriptor patterns', *Pain*, in preparation (1982).

MELZACK, R., WALL, P. D., and WEISZ, A. Z., 'Masking and metacontrast phenomena in the skin sensory system', *Exper. Neurol.*, 8(1963) 35–46.

MELZACK, R., WEISZ, A. Z., and SPRAGUE, L. T., 'Stratagems for controlling pain: contributions of auditory stimulation and suggestion', *Exper. Neurol.*, 8(1963) 239–47.

MENDELL, L. M., and WALL, P. D., 'Presynaptic hyperpolarization: a role for fine afferent fibers', *J. Physiol.*, 172(1965) 274–94.

MERSKEY, H. (Chairman) and IASP subcommittee on Taxonomy, 'Pain terms: a list with definitions and notes on usage', *Pain*, 6(1979) 249–52.

MERSKEY, H., and SPEAR, F. G., *Pain: Psychological and Psychiatric Aspects*, Baillière, Tindall and Cassell, London, 1967.

METZLER, J., 'Functional reorganization and sensory interactions in cat somatic sensory-motor and striate cortex', *Abstr. Soc. Neurosci.* 6(1980) 638.

METZLER, J., and MARKS, P. S., 'Functional changes in cat somatosensory motor cortex during short term reversible epidural blocks', *Brain Res.*, 177(1979) 379–83.

MIHIC, D., and BINKERT, E., 'Is placebo analgesia mediated by endorphine?', *Pain Abstr.*, 1(1978) 19.

MILLAR, J., and BASBAUM, A. I., 'Topography of the projection of the body surface of the cat to cuneate and gracile nuclei', *Exper. Neurol.*, 49(1975) 281–90.

MILNER, P., *Physiological Psychology*, Holt, Rinehart and Winston, New York, 1970.

MITCHELL, S. W., *Injuries of Nerves and their Consequences*, Lippincott, Philadelphia, 1872.

MORICCA, G., 'Chemical Hypophysectomy'; in J. J. BONICA (ed.), *Advances in Neurology*, Vol. 4, Raven Press, New York, 1974, 707–14.

MOUNT, B. M., 'The problem of caring for the dying in a general hospital: The palliative care unit as a possible solution', *Canad. Med. Assn J.*, 115(1976) 119–21.

MOUNT, B. M., AJEMIAN, I., and SCOTT, J. F., 'Use of the Brompton Mixture in treating the chronic pain of malignant disease', *Canad. Med. Assn J.*, 115(1976) 122–4.

MOUNTCASTLE, V.B., *Medical Physiology*, C.V. Mosby, St Louis, Mo., 1980.

MOWRER, O.H., and VIEK, P., 'An experimental analogue of fear from a sense of helplessness', *J. abnorm. Soc. Psychol.*, 43(1948) 193–200.

MULLAN, S., 'Percutaneous cordotomy for pain', *Surg. Clin. N. Amer.*, 46(1966) 3–12.

MÜLLER, J., *Elements of Physiology*, Taylor, London, 1842.

NAFE, J. P., 'The pressure, pain and temperature senses'; in C. A. MURCHISON (ed.), *Handbook of General Experimental Psychology*, Clark University Press, Worcester, Mass., 1934.

NAKAHAMA, H., NISHIOKA, S., and OTSUKA, T., 'Excitation and inhibition in ventrobasal thalamic neurons before and after cutaneous input deprivation', *Progr. Brain Res.*, 21(1966) 180–96.

NASHOLD, B. S., WILSON, W. P., and SLAUGHTER, D. G., 'Sensations evoked by stimulation in the midbrain of man', *J. Neurosurg.*, 30(1969) 14–24.

NATHAN, P. W., 'Reference of sensation at the spinal level, *J. Neurol. Neurosurg. Psychiat.*, 19(1956) 88–100.

NATHAN, P. W., 'Pain traces left in the central nervous system'; in C. A. KEELE and R. SMITH (eds.), *The Assessment of Pain in Man and Animals*, Livingstone, London, 1962, 129–34.

NATHAN, P. W., 'Results of antero-lateral cordotomy for pain in cancer', *J. Neurol. Neurosurg. Psychiat.*, 26(1963) 353–62.

NATHAN, P. W., 'Painful legs and moving toes: evidence on the site of the lesion', *J. Neurol. Neurosurg. Psychiat.*, 41(1978) 934–9.

NATHAN, P. W., and WALL, P. D., 'Treatment of post-herpetic neuralgia by prolonged electrical stimulation', *Brit. Med. J.*, 3(1974) 645–47.

NAUNYN, B., 'Ueber die Auslosung von Schmerzemfindung durch summation sich zeitlich folgender sensibelen Erregungen', *Arch. exper. Pathol. Pharmakol.*, 25(1889) 272–305.

NAUTA, W. J. H., 'Hippocampal projections and related neural pathways to the midbrain in the cat', *Brain*, 81(1958) 319–40.

NOBACK, C. R., and SCHRIVER, J. E., 'Encephalization and the lemniscal systems during phylogeny', *Ann. N.Y. Acad. Med.*, 167(1969) 118–28.

NOORDENBOS, W., *Pain*, Elsevier Press, Amsterdam, 1959.

NOORDENBOS, W., and WALL, P. D., 'The failure of nerve grafts to relieve pain following nerve injury', *J. Neurol. Neurosurg. Psychiat.*, 44(1981) 1008–73.

NORTH, M. A., 'Naloxone reversal of morphine analgesia but failure to alter reactivity to pain in the formalin test', *Life Sci.*, 22(1978) 295–302.

O'KEEFE, J., 'Spinal cord mechanisms subserving pain perception', McGill University (Master's thesis), Montreal, 1964.

O'KEEFE, J., and NADEL, L., *The Hippocampus as a Cognitive Map*, Oxford University Press, New York, 1978.

OLDS, M. E., and OLDS, J., 'Approach-escape interactions in the rat brain', *Amer. J. Physiol.*, 203(1962) 803–10.

OLDS, M.E., and OLDS, J., 'Approach-avoidance analysis of rat diencephalon',

J. Comp. Neurol., 120(1963) 259–95.

PAVLOV, I. P., *Conditioned Reflexes*, Humphrey Milford, Oxford, 1927.

PAVLOV, I. P., *Lectures on Conditioned Reflexes*, International Publishers, New York, 1928.

PEARSON, A. A., 'Role of gelatinous substance of spinal cord in conduction of pain', *Arch. Neurol. Psychiat.*, 68(1952) 515–29.

PERL, E. R., 'Afferent basis of nociception and pain: evidence from the characteristics of sensory receptors and their projections to the spinal dorsal horn'; in J. J. BONICA (ed.), *Pain*, Raven Press, New York, 1980, pp. 19–45.

PERRY, C., 'Cognitive patterns in hypnosis', Paper presented at the 88th Ann. Conf. Amer. Psychol. Assoc., Montreal, 1980.

POMERANZ, B., CHENG, R., and LAW, P., 'Acupuncture reduces electrophysiological and behavioral responses to noxious stimuli: pituitary is implicated', *Exper. Neurol.*, 54(1977) 172–8.

POMERANZ, B., WALL, P. D., and WEBER, W. V., 'Cord cells responding to fine myelinated afferents from viscera, muscle and skin', *J. Physiol.*, 199(1968) 511–32.

PRICE, D. D., and MAYER, D. J., 'Physiological laminar organization of the dorsal horn of *M. mulatta*', *Brain Res.*, 79(1974) 321–5.

PRIETO, E. J., HOPSON, L., BRADLEY, L. A., BYRNE, M., GEISINGER, K. F., MIDAX, D., and MARCHISELLO, P. J., 'The language of low back pain: factor structure of the McGill Pain Questionnaire', *Pain*, 8(1980) 11–19.

REXED, B., 'The cytoarchitectonic organization of the spinal cord in the cat', *J. Comp. Neurol.*, 96(1952) 415–95.

REYNOLDS, D. V., 'Surgery in the rat during electrical analgesia induced by focal brain stimulation', *Science*, 164(1969) 444–5.

REYNOLDS, D. V., 'Reduced response to aversive stimuli during focal brain stimulation: electrical analgesia and electrical anesthesia'; in D. V. REYNOLDS and A. E. SJOBERG (eds.), *Neuroelectric Research,* Thomas, Springfield, Ill. 1970, 151–67.

REYNOLDS, O. E., and HUTCHINS, H. C., 'Reduction of central hyperirritability following block anesthesia of peripheral nerve', *Amer. J. Physiol.*, 152(1948) 658–62.

ROBERTS, A. H., and REINHARDT, L., 'The behavioral management of chronic pain: long-term follow-up with comparison groups', *Pain*, 8(1980) 151–62.

ROBERTS, W. W., 'Fear-like behavior elicited from dorsomedial thalamus of cat', *J. Comp. Physiol. Psychol.*, 55(1962) 191–7.

ROSE, J. E., and MOUNTCASTLE, V. B., 'Touch and Kinesthesis', *Hdbk Physiol.*, 1(1959) 387–429.

ROSSI, G. F., and ZANCHETTI, A., 'The brainstem reticular formation', *Arch. Ital. Biol.*, 95(1957) 199–435.

RUBINS, J. L., and FRIEDMAN, E. D., 'Asymbolia for pain', *Arch. Neurol. Psychiat.*, 60(1948) 554–73.

RUFFINI, A., 'Les dispositifs anatomiques de la sensibilité cutanée sur les

expansions nerveuses de la peau chez l'homme et quelques autres
mammifères', *Rev. gen. Histol.*, 1(1905) 421–510.

RUSSELL, W. R., and SPALDING, J. M. K., Treatment of painful amputation
stumps', *Brit. Med. J.*, 2(1950) 68–73.

RYBSTEIN-BLINCHIK, E., 'Effects of different cognitive strategies on chronic
pain experience', *J. behav. Med.*, 2(1979) 93–101.

SANDREW, B. B., YANG, R. C. C., and WANG, S. C., 'Electro-acupuncture
analgesia in monkeys: a behavioral and neurophysiological assessment', *Arch.
int. Pharmacodyn. Ther.*, 231(1978) 274–84.

SAUNDERS, C., 'Care of the dying', *Nursing Times*, 72(1976) 3–24.

SAUNDERS, C. (ed.), *The Management of Terminal Disease*, Edward Arnold,
London, 1978.

SCHMIDT, R. F., 'The gate-control theory of pain: an unlikely hypothesis'; in
R. JANZEN *et al.* (eds.), *Pain*, Churchill Livingstone, London, 1972, pp.
124–7.

SCHOENE, W. C., ASBURY, A. L., ASTROM, K. E., and MASTERS, R.,
'Hereditary sensory neuropathy', *J. Neurol. Sci.*, 11(1970) 463–72.

SCHOENEN, J., 'Organisation Neuronale de la Moelle Epinière de l'Homme',
thesis, Faculty of Medicine, Université de Liège, 1980.

SCHREINER, L., and KLING, A., 'Behavioral changes following rhinencephalic
injury in cat', *J. Neurophysiol.*, 15(1953) 643–59.

SCHWETSCHENAU, P. R., RAMIREZ, A., JOHNSTON, J., BARNES, E.,
WIGGS, C., and MARTINS, A.N., 'Double-blind evaluation of intradiscal
chymopapain for herniated lumbar discs,' *J. Neurosurg.*, 45(1976) 622–7.

SEMMES, J., and MISHKIN, M., 'Somatosensory loss in monkeys after
ipsilateral cortical ablation', *J. Neurophysiol.*, 28(1965) 473–86.

SHEALY, C. N., MORTIMER, J. T., and RESWICK, J. B., 'Electrical inhibition
of pain by stimulation of the dorsal columns', *Anesth. Analg.*, 46(1967)
489–91.

SHEEHAN, P. W., and PERRY, C. W., *Methodologies of Hypnosis: A Critical
Appraisal of Contemporary Paradigms of Hypnosis*, Lawrence Erlbaum
Associates, Hillsdale, N.J., 1976.

SHERMAN, R. A., SHERMAN, C. J., and GALL, N. G., 'A survey of current
phantom limb pain treatment in the United States', *Pain*, 8(1980) 85–99.

SHERRINGTON, C. S., 'Cutaneous sensations'; in E. A. SCHÄFER (ed.),
Textbook of Physiology, Pentland, London, 1900, pp. 920–1001.

SHERRINGTON, C. S., *Integrative Action of the Nervous System*, Scribner, New
York, 1906.

SILVER, B. V., and BLANCHARD, E. G., 'Biofeedback and relaxation training
in the treatment of psychophysiological disorders: Or, are the machines really
necessary?', *J. behav. Med.*, 1(1978) 217–39.

SIMMEL, M. L., 'On phantom limbs', *Arch. Neurol. Psychiat.*, 75(1956)
637–47.

SIMMEL, M. L., 'The reality of phantom sensations', *Soc. Res.*, 29(1962)
337–56.

SIMONS, D. G., 'Muscle pain syndromes, Part I', *Amer. J. Phys. Med.*, 54(1975) 289–311.

SIMONS, D. G., 'Muscle pain syndromes. Part II', *Amer. J. Phys. Med.*, 55(1976) 15–42.

SINCLAIR, D. C., 'Cutaneous sensation and the doctrine of specific nerve energies', *Brain*, 78(1955) 584–614.

SINCLAIR, D. C., *Cutaneous Sensation,* Oxford University Press, London, 1967.

SJOLUND, B. H., and ERIKSSON, M. B. E., 'Endorphins and analgesia produced by peripheral conditioning stimulation'; in J. J. BONICA, D. ALBE-FESSARD and J.C. LIEBESKIND (eds.), *Advances in Pain Research and Therapy*, Vol. 3, Raven Press, New York, 1979, pp. 587–99.

SNYDER, S., 'Brain peptides as neurotransmitters', *Science*, 209(1980) 976–83.

SOLA, A. E., and WILLIAMS, R. L., 'Myofascial pain syndromes', *Neurology*, 6(1956) 91–5.

SOPER, W., 'Analgesia induced by brain stimulation: interaction of site and parameters of stimulation on the distribution of analgesic fields', McGill University (Ph.D. thesis), Montreal, 1979.

SOUREK, K., 'Commissural myelotomy', *J. Neurosurg.*, 31(1969) 524–7.

SPENCER, W. A., and APRIL, R. S., 'Plastic properties of monosynaptic pathways in mammals'; in G. HORN and R. A. HINDE, *Short-term Changes in Neural Activity and Behaviour*, Cambridge University Press, Cambridge, 1970, pp. 433–74.

SPIEGEL, E. A., KLETZKIN, M., and SZEKELEY, E. G., 'Pain reactions upon stimulation of the tectum mesencephali', *J. Neuropath. exper. Neurol.* 13(1954) 212–20.

SPIEGEL, E. A., and WYCIS, H. T., 'Present status of stereoencephalotomies for pain relief', *Confinia Neurologica*, 27(1966) 7–17.

SPILLANE, J. D., NATHAN, P. W., KELLY, R. E., and MARSDEN, C. D., 'Painful legs and moving toes', *Brain*, 94(1971) 541–56.

STERLING, P., 'Referred cutaneous sensation', *Exper. Neurol.*, 41(1973) 451–6.

STERNBACH, R. A., *Pain: A Psychophysiological Analysis*, Academic Press, New York, 1968.

STERNBACH, R. A., 'Strategies and tactics in the treatment of patients with pain'; in B. L. CRUE (ed.), *Pain and Suffering: Selected Aspects*, C. C. Thomas, Springfield, Ill., 1970, pp. 176–85.

STERNBACH, R. A., *Pain Patients: Traits and Treatment*, Academic Press, New York, 1974.

STERNBACH, R. A., and TIMMERMANS, G., 'Personality changes associated with reduction of pain', *Pain*, 1(1975) 177–81.

STERNBACH, R. A., and TURSKY, B., 'On the psychophysical power function in electric shock', *Psychosom. Sci.*, 1(1964) 217–18.

STERNBACH, R. A., and TURSKY, B., 'Ethnic differences among housewives in psychophysical and skin potential responses to electric shock', *Psychophysiology*, 1(1965) 241–6.

STEVENS, S. S., CARTON, A. S., and SHICKMAN, G. M., 'A scale of apparent intensity of electric shock', *J. Exper. Psychol.*, 56(1958) 328–34.

STEWART, D., THOMSON, J., and OSWALD, D., 'Acupuncture analgesia; an experimental investigation', *Brit. Med. J.*, 1(1977) 67–70.

SUNDERLAND, S., *Nerves and Nerve Injuries*, E. and S. Livingstone, Edinburgh, 1978.

SWANSON, D. W., MARUTA, T., and SWENSON, W. M., 'Results of behavior modification in the treatment of chronic pain', *Psychosom. Med.*, 41(1979) 55–61.

SWANSON, D. W., SWENSON, W. M., MARUTA, T., and MCPHEE, M. C., 'Program for managing chronic pain', *Proc. Staff Meetings Mayo Clinic*, 51 (1976) 401–8.

SWEET, W. H., 'Pain', *Hdbk Physiol.*, 1(1959) 459–506.

SWEET, W. H., General discussion; in J. J. BONICA (ed.), *Pain*, Raven Press, New York, 1980, 379–80.

SZASZ, T. S., 'The psychology of persistent pain: a portrait of l'homme douloureux'; in A. SOULAIRAC, J. CAHN, and J. CHARPENTIER (eds.), *Pain*, Academic Press, New York, 1968, pp. 93–113.

SZENTAGOTHAI, J., 'Neuronal and synaptic arrangement in the substantia gelatinosa Rolandi', *J. comp. Neurol.*, 122(1964) 219–39.

TAN, S.-Y., 'Acute pain in a clinical setting: effects of cognitive-behavioral skills training', McGill University (Ph.D. thesis), Montreal, 1980.

TAUB, A., 'Local, segmental and supraspinal interaction with a dorsolateral spinal cutaneous afferent system', *Exper. Neurol.*, 10(1964) 357–74.

TAUB, H. A., BEARD, M. C., EISENBERG, L., and MCCORMACK, R. K., 'Studies of acupuncture for operative dentistry', *J. Amer. Dent. Assn*, 95(1977) 555–61.

TAYLOR, C. B., ZLUTNICK, S. I., CORLEY, M. J., and FLORA, J., 'The effects of detoxification, relaxation, and brief supportive therapy on chronic pain', *Pain*, 8(1980) 319–29.

TERENIUS, L., 'Endogenous peptides and analgesia', *Ann. Rev. Pharmacol.*, 18(1978) 189–205.

TERENIUS, L., 'Endorphins in chronic pain'; in J. J. BONICA, J. C. LIEBESKIND and D. G. ALBE-FESSARD (eds.), *Advances in Pain Research and Therapy*, Vol. 3, Raven Press, New York, 1979, pp. 459–71.

THORSTEINSSON, G., STONNINGTON, H. H., STILLWELL, G. K., and ELVEBACK, L.R., 'Transcutaneous electrical stimulation: a double-blind trial of its efficacy for pain', *Arch. Phys. Med. Rehabil.*, 58(1977) 8–13.

TITCHENER, E. B., *A Textbook of Psychology*, Macmillan, New York, 1909–10.

TITCHENER, E. B., 'Notes from the psychological laboratory of Cornell University', *Amer. J. Psychol.*, 31(1920) 212–14.

TOWER, S. S., 'Pain: definition and properties of the unit for sensory reception', *Res. Publ. Assn nerv. ment. Dis.*, 23(1943) 16–43.

TRAVELL, J., and RINZLER, S. H., 'Relief of cardiac pain by local block of somatic trigger areas', *Proc. Soc. Exper. Biol. Med.*, 63(1946) 480–82.

TRAVELL, J., and RINZLER, S. H., 'The myofascial genesis of pain', *Postgrad. Med.*, 11(1952) 425–34.

TURK, D. C., and GENEST, M., 'Regulation of pain: the application of cognitive and behavioral techniques for prevention and remediation'; in P. C. KENDALL and S. D. HOLLON (eds.), *Cognitive-Behavioral Interventions: Theory, Research, and Procedures*, Academic Press, New York, 1979, pp. 287–318.

TURK, D. C., MEICHENBAUM, D. H., and BERMAN, W. H., 'Application of biofeedback for the regulation of pain: a critical review', *Psychol. Bull.*, 86(1979) 1322–38.

TURNBULL, I. M., SHULMAN, R., and WOODHURST, W. B., 'Thalamic stimulation for neuropathic pain', *J. Neurosurg.*, 52(1980) 486–93.

TWYCROSS, R., 'Clinical experience with diamorphine in advanced malignant disease', *Int. J. clin. Pharmacol. Therap. Toxicol.*, 9(1974) 184–98.

TWYCROSS, R. G., 'Relief of pain'; in C. M. SAUNDERS (ed.), *The Management of Terminal Disease*, Edward Arnold, London, 1978, pp. 65–92.

UDDENBERG, N., 'Functional organization of long, second-order afferents in the dorsal funiculus', *Exper. Brain Res.*, 4(1968) 377–82.

URBAN, B. J., and NASHOLD, B. S., 'Percutaneous epidural stimulation of the spinal cord for relief of pain', *J. Neurosurg.*, 48(1978) 323–8.

VALLBO, A. B., and HAGBARTH, K. E., 'Activity from skin mechanoreceptors recorded percutaneously in awake human subjects', *Exper. Neurol.*, 21(1968) 270–89.

VAN BUREN, J., and KLEINKNECHT, R. A., 'An evaluation of the McGill Pain Questionnaire for use in dental pain assessment', *Pain*, 6(1979) 23–33.

VAN HEES, J., and GYBELS, J. M., 'Pain related to single afferent C fibers from human skin', *Brain Res.*, 48(1972) 397–400.

VANE, J. R., 'Inhibition of prostaglandin synthesis as a mechanism of action for aspirin-like drugs', *Nature, New Biol.*, 231(1971) 232–5.

VIERCK, C. J., HAMILTON, D. M., and THORNBY, J. I., 'Pain reactivity of monkeys after lesions to the dorsal and lateral columns of the spinal cord', *Exper. Brain Res.*, 13(1971) 140–58.

VIERCK, C. J., LINEBERRY, C. G., LEE, P. K., and CALDERWOOD, H. W., 'Prolonged hypalgesia following "acupuncture" in monkeys', *Life Sci.*, 15(1974) 1277–89.

WAGMAN, I. H., and PRICE, D. D., 'Responses of dorsal horn cells of *M. mulatta* to cutaneous and sural nerve A and C fiber stimuli', *J. Neurophysiol.*, 32(1969) 803–17.

WALDER, A., Invited editorial, *Pain*, 9(1980) 1–2.

WALL, P. D., 'Excitability changes in afferent fibre terminations and their relation to slow potentials', *J. Physiol.*, 142(1958) 1–21.

WALL, P. D., 'Presynaptic control of impulses at the first central synapse in the cutaneous pathway', *Progr. Brain Res.*, 12(1964) 92–118.

WALL, P. D., 'The laminar organization of dorsal horn and effects of descending impulses', *J. Physiol.*, 188(1967) 403–23.

WALL, P. D., 'The sensory and motor role of impulses travelling in the dorsal columns towards cerebral cortex', *Brain*, 93(1970) 505–24.

WALL, P. D., 'Modulation of pain by nonpainful events'; in J. J. BONICA and D. ALBE-FESSARD (eds.), *Advances in Pain Research and Therapy*, Vol. 1, Raven Press, New York, 1976, pp. 1–16.

WALL, P. D., 'The presence of ineffective synapses and the circumstances which unmask them', *Phil. Trans. Roy. Soc. London*, Series B, 278 (1977) 361–72.

WALL, P. D., 'The gate-control theory of pain mechanisms: a re-examination and a re-statement', *Brain*, 101(1978) 1–18.

WALL, P. D., 'On the relation of injury to pain. The John J. Bonica Lecture', *Pain*, 6(1979) 253–64.

WALL, P. D., 'The role of substantia gelatinosa as a gate control'; in J. J. BONICA (ed.), *Pain*, Raven Press, New York, (1980a), 205–31.

WALL, P. D., 'The substantia gelatinosa. A gate-control mechanism set across a sensory pathway', *Trends in Neurosciences,* Sept. 1980b, 221–4.

WALL, P. D., and CRONLY-DILLON, J. R., 'Pain, itch and vibration', *Arch. Neurol.*, 2(1960) 365–75.

WALL, P. D., and DEVOR, M., 'The effects of peripheral nerve injury on dorsal root potentials and on transmission of afferent signals into spinal cord', *Brain Res.*, 209(1981) 95–111.

WALL, P. D., DEVOR, M., INBAL, R., SCADDING, J. W., SCHONFELD, D., SELTZER, Z., and TOMKIEWICZ, M. M., 'Autotomy following peripheral nerve lesions', *Pain*, 7(1979) 103–13.

WALL, P. D., and EGGER, M. D., 'Formation of new connections in adult rat brains after partial deafferentation', *Nature*, 232(1971) 542–5.

WALL, P. D., and GUTNICK, M., 'Ongoing activity in peripheral nerves. II. The physiology and pharmacology of impulses originating in a neuroma', *Exper. Neurol.*, 43(1974) 580–93.

WALL, P. D., MERRILL, E. G., and YAKSH, T. L., 'Responses of single units in laminae 2 and 3 of cat spinal cord', *Brain Res.*, 160(1979) 245–60.

WALL, P. D., NATHAN, P. W., and NOORDENBOS, W., 'Ongoing activity in peripheral nerve. I. Interactions between electrical stimulation and ongoing activity', *Exper. Neurol.*, 38(1973) 90–98.

WALL, P. D., SCADDING, J. W., and TOMKIEWICZ, M. M., 'The production and prevention of experimental anaesthesia dolorosa', *Pain*, 6(1979) 175–82.

WALL, P. D., and SWEET, W. H., 'Temporary abolition of pain', *Science*, 155(1967) 108–9.

WALL, P. D., WAXMAN, S., and BASBAUM, A. I., 'Ongoing activity in peripheral nerve. III. Injury discharge', *Exper. Neurol.*, 45(1974) 576–89.

WALL, P. D., and WOOLF, C. J., 'What we don't know about pain', *Nature*, 287(1980) 185–6.

WALTERS, A., 'Psychogenic regional pain alias hysterical pain', *Brain*, 84(1961) 1–18.

WAND-TETLEY, J. I., 'Historical methods of counter-irritation', *Ann. Phys. Med.*, 3(1956) 90–98.

WEDDELL, G., 'Somesthesis and the chemical senses', *Ann. Rev. Psychol.*, 6(1955) 119–36.

WHITE, J. C., and SWEET, W. H., *Pain and the Neurosurgeon*, C. C. Thomas, Springfield, Illinois, 1969.

WILLIS, W. D., and COGGESHALL, R. E., *Sensory Mechanisms of the Spinal Cord*, Plenum Press, New York, 1978.

WISSLER, C., 'The sun dance of the Blackfoot Indians', *Amer. Mus. Nat. Hist., Anthropology Papers*, 16(1921) 223–70.

WOLF, S., and WOLFF, H. G., 'Pain arising from the stomach and mechanisms underlying gastric symptoms', *Assn Res. nerv. ment. Dis.*, 23(1943) 289–301.

WYNN PARRY, C. B., 'Pain in avulsion lesions of the brachial plexus', *Pain*, 9(1980) 41–53.

YAKSH, T. L., 'Analgetic actions of intrathecal opiates in cat and primate', *Brain Res.*, 153(1978) 205–10.

YAKSH, T. L., and RUDY, T. A., 'Analgesia mediated by a direct spinal action of narcotics', *Science*, 192(1976) 1357–8.

ZBOROWSKI, M., 'Cultural components in responses to pain', *J. soc. Issues*, 8(1952) 16–30.

ZIMBARDO, P. G., and RUCH, F. L., *Psychology and Life*, Scott, Foresman, Glenview, Ill., 1975.

ZOHN, D. A., and MENNELL, J. M., *Musculoskeletal Pain: Diagnosis and Physical Treatment*, Little, Brown, Boston, 1976.

Index